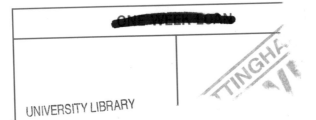

GROWTH FACTORS AND PSYCHIATRIC DISORDERS

Novartis Foundation Symposium 289

GROWTH FACTORS AND PSYCHIATRIC DISORDERS

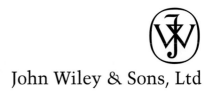

John Wiley & Sons, Ltd

Other Wiley Editorial Offices

John Wiley & Sons Inc., 111 River Street, Hoboken, NJ 07030, USA

Jossey-Bass, 989 Market Street, San Francisco, CA 94103-1741, USA

Wiley-VCH Verlag GmbH, Boschstr. 12, D-69469 Weinheim, Germany

John Wiley & Sons Australia Ltd, 33 Park Road, Milton, Queensland 4064, Australia

John Wiley & Sons (Asia) Pte Ltd, 2 Clementi Loop #02-01, Jin Xing Distripark, Singapore
129809

John Wiley & Sons Canada Ltd, 6045 Freemont Blvd, Mississauga, Ontario, Canada L5R 4J3

Wiley also publishes its books in a variety of electronic formats. Some content that appears in
print may not be available in electronic books.

Novartis Foundation Symposium 289

x + 240 pages, 26 figures, 5 tables

British Library Cataloguing in Publication Data

A catalogue record for this book is available from the British Library

ISBN 9780470516041
, ००੨ ੨ ੬੧੨੭੩ T
Typeset in 10½ on 12½ pt Garamond by SNP Best-set Typesetter Ltd., Hong Kong
Printed and bound in Great Britain by T.J. International Ltd, Padstow, Cornwall.

Contents

v

Participants

Huda Akil University of Michigan, Mental Health Research Institute, 205 Zina Pitcher, Box 720, Ann Arbor, MI 48109, USA

Yves-Alain Barde Biozentrum, University of Basel, Division of Pharmacology and Neurobiology, Klingelbergstrasse 50/70, CH-4056 Base, Switzerland

Mark Bothwell Department of Physiology and Biophysics, University of Washington, Health Science Building, Box 357290, Seattle, WA 98195-7290, USA

Nicholas J. Brandon Schizophrenia and Bipolar Research, Wyeth Discovery Neuroscience, CN 8000, Princeton, NJ 08543, USA

Andrés Buonanno Section on Molecular Neurobiology, National Institute of Child Health and Development, Bldg 35, Room 2C-1000, 35 Lincoln Drive, Bethesda, MD 20892-3714, USA

Eero Castrén University of Helsinki, Neuroscience Center, PO Box 56, Viikinkaari 4, 00014 Helsinki, Finland

Moses Chao *(Chair)* Molecular Neurobiology Program, Skirball Institute of Biomolecular Medicine, Department of Cell Biology, New York University School of Medicine, 540 First Avenue, New York, NY 10016, USA

Jonathan Flint The Wellcome Trust Centre for Human Genetics, The University of Oxford, Roosevelt Drive, Oxford OX3 7BN, UK

Jay N. Giedd Child Psychiatry Branch, NIMH, Building 10, Room 4C110, 10 Center Drive, MSC 1367, Bethesda, MD 20892-1600, USA

Stephen Haggarty Broad Institute, 7 Cambridge Center, Cambridge, MA 02142, USA

René Hen Columbia University P & S, Center for Neurobiology and Behavior, 1051 Riverside Drive, Annex, Room 767, Box 87, New York, NY 10032, USA

Daniel C. Javitt Nathan Kline Institute/New York University School of Medicine, Department of Cognitive Neuroscience and Schizophrenia, 140 Old Orangeburg Road, Room S235, Orangeburg, NY 10962, USA

René S. Kahn Universitair Medisch Centrum Utrecht, A01.126, Postbus 85.500, 3508 GA Utrecht, The Netherlands

Emine Eren Koçak *(Novartis Foundation Bursar)* Institute of Neurological Sciences and Psychiatry, Hacettepe University, Sihhiye, 06100 Ankara, Turkey

Francis S. Lee Department of Psychiatry, Weill Medical College of Cornell University, 1300 York Avenue, Room LC-903, New York, NY 10021, USA

Bai Lu Laboratory of Cellular and Synaptic Neurophysiology, Porter Neuroscience Research Center, Building 35, Room 1C-1004, 35 Convent Drive, MSC 3714, Bethesda, MD 20892-3714, USA

Dolores Malaspina NYU School of Medicine, Department of Psychiatry, 550 First Avenue, MLH-HN323, New York, NY 10016, USA

Kevin McAllister Novartis Institutes for BioMedical Research, Novartis Pharma AG, Lichtstrasse 35, Basel, CH-4056, Switzerland

Michael J. Owen Department of Psychological Medicine, Wales College of Medicine, Cardiff University, Cardiff CF14 4XN, UK

Martin C. Raff MRC LMCB, University College London, Gower Street, London WC1E 6BT, UK

Michael Sendtner Institut für Klinische Neurobiologie, Universitätsklinikum Würzburg, Zinklesweg 10, D-97080 Würzburg Germany

Pamela Sklar Massachusetts General Hospital, Harvard Medical School, Simches Research Building, 185 Cambridge Street, Boston, MA 02114, USA

Michael Spedding Institute of Research Servier, Experimental Sciences, 11 Rue des Moulineaux, FR-92150, Suresnes, France

David A. Talmage Department of Pharmacology, Centers for Molecular Medicine 548, SUNY Stony Brook, Stony Brook, NY 11794, USA

Enrico Tongiorgi BRAIN Centre for Neuroscience, Università di Trieste, Dipartimento di Biologia, Via Giorgieri, 10-34127 Trieste, Italy

Frank Walsh Discovery Research, Wyeth Research, 500 Arcola Road, Collegeville, PA 19426, USA

Chair's introduction

Moses Chao

Molecular Neurobiology Program, Skirball Institute of Biomolecular Medicine, Departments of Cell Biology, Physiology and Neuroscience, and Psychiatry, New York University School of Medicine, 540 First Avenue, New York, NY 10016, USA

Psychiatric disorders such as depression, bipolar disease and schizophrenia are debilitating mental illnesses that are influenced by many genetic and environmental factors. While little is known about the neural circuits that underlie mood disorders, genetic studies in the last three years have identified several growth factors as susceptibility genes for depression and schizophrenia, as well as learning and memory disorders. One common theme is that these disorders reflect dysregulation of neural plasticity, as well as neurodevelopment. This symposium on growth factors and psychiatric disorders will consider the pathophysiology and genetics of schizophrenia and depression, and will discuss how growth factors such as neurotrophins and neuregulins may alter synaptic plasticity on a molecular and neural systems level.

I wish to start with a historical footnote. A few weeks ago, Tom Eagleton, a prominent politician, passed away. In 1972, he ran as the vice presidential nominee with George McGovern. Eagleton was asked to step down because it was disclosed that he had suffered several bouts of serious depression. One of the comments made by McGovern in an obituary in the *New York Times* was that that no one in the 1970s knew anything about mental illness, including himself. McGovern had asked Eagleton to leave the ticket, and then lost the general election to Nixon. Over the last 35 years, much progress has been made in biomedical research, including the advent of molecular biology and the sequencing of the entire human genome. Many new insights have been generated from molecular genetics that are relevant to psychiatric disorders.

This meeting presents an opportunity to bring three different groups together: the psychiatric community, basic neuroscientists and human geneticists. These groups rarely encounter each other at meetings. The goal is to encourage cross-fertilization of these disciplines in a small, focused conference. The format of a Novartis Foundation symposium offers an excellent opportunity to foster multi-disciplinary interactions that will generate new approaches to this increasingly important topic.

The rationale for this meeting came from the realization that many complex psychiatric disorders have a genetic basis. This has been suggested by a growing number of association and linkage studies. Also, it has become clear that there are clear links to growth factors and their receptors. We will discuss the role of growth factors at length in this meeting, in particular brain-derived neurotrophic factor (BDNF) and neuregulins and their tyrosine kinase receptors, as well as members of the fibroblast growth factor (FGF) family. It is also worth noting that one of the major hypotheses to account for psychiatric illnesses is from neurodevelopmental and genetic contributions; another comes from changes in synaptic plasticity. These activities are inherent in the actions of growth factors. I am certain these themes will emerge in the papers at this meeting. The challenge for the participants is to determine the strength of these hypotheses.

My interest in this area stems from work on neurotrophic factor receptors, particularly the nerve growth factor (NGF) family, but BDNF has garnered much attention over the last few years. The original identification and cloning of BDNF was done by Yves-Alain Barde (Leibrock et al 1989). It took Yves Barde's group many years to purify the BDNF protein and to identify the gene. This trophic factor was originally identified for its trophic and differentiation properties, but it also possesses other biological activities. In the last 10 years it has become clear that BDNF exerts dramatic effects upon synaptic transmission in an activity-dependent manner, both on the presynaptic and postsynaptic sites of the synapse. This is an exciting area of research, as there are several strong connections to psychiatric disease. There are two seminal papers in this area. The first is by Eric Lander and Pam Sklar, who identified BDNF as a potential risk locus for bipolar disorder (Sklar et al 2002). A year later, Daniel Weinberger and Bai Lu (Egan et al 2003) characterized the same polymorphism in the context of BDNF release and epsodic memory in human subjects. These findings set the stage for a growing number of studies on BDNF and human behaviour.

The other finding that had an important impact on the field of psychiatry came from studies on neuregulin. Kári Stefánsson and deCODE published the original observation that proposed neuregulin as a potential risk factor for schizophrenia (Stefansson et al 2002). When this paper was published, there was scepticism about how polymorphisms in neuregulin were related to schizophrenia. Since this finding, there has been considerable attention on this issue in other populations. Many single nucleotide polymorphisms in neuregulin 1 have now provided strong genetic evidence in many diverse human populations, including Irish, Scottish and Chinese. This analysis has been complicated because the gene is very large and produces many splice variants and isoforms derived from multiple processing events. As a result, there are a large number of neuregulin proteins with different functions. The history of this protein is complex: it was designated by at least five different names. These names indicate that neuregulin proteins possess many activities, ranging from glial growth, neuronal migration, synapse formation and myelination. In this meeting, we will define several of the functions of this interesting family of proteins, which are directly relevant to the development of psychiatric illnesses.

BDNF and neuregulin are of considerable interest, but many other growth factors display similar activities and functions. I hope we can also consider these other growth factor activities. In terms of the main questions that should be considered at this meeting, the first is how strong is the evidence that growth factors and trophic factors are involved in psychiatric diseases? The mechanism of action of growth factors in psychiatric illnesses has not been explored yet, but if we consider the common signalling mechanisms of tyrosine kinase receptors, the question arises whether other growth factors are also involved in psychiatric disorders? This raises the question of specificity: do only a few trophic factors have an impact upon mental illnesses, or do they all participate in some way?

Another unanswered question concerns pharmacological treatments with antidepressants and other psychotropic drugs. Many antidepressants and psychotropic drugs require a long period of time to become efficacious. Why? BDNF levels are increased by antidepressants, but this time course differs from the clinical time course. Finally, since many of the drugs that have been introduced in the last few years are derived from previous drugs (there have been very few new pharmacological approaches), can we use the information from cellular mechanisms and signal transduction to design new approaches and new drugs for psychiatric illnesses?

The meeting will be primarily devoted to growth factors and trophic factors, and their relevance to psychiatric illnesses, but there are many other genes and proteins that have been implicated in these illnesses. During the course of the symposium we will consider some of the most relevant candidates. I hope that the topic of growth factors will act as a probe into the study of psychiatric illnesses, and that the information will be integrated to provide insights into future treatment for mood disorders.

References

Egan MF, Kojima M, Callicott JH et al 2003 The BDNF val66met polymorphism affects activity-dependent secretion of BDNF and human memory and hippocampal function. Cell 112:257–269

Leibrock J, Lottspeich F, Hohn A et al 1989 Molecular cloning and expression of brain-derived neurotrophic factor. Nature 341:149–152

Sklar P, Gabriel SB, McInnis MG et al 2002 Family-based association study of 76 candidate genes in bipolar disorder: BDNF is a potential risk locus. Mol Psychiatry 7:579–593

Stefansson H, Sigurdsson E, Steinthorsdottir V et al 2002 Neuregulin 1 and susceptibility to schizophrenia. Am J Hum Genet 71:877–892

Phenomenology, aetiology and treatment of schizophrenia

Daniel C. Javitt

Program in Cognitive Neuroscience and Schizophrenia, Nathan Kline Institute for Psychiatric Research and New York University School of Medicine, Orangeburg, NY 10962 USA

Abstract. Schizophrenia is a serious mental disorder that affects up to 1% of the population worldwide. Traditional models of schizophrenia have emphasized dopaminergic dysfunction. Over the last 15 years, however, glutamatergic models have become increasingly mainstream, and account for features of the disorder that are poorly explained by dopaminergic dysfunction alone. Glutamatergic models, such as the PCP/NMDA model, are based upon the observation that the psychotomimetic agents phencyclidine (PCP) and ketamine induce psychotic symptoms and neurocognitive disturbances similar to those of schizophrenia by blocking neurotransmission at N-methyl-D-aspartate (NMDA)-type glutamate receptors. Because NMDA receptors are located throughout the brain, information-processing deficits are observed not only in higher cortical regions, but also in sensory cortices and subcortical systems. Further, NMDA receptors are located on brain circuits that regulate dopamine release, suggesting that dopaminergic deficits in schizophrenia may also be secondary to underlying glutamatergic dysfunction. Agents that stimulate glutamatergic neurotransmission, including glycine-site agonists and glycine transport inhibitors, have shown encouraging results in preclinical studies and are currently undergoing clinical development. Overall, these findings suggest that glutamatergic theories may lead to new conceptualizations and treatment approaches that would not be possible based upon dopaminergic models alone.

2008 Growth factors and psychiatric disorders. Wiley, Chichester (Novartis Foundation Symposium 289) p 4–22

Schizophrenia is a serious mental disorder that affects up to 1% of the population worldwide, and is one of the leading causes of chronic disability. Although the causes of schizophrenia remain unknown, the disease has been extensively characterized from both a symptomatic and neurocognitive perspective, and much information has accumulated about elements such as genetic segregation and longitudinal course. Although schizophrenia was once seen as a disease affecting only a few key brain regions and regionally discrete neurotransmitter systems, more recent findings implicate widespread cortical and subcortical dysfunction, suggesting more generalized aetiology. On a neurochemical level, antagonists of N-

4

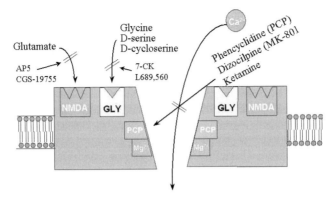

FIG. 1. Schematic model of the NMDA receptor complex. NMDA, N-methyl-D-aspartate; GLY, glycine.

methyl-D-aspartate (NMDA)-type glutamate receptors (Fig. 1), such as phencyclidine (PCP) or ketamine, uniquely reproduce the symptomatic, neurocognitive and neurochemical aspects of the disorder, suggesting that regardless of underlying aetiology, NMDA dysfunction represents a final common pathway leading from pathogenesis to symptoms.

Clinical phenomenology of schizophrenia

Schizophrenia was first described in the late 1800s by Emile Kraeplin and labelled 'dementia praecox' to distinguish it from senile dementias, such as what subsequently became known as Alzheimer's disease. Subsequent descriptions by Eugen Bleuler in the early 1900s emphasized core features of the disorder, such as blunted affect, loosening of associations, ambivalence and autistic preoccupation. Bleuler also was the first to describe the symptoms as 'positive' or 'negative' and first coined the term 'schizophrenia' to highlight the fragmentation of thought that he felt to be at the core of the disorder. Finally, in the 1950s, Kurt Schneider focused attention on the importance of 'first rank feature', such as running commentary hallucinations, thought insertion, withdrawal or broadcasting, and delusional perceptions. The current nosology of schizophrenia draws from these three foundations. Schizophrenia is viewed as a disorder that first appears in the late teens and early twenties in men, although somewhat later in women, and is associated with both a specific profile of symptoms, characteristic disturbances in neuropsychological functioning, and a characteristic clinical course. These features drive the current syndromal definition.

TABLE 1   Symptom domains in schizophrenia from the Positive and Negative Symptom Scale (PANSS)

Positive symptoms	Negative symptoms	Cognitive symptoms
Delusions	Blunted affect	Conceptual disorganization
Grandiosity	Emotional withdrawal	Difficulty in abstract thinking
Suspiciousness/persecution	Poor rapport	Mannerisms and posturing
Unusual thought content	Lack of spontaneity and flow of conversation	Disorientation
	Active social avoidance	Poor attention

Clinical symptoms

Symptoms of schizophrenia are currently divided into three main classes: positive, negative and cognitive (Table 1). Positive symptoms consist of such items as suspiciousness/persecution, grandiosity, delusions and unusual thought content and, in general, reflect features of the schizophrenia experience that are not shared by the general population. Negative symptoms, in contrast, consist of symptoms such as lack of spontaneity, social/emotional withdrawal, poor rapport and blunted affect, and reflect features of normal experience that are reduced in individuals with schizophrenia.

Finally, cognitive symptoms—which are also referred to as disorganized symptoms or autistic preoccupation—consist of such elements as conceptual disorganization, disorientation and poor attention. Rather than being fully separate symptom domains, however, such symptoms tend to co-occur within individuals and to worsen or improve in parallel. Thus, rather than reflecting different pathogenetic mechanisms, the different symptom clusters should be seen as different manifestations of the same underlying pathogenetic mechanisms.

Neuropsychological deficits

In addition to symptoms, schizophrenia is associated with characteristic neuro-cognitive deficits that represent a key component of the disorder. Although some features of the neurocognitive disturbance, such as deficits in working memory or executive processing, are emphasized more than others, deficits are widespread across neurocognitive domains and localize across brain regions (e.g. Bilder et al 2000). When tested on basic IQ tests, such as the WAIS, patients with established schizophrenia typically score about 1 standard deviation, or 15 IQ points, below the population mean. Deficits are typically present at first episode and remain relatively constant over the course of the illness.

TABLE 2 Consensus neuropsychological domains in schizophrenia, Provisional MATRICS Consensus Battery[a]

- Speed of Processing
- Attention/Vigilance
- Working Memory
- Verbal Learning
- Visual Learning
- Reasoning and Problem Solving
- Social Cognition

[a] http://www.matricsinc.org

The number of neuropsychological 'domains' that should be considered in schizophrenia remains an area of active investigation. Typical domains include such components as long-term memory, attention, executive ability, motor speed and visuospatial ability (Bilder et al 2000). Of these, long-term (declarative) memory ability is typically most affected (Bilder et al 2000). A recent NIMH-funded consensus battery for schizophrenia has suggested division of neurocognitive domains into seven components (Table 2), which, by inference, have separate neurophysiological substrates.

In general, neurocognitive deficits are apparent even in individuals presenting with an initial episode of psychosis and are stable thereafter, suggesting that cognitive decline precedes the onset of substantial symptoms (e.g. Bilder et al 2000). Both follow-back and cross-sectional data suggest that cognitive functioning may decline during the 3–4 years immediately preceding the onset of schizophrenia symptoms. For example, two studies have investigated Iowa test performance during childhood and adolescence in individuals who subsequently developed schizophrenia. Compared with the general population, such individuals showed only modest deficits even when assessed during 4th and 8th grade, but showed a marked decline in performance between 8th and 11th grade (Ho et al 2005). Similarly, individuals with prodromal schizophrenia who have not yet converted to psychosis show cognitive deficits that are intermediate between those of first-episode and control subjects, and such deficits may predict subsequent conversion to psychosis (Lencz et al 2006).

Although neurocognitive deficits appear generalized when viewed through the prism of neuropsychological testing, more focused assessment of key processes does show significant and informative variations within neuropsychological subtests. For example, patients with schizophrenia show reduced ability to learn new information, but intact ability to retain information once it has been learned. This pattern differs from the 'amnestic' syndrome that results from bilateral hippocampal damage (Bilder et al 2000), but is highly similar to effects seen following administration of NMDA antagonists (Parwani et al 2005). Overall, the pattern of cognitive dysfunction in schizophrenia closely follows the pattern observed following administration of NMDA antagonists across a variety of domains, suggesting that NMDA dysfunction may be seen as a parsimonious model of schizophrenia.

Neurochemical models of schizophrenia

The first effective treatments for schizophrenia were discovered fortuitously in the late 1950s, and subsequently shown to mediate their effects at dopamine D2 receptors. Since that time, dopamine has been the primary neurotransmitter implicated in schizophrenia, and the majority of neurochemical studies of schizophrenia continue to focus on dopaminergic mechanisms (Carlsson 1988). Neurochemical models of schizophrenia based upon dopaminergic theories have had substantial heuristic value in explaining key symptoms of schizophrenia, in particular, positive symptoms, and in guiding treatment considerations. Nevertheless, significant limitations with regard to the dopamine hypothesis remain. First, no intrinsic deficits have been observed within the dopamine system to account for the presumed hyperdopaminergia associated with schizophrenia. Second, reconceptualizations of the dopamine hypothesis propose that subcortical hyperdopaminergia may coexist with cortical hypodopaminergia, although mechanisms underlying the differential cortical and subcortical abnormalities remain to be determined. Finally, dopaminergic dysfunction, in general, accounts poorly for symptom classes in schizophrenia other than positive symptoms and for the pattern of neurocognitive dysfunction associated with schizophrenia. Thus, alternative conceptual models of schizophrenia are required.

An alternative to the dopamine model was first proposed in the early 1990s, based upon the observation that phencyclidine (PCP) and similarly acting psychotomimetic compounds induced their unique behavioural effects by blocking neurotransmission at N-methyl-D-aspartate (NMDA)-type glutamate receptors (Javitt & Zukin 1991). The ability of these compounds to transiently reproduce key symptoms of schizophrenia by blocking NMDA receptors led to the concept that symptoms in schizophrenia may reflect underlying dysfunction or dysregulation of NMDA receptor-mediated neurotransmission.

Symptom patterns following NMDA antagonist administration

In initial studies with PCP and ketamine in the early 1960s, it was noted that both agents produced what would now be considered positive, negative and cognitive symptoms of schizophrenia (Javitt & Zukin 1991). At the time, however, no formal rating scales were used. Recent studies with ketamine, however, have documented significant increases not only in positive symptoms, but also in negative and cognitive symptoms (e.g. Lahti et al 2001). Levels of symptoms during acute ketamine challenge, moreover, tend to show a similar pattern across factors as they do in schizophrenia. When patients with schizophrenia are exposed to ketamine, they also show increases in positive symptoms, as well as negative symptoms (Lahti et al 2001), suggesting that NMDA antagonists affect a brain system that is already vulnerable in schizophrenia.

Cognitive deficits following NMDA antagonist treatment

As with symptoms, initial studies conducted with PCP in the early 1960s showed deficits highly reminiscent of schizophrenia (Javitt & Zukin 1991). Studies conducted with ketamine over the last 15 years have confirmed and extended these findings. Deficits have been observed across widespread neuropsychological domains including working memory, response inhibition and executive processing (Krystal et al 2005, Umbricht et al 2000). Ketamine infusion also reproduces both the severity and type of thought disorder seen in schizophrenia with both, for example, being associated with high levels of poverty of speech, circumstantiality and loss of goal, and relatively low levels of distractive or stilted speech or paraphasias (Adler et al 1999). Thus, reduction in NMDA functioning within brain could serve as a single unifying feature to account for the otherwise complex pattern of deficit observed in the disorder.

As opposed to ketamine, administration of dopaminergic agonists such as amphetamine does not reproduce the pattern of deficit observed in schizophrenia. For example, in one recent study that directly compared effects of amphetamine and ketamine in normal volunteers, both ketamine and amphetamine induced positive symptoms and conceptual disorganization. However, only ketamine produced perceptual changes, concrete ideation or negative symptoms. Further, only ketamine induced schizophrenia-like disruptions in delayed recall. Finally, amphetamine did not induce working memory disturbances, and it significantly reversed ketamine-induced disruptions. These findings suggest that augmentation, rather than blockade, of frontal dopaminergic systems may be beneficial in schizophrenia (Krystal et al 2005).

NMDA dysfunction and sensory processing impairment

Another key difference between dopaminergic and NMDA models of schizophrenia is the predicted involvement of sensory processing. Whereas NMDA receptors are widely distributed throughout cortex, dopaminergic innervation of these regions is relatively sparse. Studies over recent years have thus assessed sensory processing deficits in schizophrenia, and have also investigated the consequence of sensory processing on higher-order cognitive dysfunction. Studies have focused mainly on auditory and visual sensory deficits, although deficits in other sensory systems have also been documented.

Auditory deficits in schizophrenia. Deficits in auditory processing have been investigated using both behavioural and neurophysiological measures. Behaviourally, patients show deficits in matching of tones following brief delay (Strous et al 1995), suggesting dysfunction of the auditory sensory memory system. This is a heuristically valuable paradigm, as underlying anatomical substrates have been well characterized in primate and human models. Lesions of auditory sensory cortex, located in superior temporal lobe, produce increases in tone matching threshold without affecting disruptive effects of distracting stimuli. In contrast, lesions of prefrontal cortex increase distractibility without affecting thresholds (Rabinowicz et al 2000). In patients with schizophrenia, increased thresholds are observed with no accompanying increase in susceptibility to either visual (March et al 1999) or auditory distraction (Rabinowicz et al 2000). Further, when equated for performance at short interstimulus interval (<1 s), patients show equivalent decay with increasing interval (March et al 1999), suggesting normal retention within the sensory memory system. These behavioural findings thus suggest dysfunctional information processing at the level of auditory sensory cortex.

Auditory function has also been assessed with event-related potentials (ERP), and especially mismatch negativity (MMN). MMN is elicited by infrequent changes in nature or pattern of repetitive auditory stimulation. Deviant stimuli may differ from standards in a number of stimulus dimensions, including pitch, duration, intensity or location. Generators for MMN have been mapped to auditory sensory cortex in the region of Heschl's gyrus (Javitt 2000). Deficits in MMN generation were first demonstrated in schizophrenia over 10 years ago and currently represent one of the best replicated neurophysiological findings in schizophrenia (Umbricht & Krljes 2005). Schizophrenia-like deficits in MMN generation can be induced by local infusion of NMDA antagonists into primate auditory cortex (Javitt 2000) and by systemic administration of NMDA antagonists in healthy volunteers (Umbricht et al 2000) (Fig. 2), suggesting that such deficits may index NMDA dysfunction at the level of auditory cortex.

More recent studies have investigated consequences of elevated tone matching thresholds to more complex forms of information processing dysfunction. Patients with schizophrenia, for example, show well-established deficits in ability to determine emotion based upon vocal modulation (prosody), which are thought to be rate-limiting in terms of functional outcome (Brekke et al 2005). The aetiology of such deficits has been poorly understood, as patients show normal emotional responses to happy or sad events, and show intact internal representation of

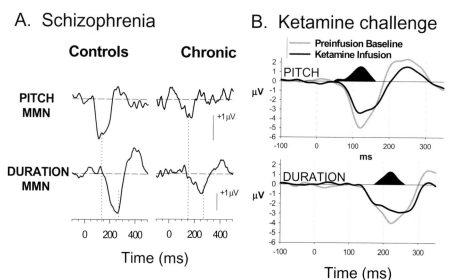

A. Schizophrenia   B. Ketamine challenge

FIG. 2.   Comparison of mismatch negativity (MMN) deficits in schizophrenia (A) vs. those observed following ketamine administration in normal volunteers. Figures are redrawn from Javitt et al (1995) and Umbricht et al (2000).

emotion (Kring et al 2003), suggesting that failure to detect emotion may be related to underlying failure to utilize sensory cues. An initial study of prosodic detection in schizophrenia demonstrated that such deficits were highly related to underlying disturbances in underlying tone matching ability (Leitman et al 2005), and extended not only to emotion detection but also to ability to detect attitudinal prosody (sarcasm) (Leitman et al 2006), as well as non-affective prosody such as the ability to differentiate statements and questions (Leitman et al 2007). Further, severity of deficit across individuals correlated highly with reduced structural integrity within auditory white matter pathways at the level of auditory cortex (Leitman et al 2007) (Fig. 3). Taken together, these findings suggest that basic deficits in NMDA receptor-mediated neurotransmission at the level of auditory sensory cortex may contribute to holistic deficits in schizophrenia such as ability to detect emotion during interpersonal interactions, and that such deficits contribute disproportionately to impaired functional outcome.

Visual processing deficits. Similar studies have been performed investigating consequences of NMDA dysfunction in the early visual system. The early visual system consists of discrete magnocellular and parvocellular pathways that differ in characteristics and function. The magnocellular pathway provides rapid transmission

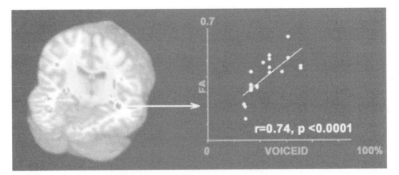

FIG. 3.   Voxelwise correlation of white matter integrity in schizophrenia, as measured by diffusion tensor imaging with deficits in voice emotion identification (VOICEID) in schizophrenia. (*Left*) Regional correlation clusters (dark grey) showing localization to subcortical and cortical auditory pathways. (*Right*) Correlation between local fractional anisotropy and voice identification in patients with schizophrenia.

of low-resolution information to cortex, in order to prime attentional systems and 'frame' the overall visual scene. The parvocellular pathway, in contrast, provides slower, higher resolution information to fill-in scene details (Chen et al 2007). NMDA receptors are located at multiple levels in the early visual system, including retina, lateral geniculate nucleus (LGN) and primary cortex. The magnocellular system, in particular, functions in a non-linear gain mode that is dependent upon NMDA receptor-mediated neurotransmission. Administration of NMDA antagonists to cat LGN produces a characteristic reduction in gain that is also observed in schizophrenia (Butler et al 2005b).

To date, deficits in visual processing have been demonstrated in schizophrenia using both steady-state (Butler et al 2005a) and transient (Butler et al 2007) visual evoked potential approaches. Further, deficits in early visual processing produce subsequent impairments on higher order processes such as object identification (Doniger et al 2002), motion processing (Kim et al 2006), face emotion recognition (Butler et al 2005a) and reading (Revheim et al 2006). Thus, as in the auditory system, basic deficits in NMDA function within subcortical and cortical systems lead to complex patterns of neuropsychological dysfunction observed in schizophrenia.

Glutamate–dopamine interactions

Finally, NMDA dysfunction may also account for impaired dopaminergic regulation in schizophrenia. Dopaminergic dysfunction has been studied most extensively using positron emission (PET) or single photon emission (SPECT) markers

of response to amphetamine. In such studies, D2 agonists are tagged with appropriate radionuclides (e.g.^{14}C,^{123}I) and the pattern of displacement is evaluated
following amphetamine administration. Across cohorts, patients with acute schizophrenia show enhanced striatal dopamine release to amphetamine challenge,
consistent with presumed dysregulation of subcortical dopamine circuits (Laruelle
et al 1999). Deficits similar to those observed in schizophrenia are observed also
in normal volunteers undergoing ketamine infusion (Kegeles et al 2000), and in
rodents treated subchronically (Balla et al 2001) with NMDA receptor antagonists,
suggesting that dopaminergic dysregulation in schizophrenia may be 'downstream'
of a primary deficit in NMDA function.

Clinical studies with NMDA agonists

In rodents (Javitt et al 2004) and primates (Linn et al 2007), effects of NMDA
antagonists may be reversed by concurrent treatment with agonists of the NMDA/
glycine site, such as glycine or D-serine, as well as more recently developed glycine
transport inhibitors, which increase brain glycine levels by blocking its removal
from the synaptic cleft by glycine type I (GLYT1) transporters (Javitt et al 1997)
(Fig. 4). Over the last decade, several small scale studies using naturally occurring
glycine-site agonists have been conducted. Several agents have been used for these
studies: glycine, D-serine and D-alanine, which function as full agonists; D-
cycloserine, which functions as a partial agonist; and sarcosine, which is a naturally
occurring glycine transport inhibitor. Across studies, the full agonists glycine and
D-serine have been found to be more effective than the partial agonist D-

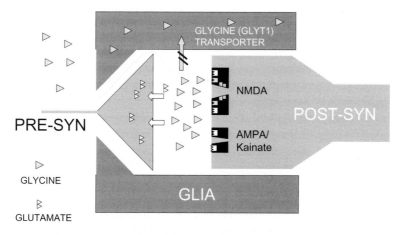

FIG. 4.   Schematic model of synaptic glycine regulation by glycine transport inhibitors.

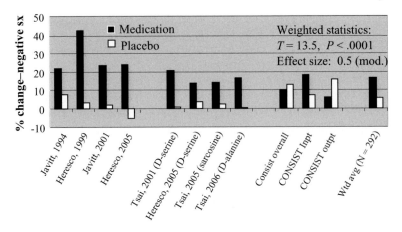

FIG. 5.   Summary of clinical trials performed to date with full NMDA agonists combined with antipsychotics other than clozapine. Further details about individual studies can be found in Javitt (2006).

cycloserine, and compounds have been found to be more effective when combined with typical or newer atypical antipsychotics (e.g. risperidone, olanzapine) than with clozapine (Javitt 2006).

Across all studies utilizing full agonists in combination with either typical or newer atypicals, involving approximately 292 patients to date, NMDA agonists have been found to produce an approximately 15% improvement in negative symptoms (Fig. 5), along with significant changes in positive and cognitive symptoms in some but not all studies. Weighted statistics show that glycine vs. placebo differences are statistically significant across studies, and are of moderate effect-size (0.5 SD units). It is worth noting that all compounds tested to date are low affinity 'agents of convenience' that could be entered easily into clinical trials because they are naturally occurring compounds. Several selective, high affinity glycine transport (GLYT1) inhibitors have been shown to have beneficial effects in preclinical paradigms and are currently under clinical development. In addition, several other glutamatergic approaches are currently being evaluated, including use of compounds that act at metabotropic and AMPA-type glutamate receptors. Whether or not such agents are effective clinically should become apparent over the next decade.

Finally, one study has evaluated effects of glycine in a limited number of individuals showing prodromal symptoms of schizophrenia. In that study, large effect-size improvement was observed, including early remission, in three of 10 subjects (Woods et al 2004). These data, if confirmed, would indicate that NMDA agonists might have a primary role in the earliest stages of schizophrenia psychosis, with potential impact across symptomatic domains.

Acknowledgements

Preparation of this manuscript was supported in part by USPHS grants K02 MH01439, R01 DA03383, and R37 MH49334, and by a Clinical Scientist Award in Translational Research from the Burroughs Wellcome Fund.

References

Adler CM, Malhotra AK, Elman I et al 1999 Comparison of ketamine-induced thought disorder in healthy volunteers and thought disorder in schizophrenia. Am J Psychiatry 156:1646–1649

Balla A, Koneru R, Smiley J, Sershen H, Javitt DC 2001 Continuous phencyclidine treatment induces schizophrenia-like hyperreactivity of striatal dopamine release. Neuropsychopharmacology 25:157–164

Bilder RM, Goldman RS, Robinson D et al 2000 Neuropsychology of first-episode schizophrenia: initial characterization and clinical correlates. Am J Psychiatry 157:549–559

Brekke J, Kay DD, Lee KS, Green MF 2005 Biosocial pathways to functional outcome in schizophrenia. Schizophr Res 80:213–225

Butler PD, Gur RC, Jalbkowcski M et al 2005a Visual processing impairment and emotion recognition dysfunction in schizophrenia. Schizophr Bull 31:352

Butler PD, Zemon V, Schechter I et al 2005b Early-stage visual processing and cortical amplification deficits in schizophrenia. Arch Gen Psychiatry 62:495–504

Butler PD, Martinez A, Foxe JJ et al 2007 Subcortical visual dysfunction in schizophrenia drives secondary cortical impairments. Brain 130:417–430

Carlsson A 1988 The current status of the dopamine hypothesis of schizophrenia. Neuropsychopharmacology 1:179–186

Chen CM, Lakatos P, Shah AS et al 2007 Functional anatomy and interaction of fast and slow visual pathways in macaque monkeys. Cereb Cortex 17:1561–1569.

Doniger GM, Foxe JJ, Murray MM, Higgins BA, Javitt DC 2002 Impaired visual object recognition and dorsal/ventral stream interaction in schizophrenia. Arch Gen Psychiatry 59:1011–1020

Ho BC, Andreasen NC, Nopoulos P, Fuller R, Arndt S, Cadoret RJ 2005 Secondary prevention of schizophrenia: utility of standardized scholastic tests in early identification. Ann Clin Psychiatry 17:11–18

Javitt DC 2000 Intracortical mechanisms of mismatch negativity dysfunction in schizophrenia. Audiol Neurootol 5:207–215

Javitt DC 2006 Is the glycine site half saturated or half unsaturated? Effects of glutamatergic drugs in schizophrenia patients. Curr Opin Psychiatry 19:151–157

Javitt DC, Zukin SR 1991 Recent advances in the phencyclidine model of schizophrenia. Am J Psychiatry 148:1301–1308

Javitt DC, Doneshka P, Grochowski S, Ritter W 1995 Impaired mismatch negativity generation reflects widespread dysfunction of working memory in schizophrenia. Arch Gen Psychiatry 52:550–558

Javitt DC, Sershen H, Hashim A, Lajtha A 1997 Reversal of phencyclidine-induced hyperactivity by glycine and the glycine uptake inhibitor glycyldodecylamide. Neuropsychopharmacology 17:202–204

Javitt DC, Balla A, Burch S, Suckow R, Xie S, Sershen H 2004 Reversal of phencyclidine-induced dopaminergic dysregulation by N-methyl-D-aspartate receptor/glycine-site agonists. Neuropsychopharmacology 29:300–307

Kegeles LS, Abi-Dargham A, Zea-Ponce Y et al 2000 Modulation of amphetamine-induced striatal dopamine release by ketamine in humans: implications for schizophrenia. Biol Psychiatry 48:627–640

Kim D, Wylie G, Pasternak R, Butler PD, Javitt DC 2006 Magnocellular contributions to impaired motion processing in schizophrenia. Schizophr Res 82:1–8

Kring AM, Barrett LF, Gard DE 2003 On the broad applicability of the affective circumplex: representations of affective knowledge among schizophrenia patients. Psychol Sci 14:207–214

Krystal JH, Perry EB Jr, Gueorguieva R et al 2005 Comparative and interactive human psychopharmacologic effects of ketamine and amphetamine: implications for glutamatergic and dopaminergic model psychoses and cognitive function. Arch Gen Psychiatry 62:985–994

Lahti AC, Weiler MA, Tamara Michaelidis BA, Parwani A, Tamminga CA 2001 Effects of ketamine in normal and schizophrenic volunteers. Neuropsychopharmacology 25: 455–467

Laruelle M, Abi-Dargham A, Gil R, Kegeles L, Innis R 1999 Increased dopamine transmission in schizophrenia: relationship to illness phases. Biol Psychiatry 46:56–72

Leitman DI, Foxe JJ, Butler PD, Saperstein A, Revheim N, Javitt DC 2005 Sensory contributions to impaired prosodic processing in schizophrenia. Biol Psychiatry 58:56–61

Leitman DI, Ziwich R, Pasternak R, Javitt DC 2006 Theory of Mind (ToM) and counterfactuality deficits in schizophrenia: misperception or misinterpretation? Psychol Med 36: 1075–1083

Leitman DI, Hoptman MJ, Foxe JJ et al 2007 The neural substrates of impaired prosodic detection in schizophrenia and its sensorial antecedents. Am J Psychiatry 164:474–482

Lencz T, Smith CW, McLaughlin D et al 2006 Generalized and specific neurocognitive deficits in prodromal schizophrenia. Biol Psychiatry 59:863–871

Linn GS, O'Keeffe RT, Lifshitz K, Schroeder C, Javitt DC 2007 Behavioral effects of orally administered glycine in socially housed monkeys chronically treated with phencyclidine. Psychopharmacology (Berl) 192:27–38

March L, Cienfuegos A, Goldbloom L, Ritter W, Cowan N, Javitt DC 1999 Normal time course of auditory recognition in schizophrenia, despite impaired precision of the auditory sensory ("echoic") memory code. J Abnorm Psychol 108:69–75

Parwani A, Weiler MA, Blaxton TA et al 2005 The effects of a subanesthetic dose of ketamine on verbal memory in normal volunteers. Psychopharmacology (Berl) 183:265–274

Rabinowicz EF, Silipo G, Goldman R, Javitt DC 2000 Auditory sensory dysfunction in schizophrenia: imprecision or distractibility? Arch Gen Psychiatry 57:1149–1155

Revheim N, Butler PD, Schechter I, Jalbrzikowski M, Silipo G, Javitt DC 2006 Reading impairment and visual processing deficits in schizophrenia. Schizophr Res 87:238–245

Strous RD, Cowan N, Ritter W, Javitt DC 1995 Auditory sensory ("echoic") memory dysfunction in schizophrenia. Am J Psychiatry 152:1517–1519

Umbricht D, Krljes S 2005 Mismatch negativity in schizophrenia: a meta-analysis. Schizophr Res 76:1–23

Umbricht D, Schmid L, Koller R, Vollenweider FX, Hell D, Javitt DC 2000 Ketamine-induced deficits in auditory and visual context-dependent processing in healthy volunteers: implications for models of cognitive deficits in schizophrenia. Arch Gen Psychiatry 57:1139–1147

Woods SW, Thomas L, Tully E et al 2004 Effects of oral glycine in the schizophrenia prodrome. Schizophr Res 70:79

DISCUSSION

Chao: It's apparent that there are many cognitive processes involved in schizophrenia. To what extent do the deficits overlap with those in other psychiatric diseases?

Javitt: We are still working on this. It's a matter of the level you choose to look at. One might think that the learning and memory deficits are shared in Alzheimer's, but when we look at what is driving learning and memory problems we see much more of an encoding failure in schizophrenia, as opposed to the retention failure that characterizes Alzheimer's. For people with amnestic syndrome, their main problem is retention. One of the interesting features of schizophrenia is that people with the disease have relatively intact retention even though their encoding is poor. Memory deficits can be a problem in many diseases, but if one looks at the exact pattern it becomes much more specific with schizophrenia. There are social communicative disorders in autism spectrum disorders, but in schizophrenia, we find that the pattern patients have reflects their inability to use tonal cues. They can use intensity cues fine: for example, they have no problem in picking up anger, because anger is conveyed by the voice getting louder. But to decode happiness requires picking up pitch variability and patients with schizophrenia are quite poor at this. It is quite likely that there are other diseases that have social communicatory dysfunction, but won't have this driven by the same level of dysfunction. We are currently in a disagreement with some members of the dyslexia community: we showed that the magnocellular dysfunction in our patients correlated with their reading deficits. Some members of the dyslexia community have been saying that in dyslexia reading deficits don't correlate with magnocellular dysfunction but instead with phonological processing deficits. This could be true, but it doesn't change the fact that we are seeing these deficits in schizophrenia being magnocellular. There are lots of conditions where there are reading deficits, but if you look at the nitty gritty of what is driving them, it could be different in each case. At a macro level there are a lot of diseases that cause cognitive dysfunction, but as you drill down to specific patterns schizophrenia will turn out to be relatively unique. The pattern will look very much like an NMDA pattern, and, to put this the other way, if you have a pattern that looks like an NMDA pattern, then I'd say you are looking at schizophrenia. It could be that schizophrenia is basically the condition that happens when NMDA function falls below a certain level.

Raff: To what extent are these cognitive and perceptive defects you see stable once the patient is clinically stable, and to what extent is there progression?

Javitt: From our work we don't have all that much direct information on this. Mismatch negativity seems to fall for the first year after people develop the illness, and then remains quite stable. Many of these processes have a normal decline with ageing. There may be some exaggerated decline in the patients, but for the most part it tracks like the normal ageing curve. The cognitive deficits seem to track the normal ageing curve.

Raff: Are the imaging findings consistent with a lack of progression?

Javitt: Yes.

Lu: Following what you said about the cognitive deficits, I guess many people have thought about working memory. Would you say that recognition memory for objects or faces is impaired in schizophrenia as well?

Javitt: Working memory does lots of different thing, but the term is used in two different ways. There is a distinction between retaining the information in the working memory system (keeping it online), versus getting it in the memory system. Some people say that memory is just keeping it in once it gets in, whereas others use the term more broadly, including the process of getting it in the definition. This is a distinction worth making, because what is impaired in schizophrenia is getting information into the working memory system. In terms of faces, people with schizophrenia have a less precise representation of face that they then feed into whatever area is responsible for holding that face information online. They will do worse in a face recognition task for this reason: it is not because they are unable to hold the memory, but because they had degraded input into the memory system.

Lu: If I can push this further, one aspect is retaining it, the other is getting it. Is that correct?

Javitt: There is encoding, retention and retrieval. Encoding seems to be impaired. Retention is relatively intact, and retrieval is hard to distinguish from encoding. In chronic patients, retention doesn't seem to be impaired, but in acute patients it might be. Then the question becomes one of circuitry. It is hard to know where the circuit is breaking down. We have done a series of tests known as a fragmented object test. We present chopped up pictures and add more and more information. We look at how many pieces people need in order to identify the object. Schizophrenia patients need more pieces. We can do this test with electrophysiology and imaging to see which parts of the brain are not doing what they should. When we look at this we see activations in visual cortex, in the lateral occipital complex, the part of the brain related to object recognition. They have reduced activation of that area of the brain. There is a lot of work looking at the circuitry there, and it turns out that in order to do this task one not only needs direct inputs into this visual area, but also inputs that go up through the dorsal ventral stream into frontal cortex, back down to hippocampus and back down to inferotemporal cortex. The patients with schizophrenia don't look like they have this normal circuit. The circuit seems to break down at early stages, at the visual/magnocellular input level. One thing that has come into the literature is the idea that areas are disconnected; that there is something physically abnormal about the connections. But nothing we have seen suggests this.

Lu: Just a comment on the glutamate hypothesis. Perhaps you could call it the NMDA hypothesis instead. NMDA receptors can be divided into different subclasses based on the NR2 subunits they contain. Two subtypes of NMDA receptors have received a lot of interests in recent years: the NR2A and the NR2B subtypes. One idea is that the NR2A is for LTP and the NR2B is for LTD. Perhaps attention should be paid to this difference. Also, as I hear more from the clinical aspect, synaptic transmission seems to be implicated. I would argue that the problem is not with synaptic transmission per se but rather synaptic plasticity (activity-dependent changes in synaptic efficacy). We may learn from studies of neurotrophins. Years ago people were looking for the effect of dumping BDNF and seeing what happens in *in vitro* systems, and they reported enhancement of synaptic transmission. This is not physiologically meaningful: if you enhanced all the glutamatergic synaptic transmission, it won't be very helpful for your cognitive functions. What is needed is the modification of a certain synapse in a use-dependent manner. This modification is what we now know as synaptic plasticity. NMDA receptor fits a lot better into the plasticity theory than the glutamate transmission theory.

Javitt: I agree, but I am concerned that some of the features of NMDA receptors in synaptic transmission get overlooked. They do a lot of things, and one of them is to activate cascades, initiating plasticity. But some of the curves, such as in the magnocellular system, are non-linear gain curves, and require a receptor such as NMDA that has a voltage dependence in order to generate those curves. You don't need NMDA receptors to do it—you can do it with a combination of other receptors—but NMDA receptors are a one-stop shop for generating these curves. Even the slow channel kinetics of NMDA receptors are taken advantage of by the visual system for processing motion. I think the difference between 2B and 2A is critical. In terms of behavioural tests, we know of some that are much better for looking at LTP than LTD. If we could come up with LTD tasks that could be applied in patients, this would be very interesting. It's possible that these processes are also impaired.

Barde: You asked for an explanation of how to link NMDA with growth factors. Probably the best way to drive the expression of the BDNF gene is by synaptic activation of the NMDA receptors. This was shown nicely by Hilmar Bading and colleagues (Hardingham et al 2002). Regarding the effects of BDNF in the brain, a student in our lab, Stefanie Rauskolb, managed to generate a mouse that is essentially lacking BDNF through the entire nervous system. We generated this mouse mostly to look at the morphological effect of deprivation of BDNF. Perhaps not so surprisingly, mice can reach several months of age. Their brains are smaller, but this is not because there are fewer neurons. The main differences are due to changes in volume of the axons, and presumably of the myelin sheath as a consequence. It is not so much the dendritic aborization that is decreased, though this is what has been mostly looked at so far. In terms of what happens to the volume of the brain, this can be linked up: if there is less synaptic inactivation of the NMDA receptor, there is less transcription of the BDNF gene, and axons will be smaller and less myelinated.

Javitt: Conversely, if you had less BDNF, would you expect this to affect NMDA transmission?

Barde: Perhaps, by the activation of expression of NMDA receptors.

Flint: You presented quite a lot of psychological data. You put these in the context of dopamine and NMDA. Do you think your neuropsychological data support the connectionist ideas that Chris Frith and others have put forward about schizophrenia (McGuire & Frith 1996)?

Javitt: They certainly support connectionist concepts, if you think of connectionism as being functional rather than purely structural. Within the same anatomy we can get either intact or impaired function, depending on how we manipulate our test conditions. It doesn't seem that any one pathway is abnormal or normal; it is in a sense what you are driving it to do. If you think the hippocampus is encoding information or retaining information, it is the same neurons that retain and encode, but they seem to be able to retain and not encode. I would break it down functionally.

Flint: I'm addressing more specifically the idea that there are internally and externally generated bits of information, and tying these bits together is a problem in schizophrenia.

Javitt: Absolutely: I just wouldn't over-emphasize this as being the problem. These pathways are needed to tie information together.

Flint: Chris Frith's idea would be that this is the key problem (McGuire & Frith 1996).

Javitt: I would say it is one of many problems.

Owen: Do you think all patients with schizophrenia have cognitive impairment? Is it a necessary feature of the disorder? I'm talking about an impairment compared with their expected trajectory.

Javitt: That seems to be what is coming out of the literature. Jim Gold has argued this forcefully (Wilk et al 2005): if you have schizophrenia you are reduced compared with what you would be expected to have from your family and background. This isn't to say that some people don't have normal or even high IQ with schizophrenia.

Malaspina: Something as elementary as pain threshold is abnormal in many people who have schizophrenia early on. I'd advance the idea that schizophrenia is a syndrome: it may be that a large proportion of cases share a similar aetiology, but several different pathophysiologies.

Tongiorgi: I have a question about the imaging. Have you or others tried to do imaging of the NMDA receptors in the brains of patients? If so, does this correlate with the striking asymmetry in the brain?

Javitt: I wish we had a functional probe of NMDA receptors. There are some ligands out there that people are developing which bind to the PCP site that binds in the channels. There is some controversy about how effective they are. I don't have access to them. There is some post-mortem work with NMDA receptors (Meador-Woodruff et al 2003) showing reductions of NMDA expression, in particular in thalamus, which might go along with some of these findings.

Tongiorgi: Is there any idea about the difference between the two hemispheres, in terms of functionality? Is there a hypothesis about the biological basis of this?

Javitt: What I showed isn't really hemispheric asymmetry, although there are people who are strong advocates of this. Depending on how we do the tests we can find deficits in left hemisphere or right hemisphere.

Buonanno: You initially seem to suggest that ketamine could have an effect on parvalbumin GABAergic neurons, but then you seem to be discussing more the issue of function in these neurons. Those two ideas could be put together: a very small change in a selected population of inhibitory neurons that could regulate rhythmic function could be difficult to observe at the level of anatomy, but nevertheless be functionally significant. You don't even need a problem in the glutamatergic synapse: it could just be affecting the way that glutamate signalling is gated. Is that consistent with what you are saying? Or do you think there is no change in any of the cell numbers?

Javitt: The hardest findings are the GAD67 parvalbumin reductions. What drives them? It's a bit of a chicken and egg argument. Do you need to postulate another pathology, or would NMDA dysfunction by itself be enough to cause what we see in postmortem studies? These studies are examples of postmortem changes that potentially could be ascribed to NMDA function. It doesn't mean that there is not an 'egg' approach to it too: if there is a primary GABAergic deficit that affects NMDA function, it wouldn't produce the syndrome of schizophrenia that we see. I don't want anyone to think I am suggesting that NMDA receptors themselves are driving this. I just see them as a point of confluence: just as too little dopamine may cause Parkinson's, too little NMDA may cause schizophrenia. It could be factors such as glutathione reductions, homocysteine elevations, kainic acid elevations, reduced GABA or genetic abnormalities play in to a final common pathway. Which will be chickens and which will be eggs? BDNF, for example, may be a chicken because NMDA may cause changes in BDNF, whereas other things might be eggs in that they cause the glutamate changes.

Buonanno: Isn't this why the genetics is critical?

Javitt: We have to believe the genetics is the egg.

References

Hardingham GE, Fukunaga Y, Bading H 2002 Extrasynaptic NMDARs oppose synaptic NMDARs by triggering CREB shut-off and cell death pathways. Nat Neurosci 5:405–414

McGuire PK, Frith CD 1996 Disordered functional connectivity in schizophrenia. Psychol Med 26:663–667

Meador-Woodruff JH, Clinton SM, Beneyto M, McCullumsmith RE 2003 Molecular abnormalities of the glutamate synapse in the thalamus in schizophrenia. Ann N Y Acad Sci 1003:75–93

Wilk CM, Gold JM, McMahon RP, Humber K, Iannone VN, Buchanan RW 2005 No, it is not possible to be schizophrenic yet neuropsychologically normal. Neuropsychology 19:778–786

Genetic variants in major depression

Jonathan Flint, Sagiv Shifman, Marcus Munafo* and Richard Mott

*Wellcome Trust Centre for Human Genetics, University of Oxford, Roosevelt Drive, Oxford OX3 7BN and *Department of Experimental Psychology, University of Bristol, 8 Woodland Road, Bristol BS8 1TN, UK*

Abstract. Major depression is one of the most common and most debilitating disorders in the world. A wealth of data indicate that additive genetic effects contribute to at least 30% of the variance in liability to major depression, yet attempts to identify the molecular basis of susceptibility using standard family based linkage and genetic association methodologies have had limited success. Alternative approaches have recently been advocated, such as the inclusion of gene by environment interactions and the use of endophenotypes. Our own data indicate that the genetic architecture of affective illness is more complex than expected. A whole genome association study of neuroticism, a personality trait that shares many of the same susceptibility loci as depression, reveals that the individual effect sizes are less than 1%. Larger sample sizes and more sophisticated analytical approaches will be needed than have hitherto been applied.

2008 Growth factors and psychiatric disorders. Wiley, Chichester (Novartis Foundation Symposium 289) p 23–42

In this paper I will review progress in mapping the genetic basis of major depression (MD). I deal here with non-psychotic affective illness and I have not reviewed the large literature on bipolar disorder. I discuss first the attempts that have been made to identify loci using human linkage and association strategies. In common with other complex traits, I show that MD has been largely resistant to genetic dissection. I consider explanations of why this is so.

Family based studies of MD

Major depression (MD) is one of the leading causes of disability in the world. Since the 1990s, when it was forecast to become the second leading cause of disability worldwide (after ischaemic heart disease) by 2020 (Murray & Lopez 1996), prevalence estimates have only added to evidence of the disorder's importance (Alonso et al 2004a). Lifetime prevalence estimates typically vary from 8% to 12% (Alonso et al 2004b, Kessler et al 2003). MD is not only common, but it is also associated with considerable morbidity (Penninx et al 2001), mortality (Schneider et al 2001) and substantial economic costs (Scott et al 2003).

Family, adoption and twin studies concur in identifying a significant heritable component to MD. A meta-analysis of high-quality twin studies concluded that the variance in liability to MD is mostly due to individual-specific environmental effects (58%–67%) and additive genetic effects (31%–42%) (Sullivan et al 2000). Very similar figures were obtained by a recent study of over 40 000 twins, which estimated the heritability of MD to be 0.38 (Kendler et al 2006a). Notably, the relative risk in first degree relatives for MD is only ~2.8 (Sullivan et al 2000) suggesting that the effect size attributable to individual genetic variants is likely to be small.

Despite the condition's prevalence and the important aetiological role of genetic susceptibility, it has attracted relatively few molecular genetic investigations. To date there have been four whole genome linkage scans (Abkevich et al 2003, Holmans et al 2004, McGuffin et al 2005, Zubenko et al 2003). Three of these reported genome-wide significant linkage signals, but disagreed about their location (each study reporting a single significant locus, on, respectively, chromosomes 2q, 12q and 15q). The fourth study (McGuffin et al 2005) was unable to detect any locus that exceeded a genome wide-significant threshold, but provided some support for loci on 12q and 15q.

Capitalizing on the additional power to be gained from using quantitative traits rather than dichotomous classifications and working with samples from the extremes of a large population, we and others have mapped a personality trait, neuroticism, genetically related to depression (Fullerton et al 2003, Nash et al 2004). The genetic studies were carried out on the basis of a considerable body of data indicating that neuroticism would serve as an effective proxy phenotype for depression, one that shares many of the same genetic loci but is considerably quicker, and cheaper, to measure (neuroticism is assessed with a self-administered personality questionnaire, which, in the version developed by Hans Eysenck, has 23 neuroticism response items [Eysenck & Eysenck 1975]). The degree of neuroticism has been found to predict the onset and subsequent episodes of MD (Boyce et al 1991) and is associated with symptoms of depression and anxiety in the general population (Jylha & Isometsa 2006). Large population-based twin studies have found a substantial genetic correlation between the two conditions (Fanous et al 2002, Kendler et al 2006b). The largest study (of almost 21 000 twins) estimated the genetic correlation to be between +0.46 and +0.47 (Kendler et al 2006b). Consequently finding quantitative trait loci (QTL) that contribute to variation in neuroticism is expected to be a step towards identifying at least some of the loci that are responsible for genetic susceptibility to MD (Flint 2004).

In order to generate a human sample collection suitable for the genetic analysis of neuroticism, we posted over 200 000 Eysenck Personality Questionnaires (EPQ)

(Eysenck & Eysenck 1975) to individuals over the age of 30 resident in southwest England. We collected 34 000 sibling pairs (Martin et al 2000) and, by contacting respondents with personality scores in the extremes of the EPQ distribution, obtained DNA samples from 561 families suitable for linkage mapping (Risch & Zhang 1995). This approach identified five loci that exceeded a 5% genome-wide significance threshold (Fullerton et al 2003), some of which have been found by other groups: QTLs on chromosome 1 have been reported now by five groups (reviewed in Fullerton 2005).

The genetic effects we found were small. The extremely large sample needed to detect them makes additional fine-mapping and gene identification steps extremely difficult. Despite the success of the initial mapping, further progress in molecular identification of the responsible variants has been slow. As we will see below, this is almost certainly due to the complex genetic architecture responsible.

Genetic association studies of MD

As with other psychiatric illnesses, many genetic association studies of MD have been performed, mostly investigating the involvement of candidates suggested by pharmacological and hormonal hypotheses of the origins of depression (serotonin transporter, serotonin 2A receptor, tyrosine hydroxylase, tryptophan hydroxylase 1 and catechol-O-methyltransferase) (reviewed in Levinson 2006). In common with the findings for other psychiatric diseases, the results have been largely inconclusive. A single meta-analysis has been reported, which found no evidence for the involvement of the serotonin receptors or transporter (Anguelova et al 2003). A potentially important finding that a hypomorphic allele of a brain specific tryptophan hydroxylase (TPH2) (Zhang et al 2004) is associated with severe depression (Zhang et al 2005) was followed by a series of reports that not only failed to replicate the finding, but could not detect the polymorphism (Glatt et al 2005, Van Den Bogaert et al 2005, Zhou et al 2005). There is also a single report, which analysed two independent samples, that FKBP5, a glucocorticoid receptor-regulating co-chaperone of HSP90, is associated with response to antidepressants and susceptibility for depression (Binder et al 2004).

There is a much larger literature of genetic association studies of neuroticism, although devoted to a remarkably small number of genes. Most interest has focused on the serotonin system, and no other variant in psychiatric genetics, indeed perhaps in all genetics, has been as extensively studied by association as a length polymorphism, 5HTTLPR, situated approximately 1 kb upstream of the serotonin transporter gene (SLC6A4). Differences in the number and sequence of a short (20–23 bp) motif give rise two common length alleles: a short (*s*) allele, consisting of 14 repeat elements (40% frequency in most populations), and a long (*l*) allele that consists of 16 repeats (Lesch et al 1996). The *s* allele is associated with decreased SLC6A4 transcription relative to the *l* allele (Lesch et al 1996).

More than 100 studies have investigated whether the 5HTTLPR polymorphism contributes to variation in personality (Anguelova et al 2003) but consensus about the potential importance of the polymorphism is not matched by a similar level of agreement in reported results. Meta-analyses of the available data find that the effect attributable to the locus is either small or non-existent (Munafo et al 2003). If the 5HTTLPR does exert some influence over neuroticism then a sufficiently large sample should detect its impact. We used our cohort of extreme scoring neuroticism individuals and also genotyped a sample of 5000 individuals selected from a population of 20921 individuals of the Norfolk cohort of the European Prospective Investigation into Cancer (EPIC-Norfolk) (Day et al 1999). Power calculations showed that either population would detect an effect accounting for just 0.5% of phenotypic variation. We found no evidence to indicate the involvement of the variant in neuroticism.

Alternative explanations

Even the most enthusiastic supporters of genetic approaches to psychiatric illness would admit that success has been limited. Over the years there have been a number of attempts to explain the relative failure.

The first possibility is that the genetic effect is easier to detect in an interaction than as a main effect. Suppose there are many independent effects, each of which increases susceptibility to depression by a small amount, for example by just 2%. Suppose also that some combinations of effect do not simply increase susceptibility additively: when two such effects are present, the risk might increase 10% rather than 4%. These effects could both be genetic, in which case the interaction is said to be epistatic, or they could be a mixture of environmental and genetic: the effect of a particular genotype will only be manifest given a particular environment. The latter seems particularly likely given that the relationship between depression and known environmental stressors, such as loss of a parent or physical, emotional or sexual abuse, is not straightforward. There is indeed some evidence that the serotonin transporter exerts an effect on depression in this way (Caspi et al 2003), though it remains to be seen whether the findings of gene by environment effects will be any more robust than the reports of main effects.

Historically, the detected effects size of early reports of positive genetic associations are much larger than subsequent findings: for example there is clear evidence of publication bias for associations between alcoholism and a genetic variant in the dopamine D2 receptor gene (Munafo et al 2006). The initial report of the association between neuroticism and the 5HTTLPR polymorphism is larger than subsequent findings; the same appears to be true for the initial report of a gene by environment interaction between the 5HTTLPR polymorphism and depression (Caspi et al 2003) when compared to attempts at replication (Gillespie et al 2004, Surtees et al 2006).

Second, genetic association studies have been constrained by the limited number of candidates so far tested. Simply put, we have tested the wrong candidates. It is possible that more robust associations are waiting to be found. Completion of the HapMap project (Altshuler et al 2005) and the advent of cheap high throughput genotyping strategies make it possible to investigate whether this is the case. Approximately 7 million single nucleotide polymorphisms (SNPs) with frequencies above 5% in the human population have been identified (Kruglyak & Nickerson 2001) and due to the absence of historical recombination between neighbouring SNPs, one variant can serve as a proxy for several others, thereby reducing the required number of genotypes. By careful choice, a systematic analysis of genomic variation can be achieved by choosing an optimal set of several hundred thousand SNPs (Pe'er et al 2006) a number that is well within the capacity of current genotyping platforms.

Whole genome association is still an expensive option, but costs can be reduced by pooling equal amounts of DNA from each individual, separately for cases and controls, and estimating allele frequencies from the DNA pools (this is referred to as allelotyping). Recent studies have shown the feasibility and accuracy of estimating SNP allele frequencies in DNA pools using microarrays containing thousands of SNPs (Meaburn et al 2006), which makes it possible to carry out whole genome association studies in a cost-effective way.

We performed a whole genome analysis of pooled DNA from 2054 individuals from our community sample and attempted to replicate the results of the most significant SNPs in an independent sample. By using eight pools with five replicates of each, we were able to retain between 21% and 94% (depending on the effect size and threshold used) of the power from genotyping 452 574 SNPs individually. Simulation indicated that our study had ~80% power to identify neuroticism loci in the genome with odds ratio (OR) >2, and ~50% power to identify small effects (OR = 1.5). Only one SNP (rs702543) showed a statistically significant association in the replication. The SNP is located in the phosphodiesterase 4D, cAMP-specific (PDE4D) gene, in an intron between exon D3 and D8. We detected association with a P value of 0.00081 in the original sample, a P value of 0.00078 in a replication sample and a combined P value = 2×10^{-6}. The SNP was genotyped in three other laboratories, on related, but not identical, phenotypes. In each case the direction of allelic effects was the same as in our sample, but the test reached statistical significance in only one additional cohort. Most importantly for the argument here, the effect of the SNP was small: it accounted for only 0.6% of the variance of neuroticism in the population.

Our linkage study on the same cohort failed to find any large effect loci (explaining more than 5% of the variance) and, given that we had approximately 50% power to detect an odds ratio of 1.5 (which is equivalent to a locus explaining 0.5%–1% of the variance) and failed to find any loci accounting for more than 1% of the variance, the 40% additive genetic variance of neuroticism almost certainly arises from many loci explaining much less than 1%. These results strongly suggest that the current failure to obtain robust results is because of low power. For effects of the magnitude we think likely to exist for neuroticism, and therefore for MD, sample sizes of thousands will be needed to obtain robust results (Flint & Munafo 2007).

An alternative strategy is to find a phenotype, related to MD, for which the effect sizes are likely to be large. There has been enthusiasm for investigating endophenotypes, which lie in the gap between gene and disease process, can be objectively measured (ideally in a reliable fashion) (Gottesman & Gould 2003), and are closer to the site of genetic action, so that a genetic approach will be more easily rewarded with success. Endophenotypes are assumed to have a relatively simple genetic architecture because there are relatively few pathways from gene to phenotype. The consequence is that sequence variants interact relatively directly with the phenotype so the correlation should be easier to detect.

For example, Hariri and colleagues reported that the 5HTTLPR polymorphism is associated with the response of the amygdala to fearful stimuli (Hariri et al 2002). In a comparison of two groups of 14 individuals, carriers of the *s* allele were found to exhibit an increased amygdala fearful response compared with those homozygous for the *l* allele: the means of the two groups were 0.28 (standard deviation 0.22) and 0.03 (standard deviation 0.19) with respect to %BOLD signal change for fearful stimuli compared to neutral stimuli. This is equivalent to an effect size of 40% of phenotypic variance. Results from the same authors indicate that the figure is too large: a subsequent study of 92 individuals (including 19 from the first study) carried out by the same group showed a significant effect, but with reported mean values of 0.16 and 0.03 for the two groups (Hariri et al 2005), equivalent to an effect size of just over 10% of the phenotypic variance. Nevertheless, 10% is considerably larger than the figure of less than 1% inferred from our whole genome association study.

The likelihood that endophenotypes do indeed have much larger effect sizes is thrown into doubt by a number of observations. First, we carried out meta-analyses of a number of studies that have used endophenotypes and found that the effect sizes are no larger than those found for main effects. Because endophenotypes typically are difficult to collect, sample sizes are small and attempts at replication few. We were only able to analyse studies that had looked at the variants in the COMT gene, long regarded as a promising candidate gene for schizophrenia, as it is the gene coding for the catechol-*O*-methyltransferase enzyme, which inactivates catechols at postsynaptic sites in the human brain. COMT contains a functional polymorphism, a SNP at position 158/108 that results in a change from valine (Val) to methionine (Met) (Chen et al 2004). We found no evidence that the effect sizes in the three endophenotypes we examined (two psychological measures and one electrophysiological) was any larger than those reported for genetic effects on the relevant disease, in this case schizophrenia (Flint & Munafo 2007).

Second, work on model organisms now provides a thorough picture of the genetic architecture of complex traits. We have now analysed by whole genome association over 100 phenotypes in the mouse, including assays of physiology, immunology, haematology and biochemistry of the animals, as well as behavioural measures. Our analysis was carried out using over 2000 animals in a population with limited genetic diversity (compared to a human fully outbred population) so that the effect sizes of individual loci will be relatively increased. Figure 1 shows the distribution of effect sizes obtained for all phenotypes. The median effect size is 2.5%; only ten loci had effect sizes greater than 5%. There was no evidence that phenotypes could be differentiated by effect size: the genetic architecture of all phenotypes was remarkably uniform. Although these results were obtained in the mouse, it is difficult to believe that the genetic architecture of similar traits will

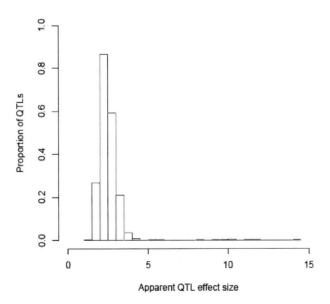

FIG. 1.   Effect size, expressed the percentage of the total phenotypic variance explained, of 843 quantitative trait loci in the mouse.

be different in our own species. The findings argue against the existence of phenotypes with larger genetic effect sizes.

Conclusion

I have reviewed evidence for the presence of substantial genetic effects on affective disorder. Current genetic strategies have not proven to be particularly successful. Neither linkage nor genetic association has yet revealed much about the biology of the condition. The reasons for this are, I argue, intrinsic to the genetic architecture of the condition, which is much more complicated than expected. Our data from a whole genome association study of neuroticism indicates that the effect sizes of individual loci explain less than 1% of the phenotype. While the inclusion of interaction effects, interactions that are either with the environment or with other genetic loci, may help gene identification, the approach is by no means a guaranteed panacea. Furthermore, attempts to use surrogate phenotypes that have a simpler, more tractable genetic architecture, are also unlikely to be helpful, since there is little evidence that the effect sizes of loci underlying endophenotypes are any larger than those of the disease phenotype. This is not to say that genetic methods will not prevail: only that larger sample sizes and more sophisticated analytical approaches will be needed than have hitherto been applied.

Acknowledgements

This work was supported by the Wellcome Trust.

References

Abkevich V, Camp NJ, Hensel CH et al 2003 Predisposition locus for major depression at chromosome 12q22–12q23.2. Am J Hum Genet 73:1271–1281
Alonso J, Angermeyer MC, Bernert S et al 2004a Disability and quality of life impact of mental disorders in Europe: results from the European Study of the Epidemiology of Mental Disorders (ESEMeD) project. Acta Psychiatr Scand Suppl:38–46
Alonso J, Angermeyer MC, Bernert S et al 2004b Prevalence of mental disorders in Europe: results from the European Study of the Epidemiology of Mental Disorders (ESEMeD) project. Acta Psychiatr Scand Suppl:21–27
Altshuler D, Brooks LD, Chakravarti A, Collins FS, Daly MJ, Donnelly P 2005 A haplotype map of the human genome. Nature 437:1299–1320
Anguelova M, Benkelfat C, Turecki G 2003 A systematic review of association studies investigating genes coding for serotonin receptors and the serotonin transporter: I. Affective disorders. Mol Psychiatry 8:574–591
Binder EB, Salyakina D, Lichtner P et al 2004 Polymorphisms in FKBP5 are associated with increased recurrence of depressive episodes and rapid response to antidepressant treatment. Nat Genet 36:1319–1325

Boyce P, Parker G, Barnett B, Cooney M, Smith F 1991 Personality as a vulnerability factor to depression. Br J Psychiatry 159:106–114

Caspi A, Sugden K, Moffitt TE et al 2003 Influence of life stress on depression: moderation by a polymorphism in the 5-HTT gene. Science 301:386–389

Chen J, Lipska BK, Halim N et al 2004 Functional analysis of genetic variation in catechol-O-methyltransferase (COMT): effects on mRNA, protein, and enzyme activity in postmortem human brain. Am J Hum Genet 75:807–821

Day N, Oakes S, Luben R et al 1999 EPIC-Norfolk: study design and characteristics of the cohort. European Prospective Investigation of Cancer. Br J Cancer 80 Suppl 1:95–103

Eysenck HJ, Eysenck SBG 1975 Manual of the Eysenck Personality Questionnaire. Educational and Industrial Testing Service, San Diego, CA

Fanous A, Gardner CO, Prescott CA, Cancro R, Kendler KS 2002 Neuroticism, major depression and gender: a population-based twin study. Psychol Med 32:719–728

Flint J 2004 The genetic basis of neuroticism. Neurosci Biobehav Rev 28:307–316

Flint J, Munafo MR 2007 The endophenotype concept in psychiatric genetics. Psychol Med 37:163–180

Fullerton J 2005 New approaches to the genetic analysis of neuroticism and anxiety. Behav Genet 36:147–161

Fullerton J, Cubin M, Tiwari H et al 2003 Linkage analysis of extremely discordant and concordant sibling pairs identifies quantitative-trait loci that influence variation in the human personality trait neuroticism. Am J Hum Genet 72:879–890

Gillespie NA, Whitfield JB, Williams B, Heath AC, Martin NG 2004 The relationship between stressful life events, the serotonin transporter (5-HTTLPR) genotype and major depression. Psychol Med 35:101–111

Glatt CE, Carlson E, Taylor TR, Risch N, Reus VI, Schaefer CA 2005 Response to Zhang et al (2005): loss-of-function mutation in tryptophan hydroxylase-2 identified in unipolar major depression. Neuron 45:11–16. Neuron 48:704–705; author reply 705–706

Gottesman, II, Gould TD 2003 The endophenotype concept in psychiatry: etymology and strategic intentions. Am J Psychiatry 160:636–645

Hariri AR, Mattay VS, Tessitore A et al 2002 Serotonin transporter genetic variation and the response of the human amygdala. Science 297:400–403

Hariri AR, Drabant EM, Munoz KE et al 2005 A susceptibility gene for affective disorders and the response of the human amygdala. Arch Gen Psychiatry 62:146–152

Holmans P, Zubenko GS, Crowe RR et al 2004 Genomewide significant linkage to recurrent, early-onset major depressive disorder on chromosome 15q. Am J Hum Genet 74:1154–1167

Jylha P, Isometsa E 2006 Temperament, character and symptoms of anxiety and depression in the general population. Eur Psychiatry 21:389–395

Kendler KS, Gatz M, Gardner CO, Pedersen NL 2006a A Swedish national twin study of lifetime major depression. Am J Psychiatry 163:109–114

Kendler KS, Gatz M, Gardner CO, Pedersen NL 2006b Personality and major depression: a Swedish longitudinal, population-based twin study. Arch Gen Psychiatry 63:1113–1120

Kessler RC, Berglund P, Demler O et al 2003 The epidemiology of major depressive disorder: results from the National Comorbidity Survey Replication (NCS-R). JAMA 289:3095–3105

Kruglyak L, Nickerson DA 2001 Variation is the spice of life. Nat Genet 27:234–236

Lesch K-P, Bengel D, Heils A et al 1996 Association of anxiety related traits with a polymorphism in the serotonin transporter gene regulatory region. Science 274:1527–1530

Levinson DF 2006 The genetics of depression: a review. Biol Psychiatry 60:84–92

Martin N, Goodwin G, Fairburn C et al 2000 A population based study of personality in 34,000 sib-pairs. Twin Res 3:310–315

McGuffin P, Knight J, Breen G et al 2005 Whole genome linkage scan of recurrent depressive disorder from the depression network study. Hum Mol Genet 14:3337–3345

Meaburn E, Butcher LM, Schalkwyk LC, Plomin R 2006 Genotyping pooled DNA using 100K SNP microarrays: a step towards genomewide association scans. Nucleic Acids Res 34:e27

Munafo MR, Clark TG, Moore LR, Payne E, Walton R, Flint J 2003 Genetic polymorphisms and personality in healthy adults: a systematic review and meta-analysis. Mol Psychiatry 8:471–484

Munafo MR, Matheson IJ, Flint J 2007 Association of the DRD2 gene Taq1A polymorphism and alcoholism: a meta-analysis of case-control studies and evidence of publication bias. Mol Psychiatry 12:454–461

Murray CJL, Lopez AD 1996 The global burden of disease: a comprehensive assessment of mortality and disability from diseases, injuries and risk factors in 1990 and projected to 2020. Harvard School of Public Health on behalf of the World Health Organization and the World Bank (Global Burden of Disease and Injury Series, Vol. I). Cambridge, MA,

Nash MW, Huezo-Diaz P, Williamson RJ et al 2004 Genome-wide linkage analysis of a composite index of neuroticism and mood-related scales in extreme selected sibships. Hum Mol Genet 13:2173–2182

Pe'er I, de Bakker PI, Maller J, Yelensky R, Altshuler D, Daly MJ 2006 Evaluating and improving power in whole-genome association studies using fixed marker sets. Nat Genet 38:663–667

Penninx BW, Beekman AT, Honig A et al 2001 Depression and cardiac mortality: results from a community-based longitudinal study. Arch Gen Psychiatry 58:221–227

Risch N, Zhang H 1995 Extreme discordant sib pairs for mapping quantitative trait loci in humans. Science 268:1584–1589

Schneider B, Muller MJ, Philipp M 2001 Mortality in affective disorders. J Affect Disord 65:263–274

Scott J, Palmer S, Paykel E, Teasdale J, Hayhurst H 2003 Use of cognitive therapy for relapse prevention in chronic depression. Cost-effectiveness study. Br J Psychiatry 182:221–227

Sullivan PF, Neale MC, Kendler KS 2000 Genetic epidemiology of major depression: review and meta-analysis. Am J Psychiatry 157:1552–1562

Surtees PG, Wainwright NW, Willis-Owen SA, Luben R, Day NE, Flint J 2006 Social adversity, the serotonin transporter (5-HTTLPR) polymorphism and major depressive disorder. Biol Psychiatry 59:224–229

Van Den Bogaert A, De Zutter S, Heyrman L et al 2005 Response to Zhang et al (2005): loss-of-function mutation in tryptophan hydroxylase-2 identified in unipolar major depression. Neuron 45, 11–16. Neuron 48:704; author reply 705–706

Zhang X, Beaulieu JM, Sotnikova TD, Gainetdinov RR, Caron MG 2004 Tryptophan hydroxylase-2 controls brain serotonin synthesis. Science 305:217

Zhang X, Gainetdinov RR, Beaulieu JM et al 2005 Loss-of-function mutation in tryptophan hydroxylase-2 identified in unipolar major depression. Neuron 45:11–16

Zhou Z, Peters EJ, Hamilton SP et al 2005 Response to Zhang et al (2005): loss-of-function mutation in tryptophan hydroxylase-2 identified in unipolar major depression. Neuron 45, 11–16. Neuron 48:702–703; author reply 705–706

Zubenko GS, Maher B, Hughes HB 3rd et al 2003 Genome-wide linkage survey for genetic loci that influence the development of depressive disorders in families with recurrent, early-onset, major depression. Am J Med Genet B Neuropsychiatr Genet 123:1–18

DISCUSSION

Chao: This is a provocative paper. You cast human genetics as a dismal science just like economics. Is that what you really believe?

Flint: No, it's not a dismal science. This was an attempt to get some discussion on this issue. There has been some weak thinking about this. The fundamental issue was that in mounting the studies that we have done, how optimistic have we been in what we are expecting to find, and how much have we been relying on negative answers? There is a problem here in terms of how willing we are to publish negative results. Most of us in this field know that you do quite a lot of work, type a gene, get a negative result and you can't get this published in high-profile journals, or indeed published at all in many cases. There is an issue here about whether some of the progress in the field has been held back by people not really going at this. There are some positive findings out there, but they get overblown: the general picture is not as optimistic as some people think. I have heard it said that 2007 is the year of genome-wide association studies. Francis Collins has indicated that NIH will be directing funding to this because these studies work. In some cases they do. But in some conditions they haven't produced positive results. This is not to say that they can't do, but it is not as rosy a picture as some people would like to see. We are going to have to deal with some of the problems that the negative studies throw up if we are really going to make advances.

Akil: You made the point that contributing factors for females are different from those in males. Presumably, there are different paths to depression. True heterogeneity exists, but I haven't seen this in the equation. Is there room to go back and look for different subtypes and paths? Is this a way out?

Flint: The issue here is that you then hit all those problems, including multiple testing and data dredging that we have already seen. I agree that there's no point avoiding these sorts of issues, but how do you then go about publishing a study when you have put all these analyses in, and come up with some P value that is no longer significant? It is a cultural issue. So much of this work has been driven by our belief that many of these conditions behave like Mendelian disorders. They don't. They are conceptually different.

Akil: It is like starting with fever, and asking what is the genetics of fever. I have another question. I like your animal work, in part because this is the sort of approach I am also taking. I think recombinant inbred mouse strains have biased things. It is good to start from an outbred population and see what the situation actually looks like. I like the fact that you identify a lot of different phenotypic traits. We have done a lot of projection in humans: we have identified variables that we think are important and have taken what is in effect a candidate approach to phenotyping. We might take an unbiased approach to the genes or proteins, but we are presupposing what matters in brain function in a way that we don't understand. Should we take an equally agnostic and broad view in phenotyping human traits, finding high-throughput ways of phenotyping? Our current approach is lopsided.

Flint: That is a good idea. A number of people have been pushing this approach. Nelson Freimer and others have argued for a human phenome approach (Freimer & Sabatti 2003) Some of the studies underway have done precisely this. There is a collection of groups working on a large population in Sardinia, similar to what we have done in the mouse population. They are asking questions about how all these phenotypes interrelate (Pilia et al 2006).

Akil: Take substance abuse as an example. People say there is a syndrome called behavioural under-control, or novelty seeking, or impulsivity. Let this re-cluster on its own, rather than assume you know how novelty seeking/sensation seeking etc. correlate with each other. We should have as few assumptions as possible.

Flint: We have looked at this. We don't have the analysis on the data set from the mouse, but we have done this on F2 crosses. We have taken the different measurements on our anxiety phenotypes, and looked at how many have a common genetic basis. The initial analysis suggested that many of them do have. Subsequent work has made me less willing to accept this, primarily because when we take the individual effects apart, the F2 analysis gives us half a chromosome to look at, and we've often made the assumption that there might be one or two effects. We increasingly find that it might be 10 or 20. In its extreme form, if we repeated some of these experiments at different times of day we find different genetic localizations.

Spedding: I liked what you said, because Michael Rutter, one of the great scientists working on nurture, is so involved with the Novartis Foundation. Animal experiments show that if you swap BALB/c and C57BL mice strains at the fetal level they have the behavioural traits of the mothers and not of the genetic background (Holmes et al 2005). Furthermore, in transgenic animals we underestimate how much we change the mother–pup relationship. C57BL have completely different suckling. This is one of the major ways to separate them. One of the things I believe about twin studies is that they involve children being brought up in a very different way. You have come back with the strongest nurture aspect I have heard.

Sendtner: Many people don't know how to deal with the effects of genetic background. Now, most results from association studies are picked up to make mouse models, and then people look in mouse models for comparable effects. The example you brought up for the serotonin transporter polymorphism generates a specific phenotype in a mouse model. The BDNF gene polymorphism also results in specific changes. When people then compare these mice with patients that have been genetically analysed, these results do not match or come together, probably because there are other modifier genes in humans that are not variable in inbred mouse lines. Therefore, one has to be careful in predicting from results with inbred mice what this could mean for the human situation where there isn't this inbred genetic background.

Flint: The experiment I described is using outbred animals. What we need to consider in the knockouts is that the genetic variability has been reduced to such an extent that these two situations are not comparable. There's a lot of argument about how this works. The issue revolves around what the assumption is about the degree of genetic effects. In a cross between two strains we are introducing an unknown number of modifiers and interactions. None of this we have much control of. The critical question becomes what is the effect size attributable to the mutation? Sometimes, the modifier effects can completely compensate for the effect of the mutations. This is not to say that the mutation doesn't have an effect. You would be throwing too much information away if you said it was just because of background effects. There are two lines that can be taken on this. One is to say that there is a disease model, I knocked out a disease gene, put it on a different background and the disease goes away: this should give me some clues on how to cure the disease. Then you are into the problem of identifying the modifiers. The other approach is to say we will ignore this, and find out what this gene is doing in this particular background. I don't care at this stage what those effects are. This is the way I would conceptualize it.

Malaspina: On the basis of much of our work on twin studies, as we become aware of the great extent of the effects of the fetal environment on development, it is important to point out that twins have a very different intrauterine environment to singletons. They have different glucocorticoid exposures and dramatically different oestrogen exposures. One of the problems in the field may be that we have overestimated heritability because of the twin study potential fallacy.

Javitt: We have been slow in our group in getting into genetics. I felt bad about this, but now I realize we were appropriately cautious. However, I am not clear whether this is a conceptual issue or a methodological issue. We assume that if there is an inherited genetic liability, there should be genes somewhere that are changing. But this may be wrong.

Flint: I started off by saying that there is heritability here. I don't think there's any argument about the size of it. We can argue about how it operates, but the results across phenotypes are robust. The issue that I sort of skirted around is the conceptual one, which is that we come out of a tradition of dissecting things out gene by gene as if they were individually acting in a Mendelian fashion. This approach has worked, which is why we use it. There are some issues about background effects, but it is essentially a productive strategy. The question then is how many complex traits can be modelled in this sort of framework? A certain amount probably can, and additive models explain most of what is going on in the heritability in twin studies. If you carry out a study in which you have mapped 1000 or so genetic effects, taking into account a number of different covariates, how much of this will stand up to complete replication, done in a different laboratory with different gene–environment interactions? Probably enough to get us some genes we can work with, but not that much. Should we just say that is a complete mess? No, we should be seeing our ideas of how genes impact on organisms being conceptualized in a slightly different way. The sort of people we need to talk to are those working on the physics of complex systems and mathematicians. Looking for gene by gene interactions causes geneticists to throw their hands up, because if you do a whole genome association study with 1 million SNPs there is an appalling explosion of interactions that you can't deal with. But I know mathematicians who approach this problem in a conceptually different way: this is a geometric problem, let's see what shape it looks like. If you have a single shape you have a single test. Then you have a much more powerful system to understand what is going on in this. We don't have many concepts like this in genetics.

Raff: In diseases where complexity seems to be defeating you, history says it is sometimes helpful to study high density families. Are there such families with neuroticism, for example?

Flint: No is the short answer. The classic experiment to knock this one on the head is the mutagenesis. The mouse people came to this problem, similar to the mess that was occurring in complex trait analysis. Their answer was to try to turn these complex traits into Mendelian traits. If you want to model schizophrenia, what is it in mice? Pre-pulse inhibition. We'll give ENU to mice, screen them and find the mouse with a mutation that disrupts pre-pulse inhibition and then we'll have sorted schizophrenia. Depression? We can do that by dropping the mouse into a bucket of water and see whether it floats. And so on. There was a paper by Nadeau and Frankel in *Nature Genetics* asserting that this was the way ahead (Nadeau & Frankel 2000). There was lots of excitement and funding, but no genes. We looked at this a few years ago. MRC Harwell have screened 10 000 mice with pre-pulse inhibition and they couldn't find a single animal with a segregating mutation. We looked at one of the phenotypes: running about in a maze. They'd screened 6000 of these animals but nothing had been cloned. I asked them what they thought the problem was and they replied that the genes weren't fully penetrant. So I looked at the data and there was a huge effect of 10%. We mapped the gene and it turns out to be quite an interesting gene, but it is not like a segregating mutation within a family. If this gene was having an effect on anxiety in human pedigrees the modifiers would wipe it out. The major problem is that the phenotypes at this sort of level can't be seen. They don't exist.

Sklar: I agree with your assessment of where we are in the field, and the complications and problems. But there is a more nuanced view of where we stand in the whole genome scan field that might give non-geneticists a slightly more balanced view. We are really just beginning. Whole genome association studies test the hypothesis that there are variants that exert modest effects on complex genetic diseases, this has not been tested before. In your particular case depression is a potentially good disease to study because there are more people available and thus there is the potential to increase the power of a study to detect modest effect, but of the psychiatric syndromes it is one of the least heritable. Schizophrenia, bipolar disease and autism are each more heritable. Whole genome association studies from these diseases are in process and we do not know what the results will show. For other, equally complex genetic diseases, albeit ones with more easily measured phenotypes, in the next few months there will be lots of consistent strong genes published for the likes of diabetes, Crohn's disease and inflammatory bowel disease. There is no theoretical reason why there might not be some for psychiatric disease. It is a hypothesis that is in the process of being tested. What is critical is a conservative interpretation of the data, requiring the sorts of replication that give people confidence.

Akil: I echo what you are saying. We collaborate with Mike Boehnke who was involved in the diabetes study. If each person did their own analysis they each had one set of results and they were disparate from each other, but when they pooled their data they came up with different results that were replicated across the various studies. Having parallel studies and then bringing the work together for replication is important. Even if they started with what they thought was genome-wide significance, the top genes fell out and new genes emerged from coming together. This makes the data sharing important. The fact that there aren't enough samples, as in bipolar disease, is significant. What everyone is doing in bipolar needs to come together. This might not be enough. This is where the clinicians are so important. I think the jury is out, especially if heterogeneity has to be taken into account. The dimensions of heterogeneity will be interesting. Is it cyclicity, onset, psychosis or something else that needs to be taken into account? For how many of these do we split the sample and lose power?

Owen: I agree with a lot of this. One of the problems this field has had has been naïvety and optimism leading to boom and bust. There is another danger: the tendency of high profile journals to publish weak genetics bolstered by a bit of biology that seems plausible. We don't understand enough about the biology of these disorders to be able to rescue weak genetics. Then, geneticists like myself or Jonathan Flint come along and do a massive failure to replicate study and the same journals won't even send it out for review.

Heritability is one of the best clues that we have as to the pathophysiology of these disorders. Human genetics is essentially a technology-led process. The new genotyping technology means that we are now able to answer the next set of questions, and we need to see what these whole-genome association studies are going to produce. Already, results are reasonably encouraging from some of the non-psychiatric complex disorders. We might be hopeful that one or two of our psychiatric disorders might have some sufficiently low-hanging fruit. The Mendelian background of genetics has served us poorly. We must start to think differently about the causes of common diseases. As many others have, we have just been doing some of these whole-genome studies. The tide of positive data makes us realize that we have to conceptualize, test and manage it in a different way. Several people have mentioned the need for sharing large samples. This is right, but the worry for me is that this sets up the next challenge: defining the phenotype. As you start to set up bigger studies, the net of cases starts to expand. Without good ways of defining the phenotype for genetic studies, just as we gain power with larger samples we may reduce power with greater heterogeneity.

Tongiorgi: I'd like to add some positivity to this negative picture. Can you expand your ideas on the analysis of the genetic architecture of the behaviour. You said these are restricted to narrow localization. Is this a good tool to work on?

Flint: Yes, that is the fundamental reason why we set this study up, to see whether this approach would work. For many of these phenotypes, perhaps two or three genes are implicated genetically. This is helpful and we can look at these genes. We have looked at expression variation, sequence variation, and what is known about these genes. It is not easy. It is potentially productive but the experiments that we have carried out over the last few months have made us realize that it is even more difficult than we initially thought.

Tongiorgi: Is it difficult to find the proper genes, or is it difficult to select the phenotype?

Flint: The fundamental problem is what is the test to show that this gene is involved in the phenotype? We don't have a gold standard for sorting this out. We have thought about this and have various ways of doing it with mouse crosses, but there are other problems associated with that.

Buonanno: In your test, how do you know you have not biased the test for genes that are involved in many processes throughout the body? Would this affect the way you do genetic analysis? In other words, you were looking at very different tests in different tissues. Is this biasing your test for genes that are expressed in many processes in many tissues?

Flint: We started off with some fairly standard mouse models of human disease: asthma, diabetes, obesity and anxiety/depression. We asked whether these were heritable, then we carried out what is essentially an association study (but with a rather specific design so that we don't have the problems we get in human genetics), and then we tried to find out what these genes were. I don't think this is creating bias.

Buonanno: Let's take actin as an example. This will associate with almost every cell process. If we try any test: learning, memory, wound healing or anything—actin will show association with all of these assays.

Flint: There are two layers to this. The first is which genes you allow there to be variation in. One of the issues we don't understand about quantitative traits is the following: if we mutagenize, we know we can alter every nucleotide and get an effect, with the exception of lethals. There is a subset of alterations in the genome that lead to quantitative variation. We don't know what the parameters are that set that. It varies from population to population. To what extent this reflects biology isn't understood fully. There is a more fundamental issue here: how do we see genetic variation in general leading to phenotypes. Is it linear? Is it pleiotropic? When we analyse the data how do we take this into account? I think we need a more sophisticated analysis, but I'm a psychiatrist and I need a mathematician to help here.

Lee: I am just trying to find a positive spin on this! To increase effect size, could you use drug responses as a readout?

Flint: Pharmacogenomics. It is the same issue. There are going to be some larger effects when you have a mutation. The extent to which you get modifiers that wipe this out will depend on lots of things. The only analysis people have carried out genome wide across a whole set of analysis shows a small number of large effects, and then 900 or so small effects. This pattern is repeated for every phenotype.

Raff: I'd like to carry on this discussion but change it a bit to consider candidate gene approaches. If you had some clue about the neurobiological basis of narcissism, for example, you could sequence candidate genes in affected individuals in multiplex families. This approach has been useful in autism. Is the future to try to move the neurobiology to a point where you could sensibly choose such candidate genes?

Flint: I'll be positive about whole gene association studies: they will work. They won't deliver everything. With diabetes, which has heritability higher than depression, the effects sizes that are coming out are not huge but some 10 genes have been identified. Someone will get a big enough sample for schizophrenia and depression such that we will find some genes, but not very many. Personally, I like the idea of taking apart the neurobiology. A classic way of doing this is to take one allele, such as serotonin, which we know is involved at one level. We also know the BDNF hypothesis has a lot to do with it. This gives us a neurogenesis hypothesis which can be tested specifically, yielding a phenomenon that can be teased apart at a molecular level. This leads to a question: why bother at all with the molecules in the human population? If you have a mechanism that you understand, does it matter what genes are involved? Can't you just treat patients on the basis of the pathogenesis? The molecules are a way in, but once you have the mechanism you don't really need to go back for the molecules.

Raff: I guess it is a question of time and cost effectiveness. What will give the useful answers fastest? If you were a funding agency, where would you put your money? Is it in genome-wide linkage association studies or candidate gene approaches?

Flint: It seems a lot cheaper to fund René Hen to sort out neurogenesis than to do genome studies in 20 disorders.

Sklar: The problem is that then you have put your money down on the neurogenesis hypothesis. This sounds nice, but before this there was the dopamine hypothesis. In the fullness of time the only format for finding something that you did not think you were looking for is a genetic study.

Flint: I think that there are now other ways ahead. Most of the work that has pushed the neurogenesis hypothesis has been our ability to modify mice at a molecular level. It is this technology applied to an old problem that has led to these advances.

Sklar: With next generation sequencers it might be possible to do the experiment you might like to do—to sequence 1000 patients. It is practically not doable for the near foreseeable future.

Talmage: To some extent, the issue is what question do you want to answer? If you want to understand the genetic structure, then I see a dark future. If you want to figure out what might be broken so that you can treat it, the high-effect genes give a way of getting at that. The dopamine hypothesis may not explain the aetiology of schizophrenia, but drugs that target this pathway are effective for some of the symptoms.

Walsh: What are we trying to do? We want to understand the pathophysiology of depression by genetic means, and this is interesting, but what we are really interested in is how to treat these dreadful conditions. Different companies are looking for tools beyond the SSRIs that act on the serotonin and noradrenaline transporters. These are effective agents but they have limitations. They take three weeks to show efficacy, not everyone responds and there are side effects. There is huge interest in different approaches. One of the genes you mentioned, PDE4 is an attractive target, and I suspect that whenever these studies are published, because of the need and desire to move out of the serotonergic environment, companies and academics will study this target in detail.

Akil: A compromise vision of where we might go is the neuroscience parallel of systems biology that people talk about at the cellular level in other fields. These involve cascades of signalling events. We haven't said much about the genetics of tuning circuitry. Take the caspase study: what this tells us is that some people have differential stress vulnerability, so it is the genetics of their stress system that is being inherited. But there are many ways that you can fine-tune stress responsiveness, neuronally, developmentally and genetically. It could be CRH, glucocorticoid, mineralocorticoid or something else in the hippocampus. There might be a systems phenotype of whether you have a highly active or a subreactive or retunable system. Instead of looking at CRH, for example, by itself, if I knew enough about the genetics of that system in families I could come up with some answers. It would be heterogeneous even at the level of that system, but it would still have a final common path that could genetically be tuned very differently.

Castrén: The brain is the neural network that makes us think and feel. It is not that there will be neurotransmitters or a gene that will allow me to stand up and give a talk. The genes that we are looking at are, in a way, tools for building up a neural network. If you have worse tools, you might need to use another tool that is not as good at doing the job. Depending on the tools you have, the whole thing can be built up normally or in a more fragile state. I'd like to go back to Daniel Javitt's presentation on NMDA receptors. Many years ago we used to work on the finding we stumbled across when we looked at BDNF expression after injection of NMDA receptors. There are circumscribed brain areas where BDNF mRNA jumps up. These are the areas that were partially described by John Olney, retrosplenial cortex or posterior cingulated cortex. There is also work by Frank Sharp who used gene expression of c-Fos and HSP70 to look at brain areas that are affected by relatively small doses of these drugs. They are differently affected. There seems to be a circumscribed circuit or network that is particularly vulnerable to NMDA receptor antagonist expression. It was not an effect that you would get in every place with an NMDA receptor. It seems that based on the structure of the circuit, inhibitory interneurons are part of this story, as well as the inputs from thalamus to cortex. This is important in how the network is built up. Perhaps the construction of the network during development can become malfunctional, leading to a tendency for this network to fire up by itself. In my view, it would be interesting to characterize this network. What are the neurons involved in this network? Perhaps we could do post-mortem studies to see whether these particular neurons are affected in those people. The brain is not just synapses piled on top of each other. It is a complex structure that is mediating information exchange. This is what is wrong in many psychiatric disorders. It is not failure of just one synapse, receptor or transmitter.

Sendtner: When people try to investigate higher brain function, they always tend to break down the system into simpler, Mendelian concepts in order to get druggable targets. But when one goes back to the complexity at the genetic level, there are two interpretations. One is that there is a high number of modifiers, and the other is that there are several or many completely independent disease mechanisms that result in the same phenotype. There are other diseases such as motor neuron disease where this becomes apparent. It has an impact on drug development, because a drug could work in one patient but not another with a different disease mechanism. When meta-analysis is done on 10 000 patients with depression, and you look at the genetics, can you get information on whether depression is one disease mechanism with a high number of modifiers or is caused by several distinct disease mechanisms?

Flint: This is a point that was raised earlier, about genetics being used to sort out mechanism. This requires an agnostic view about how the condition arose. When we diagnose, we look for a set of symptoms. Let's suppose we collected a large number of people and we collected all the additional information about their background, environment and had them fully genotyped. Then we could perhaps start to carry out the analysis you suggest. Analytically this will be a challenge, but it is potentially possible.

Sendtner: Are there means to subdivide patients in the clinic?

Flint: No.

Javitt: What often happens at these meetings is that discussion gets diffused and people go past the idea that there can be genes of large effect, or that there can be aetiological mechanisms that by themselves explain an illness. For example, narcolepsy was a genetic triumph, and the transmitter system involved was discovered. Huntingtons has a pleiomorphic presentation, but it is caused by a single gene. Syphilis causes a clinical picture that looks very much like schizophrenia—it was once called temporary paresis of the insane. The characteristic symptoms of neurosyphilis are extremely heteromorphic—insanity and paresis—but all symptoms ultimately resulted from a single aetiological factor, the syphilis treponeme. I wouldn't discount the fact that there may be some specific strong causes that are being washed out by the heterogeneity. As we increase the degrees of freedom, we wash out our effect. The problem with genetics now is that we have to do analyses across widely different populations and across the entire genome. The denominator, not the numerator, is the problem. If we look at syphilis, antibiotics have cured a chunk of what we used to consider mental illness or schizophrenia, because we peeled off that subdiagnosis. It could be that there are other types of distinct subpopulations out there, which if we could isolate them, we would be able to intervene in. One of the problems in the phenotype business is that we don't have enough well characterized patients.

References

Freimer N, Sabatti C 2003 The human phenome project. Nat Genet 34:15–21

Holmes A, le Guisquet AM, Vogel E, Millstein RA, Leman S, Belzung C 2005 Early life genetic, epigenetic and environmental factors shaping emotionality in rodents. Neurosci Biobehav Rev 29:1335–1346

Nadeau JH, Frankel WN 2000 The roads from phenotypic variation to gene discovery: mutagenesis versus QTLs. Nat Genet 25:381–384

Pilia G, Chen WM, Scuteri A et al 2006 Heritability of cardiovascular and personality traits in 6,148 Sardinians. PLoS Genet 2:e132

Neurotrophins in depression and antidepressant effects

Eero Castrén and Tomi Rantamäki

Neuroscience Center, University of Helsinki, PO Box 56, 00014 Helsinki, Finland

Abstract. Neurotrophins are important regulators of neuronal plasticity in the developing and adult brain. In particular, brain-derived neurotrophic factor (BDNF) and its receptor TrkB are implicated in these functions. The synthesis and release of BDNF is regulated by neuronal activity, and synaptic reorganization mediated by BDNF is thought to be a critical process which shapes neuronal networks to code optimally for environmentally relevant information. Recent evidence links neuronal plasticity and neurotrophin signalling in mood disorders. A polymorphism in the BDNF gene has been associated with depression and bipolar disorder. BDNF levels are reduced in postmortem brain samples and in the blood of depressed patients, and these reductions are reversible by successful antidepressant treatment. Furthermore, BDNF signalling plays a critical role in the mechanism of antidepressant drug action; at least in rodents, BDNF signalling appears to be both necessary and sufficient for the behavioural effects produced by antidepressant drugs. These data suggest that neurotrophin-mediated neuronal plasticity is a critical factor in mood disorders and in their therapy. Antidepressant treatments may, through enhanced BDNF signalling, improve the ability of critical brain circuits to respond optimally to environmental demands, a process that may be critical in the recovery from depression.

2008 Growth factors and psychiatric disorders. Wiley, Chichester (Novartis Foundation Symposium 289) p 43–59

The neurotrophins, nerve growth factor (NGF) and brain-derived neurotrophic factor (BDNF), were originally discovered through their ability to support survival of peripheral neurons during development. The other two members of the neurotrophin family, neurotrophin 3 (NT3) and neurotrophin 4 (NT4) were subsequently found through their homology to NGF and BDNF (Huang & Reichardt 2001, Lu et al 2005). The neurotrophic hypothesis of neuronal development was formulated several decades ago, and has subsequently been largely confirmed by genetic studies (Huang & Reichardt 2001). It states that neurons, which are initially made in excess, compete for access to the neurotrophic factors that are produced by the target cells in limiting amounts (Levi-Montalcini 1987). However, it is important to note that the physiological role of neurotrophins is not merely to keep neurons alive, but to *select* from competing neurons those which have established the best connections with the target tissue, and thereby *optimize* the numbers of neurons required for target innervation. Therefore, neurotrophins act as 'selector factors' during the peripheral nervous system (PNS) development.

It has recently become evident that neurotrophins play a critical role in the regulation of neuronal plasticity in the adult brain (Huang & Reichardt 2001, Lu 2003, Lu et al 2005). BDNF induces 'anabolic' plastic responses, such as neuronal survival, axon branching and elongation, dendritic sprouting, synaptogenesis and long-term potentiation (LTP) by activating TrkB receptor tyrosine kinase (Lu et al 2005). Ligand-induced homodimerization of TrkB receptors leads to TrkB autophosphorylation and activation of intracellular signalling pathways. In contrast, recent evidence suggests that the opposite 'catabolic' plastic responses, such as cell death, process withdrawal, synaptic loss and long-term depression, are mediated by the activation of the p75 neurotrophin receptor, predominantly by the pro-form of BDNF (Lu et al 2005).

Similarly to the role of neurotrophins as the selector factors in the developing PNS, BDNF is considered to play a critical role in the selection of the synapses that optimally reflect environmental input in the central nervous system (CNS). Synthesis and release of BDNF is induced by neuronal activity and the subsequent TrkB activation leads to the stabilization of axonal and dendritic branches (Cohen-Cory 2002) and strengthening of active synaptic connections (Lu 2003). Through this activity-dependent plasticity process, the overall shape of neurons, and thereby the connectivity within networks, is sculptured over time to optimally reflect the external input. It is important to stress that the critical factor in this selection process is not the absolute amount of BDNF, but which synapses get it. Excess exogenous BDNF, which floods entire brain areas, will eliminate the activity-based competition and gradually deteriorate the information processing within networks. Indeed, excess BDNF prevents the activity-dependent segregation of the eye-specific columns in the developing visual cortex (Cabelli et al 1995). Analogously to the actions of BDNF, TrkB receptor functions are regulated in an activity-dependent manner. In the plasma membrane, TrkB is primarily located in the synaptic sites and, upon neuronal activity, a pool of TrkB receptors are further enriched to the sites of activity (Lu et al 2005). Neuronal activity further regulates the synthesis and the intracellular targeting of TrkB receptors (Lu et al 2005). Therefore, both BDNF release and TrkB receptor expression must take place in a co-ordinated fashion at the relevant synaptic sites for the optimal synaptic response to occur.

Mood disorders and neuronal plasticity

Recent evidence implicates neuronal plasticity in the pathophysiology of mood disorders and in the recovery from depression (Berton & Nestler 2006, Castrén

et al 2006, Duman & Monteggia 2006). Depression and stress have been connected to neuronal degeneration in certain brain areas, such as the hippocampus
and prefrontal cortex. The volume of these brain areas has been found to be
reduced in depression without a reduction in cell numbers, which suggests that
neuronal connectivity is compromised (Drevets 2001). This degeneration appears
to be at least partially reversible by successful treatment. Significantly, depression
is often associated with clinical symptoms linked to impaired information processing (e.g. short-term memory) (Berton & Nestler 2006), suggesting that neuronal
plasticity is compromised in patients. Furthermore, stress and adverse life events
during early development are associated with reduced hippocampal size and
increase the risk of depression in adulthood (Caspi & Moffitt 2006), which suggests
that mood disorders may have a developmental component.

Mood disorders and neurotrophins

The central role of neurotrophins in brain development and plasticity has focused
interest on neurotrophins, and particularly BDNF, in the pathophysiology of mood
disorders (Castrén et al 2006, Duman & Monteggia 2006). Several studies have
suggested that BDNF signalling may be altered in depression. BDNF protein levels
have been found to be reduced in postmortem samples of depressed patients, and
antidepressant treatment appears to increase the levels back to the normal range
(Chen et al 2001, Karege et al 2005). Reduced BDNF levels have also been found
in blood samples of depressed patients and here, too, the BDNF protein seems to
be restored to normal levels after successful treatment (Gervasoni et al 2005,
Shimizu et al 2003). It is currently unclear to what extent the reduced BDNF levels
associated with depression and stress are reflected in the activity status of TrkB
receptors and signalling cascades in the brain.

There are several polymorphic loci in the human BDNF gene. In particular, the
G/A polymorphism at nucleotide 196, which produces either valine or methionine
in position 66 within the prodomain of BDNF protein, has been intensively investigated in neuropsychiatric disorders (for review see Post 2007). While the Val66
BDNF is normally transported to synaptic sites and released upon neuronal activation, the transport of the Met66 BDNF appears to be abnormal and activity-
dependent release of Met66 BDNF is reduced (Egan et al 2003). The Met66 allele
is associated with poor episodic memory (Egan et al 2003), which is consistent
with the critical role of activity-dependent BDNF release in synaptic plasticity.
Furthermore, Met66 BDNF is associated with eating disorders, neuroticism and
obsessive-compulsive disorder (for review see Post 2007), all disorders that respond
to antidepressant drug treatment. Interestingly, the Val66 allele has been found as
a risk allele for bipolar disorder (Post 2007). These findings are consistent with
the critical role of neuronal plasticity in the pathophysiology of a variety of

neuropsychiatric disorders and the central role of BDNF as a mediator of neuronal plasticity.

Studies in experimental animals have provided further evidence for the role of neurotrophic factors in mood disorders. Because there is no widely accepted rodent model of depression, research has concentrated on the use of stress, either in adulthood or during development, as a depression model (Berton & Nestler 2006). Repeated stress during the perinatal period or in adults produces long-lasting changes in behaviour, reduces hippocampal volume and diminishes neurogenesis in the dentate gyrus. Furthermore, stress impairs hippocampal connectivity and inhibits LTP between the hippocampus and prefrontal cortex (Rocher et al 2004). All of these changes can be reversed by chronic treatment with antidepressant drugs. Neonatal maternal separation acutely reduces BDNF mRNA levels in the hippocampus (Kuma et al 2004, Roceri et al 2002) and poor postnatal maternal care, which is associated with increased anxiety-related behaviour in adulthood, reduces BDNF mRNA levels in the adult brain (Liu et al 2000). Chronic stress in adult animals decreases BDNF mRNA expression in the hippocampus (Smith et al 1995, Tsankova et al 2006). Tsankova et al (2006) recently showed that the reduced BDNF mRNA levels are at least partially produced by changes in the chromatin structure, in particular increased methylation of the histone tails in the BDNF promoter region. Antidepressant drugs restore the stress-induced decrease in BDNF mRNA but, remarkably, instead of reversing the suppressive histone hypermethylation, they increase histone acetylation, thereby rendering the BDNF promoter region more accessible to the transcription machinery (Tsankova et al 2006). These important findings suggest that stress and antidepressant treatment produce specific and differential long-term modifications in the chromatin structure, and that different modifications can occur independently and functionally counteract each other.

Adult neurogenesis in the hippocampal dentate gyrus is also influenced by environmental stimuli, such as enriched environment, stress and antidepressant drugs, and there is evidence that increased neurogenesis is necessary for the beneficial behavioural effects of antidepressant drugs (Dranovsky & Hen 2006). We have investigated the role of neurotrophins in antidepressant-induced neurogenesis. While reduction of BDNF levels (BDNF$^{+/-}$ mice) or inhibition of TrkB signalling (dominant negative TrkB overexpressing TrkB.T1 mice) does not affect antidepressant-induced neuronal proliferation, the long-term survival of the newborn neurons was severely reduced when BDNF signalling was compromised (Sairanen et al 2005). Importantly, we observed that neuronal apoptosis was increased simultaneously with the increase in neurogenesis in antidepressant-treated mice, indicating that neuronal turnover, and not neurogenesis per se, was increased in response to antidepressant drugs (Sairanen et al 2005). These observations are consistent with the role of neurotrophins as selector factors and suggest that enriched environment and antidepressants increase the number of neurons available for selection, thereby enhancing the adaptability of the hippocampus.

Neurotrophins and antidepressant drug action

The most consistent evidence for the role of neurotrophins in mood disorders comes indirectly through the evidence for their critical role in the mechanism of antidepressant treatments. In rodents, the current evidence suggests that TrkB signalling is both necessary and sufficient for antidepressant action (Castrén et al 2006, Duman & Monteggia 2006). Electroconvulsive shock treatment (ECT), which is the most effective antidepressant treatment known, strongly elevates BDNF mRNA levels both acutely and chronically, and repeated treatment also increases BDNF protein levels (Duman & Monteggia 2006, Nibuya et al 1995). Repeated, but not acute, treatment with essentially all known antidepressant drugs increases the expression of BDNF and TrkB mRNA in the hippocampus, however, BDNF protein is increased by only some antidepressants (Duman & Monteggia 2006, Nibuya et al 1995). Importantly, both acute and chronic treatment with a variety of antidepressants belonging to different pharmacological classes (tricyclic, serotonin and noradrenaline selective drugs, lithium) activates TrkB receptor auto-phosphorylation (Rantamäki et al 2006, 2007), which indicates that changes in BDNF synthesis lead to increased release of BDNF at the synaptic sites. Antide-pressant-induced TrkB receptor activation leads specifically to the activation of the PLCγ signalling pathway and the transcription factor CREB (cAMP-related element binding protein) (Fig. 1) (Rantamäki et al 2007, Saarelainen et al 2003). This signalling pathway might further regulate the release and synthesis of BDNF itself. Taken together these data suggest that TrkB mediated neurotrophin signal-ling is an early effect of antidepressant treatments and initiates a plastic response that gradually leads to behavioural treatment response.

The idea that BDNF signalling is a critical mediator of the antidepressant drug effect was recently tested in transgenic mouse models and behavioural paradigms sensitive to antidepressant drugs. The behavioural effects of imipramine and fluox-etine were prevented in the forced swim test (FST) in transgenic mice with reduced BDNF levels (BDNF$^{+/-}$ mice) and in mice overexpressing a dominant-negative TrkB receptor (TrkB.T1) (Fig. 2) (Saarelainen et al 2003). The similarity of the phenotype observed in both mice targeting the ligand and the receptor strongly suggests that signalling through this pathway is critical for the antidepressant effect. Subsequently, it has been shown that the behavioural effects of desipramine are also prevented in mice with a forebrain-specific knockout of the BDNF gene (see Duman & Monteggia 2006). Interestingly, although the clinical effects of antidepressants require long-term treatment, the behavioural effects of antidepres-sants in the FST (and their absence in BDNF-TrkB mutant mice) are elicited by

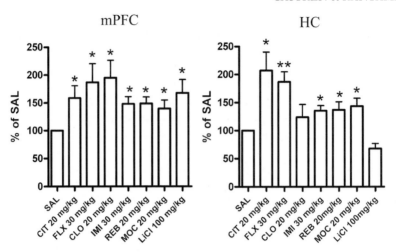

FIG. 1.   TrkB signalling is rapidly activated by a variety of antidepressant treatments. Acute treatment (30–60 min) with pharmacologically different antidepressant drugs and the anti-manic agent lithium all induce the autophosphorylation response of the TrkB receptor in the mouse medial prefrontal cortex (mPFC) and hippocampus (HC, lithium produces a significant reduction). Data shown as % ± SEM of control increase or decrease in the phosphorylation levels of TrkB catalytic domain. *p < 0.05, **p < 0.01. SAL, saline; CIT, citalopram; FLX, fluoxetine; CLO, clomipramine; IMI, imipramine; REB, reboxetine; MOC, moclobemide; LiCl, lithium chloride. Modified with kind permission of Springer Science and Business Media, from Rantamäki et al (2006, 2007).

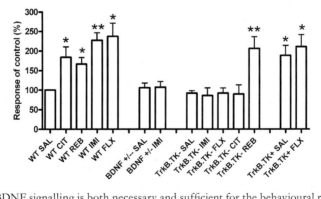

FIG. 2.   BDNF signalling is both necessary and sufficient for the behavioural responses produced by antidepressants. Acute behavioral effects of wild-type (WT), BDNF heterozygote and TrkB mutant mice with or without prior antidepressant treatment in the forced swim test. Data shown as % ± SEM of control increase or decrease in antidepressant-like response (reduced immobility or increase latency to immobility). *p < 0.05, **p < 0.01. SAL, saline; CIT, citalopram; FLX, fluoxetine; IMI, imipramine; REB, reboxetine; TrkB.TK−, truncated dominant-negative TrkB overexpressing mice; TrkB.TK+, full-length TrkB overexpressing mice. (Modified with kind permission of Springer Science and Business Media, from Koponen et al 2005, Rantamäki et al 2007, Saarelainen et al 2003.)

acute treatment. This observation suggests that the activation of TrkB autophos-phorylation, which is induced by antidepressants within a similar time frame, may be a critical initial component of behavioural antidepressant treatment. Indeed, TrkB autophosphorylation is not induced in the same TrkB.T1 overexpressing mice that fail to respond to imipramine treatment (Saarelainen et al 2003). However, we have recently observed that although reboxetine, a noradrenaline-selective uptake inhibitor, robustly activates TrkB autophosphorylation, its effects are normal in TrkB.T1 overexpressing mice (Rantamäki et al 2007), suggesting a pos-sible dissociation between the TrkB autophosphorylation response and behav-ioural antidepressant effects (Fig. 2). Nevertheless, together these data strongly argue that the activation of TrkB signalling is required for the behavioural effects of antidepressant drugs, at least in rodents, and that TrkB signalling may play a critical role early in the process which ultimately leads to clinical antidepressant effects.

Both genetic and stereotaxic injection experiments suggest that the activation of TrkB signalling is not only necessary, but also sufficient for the behavioural effects of antidepressants. Injection of BDNF directly into the midbrain area or hippocampus induces a behavioural response which is similar to that observed after antidepressant drug treatment (Berton & Nestler 2006, Duman & Monteggia 2006). Furthermore, mice that overexpress the functional TrkB receptor postna-tally in neurons and show increased basal TrkB signalling, show an antidepressant-like behaviour in the FST (Koponen et al 2005) (Fig. 2). The antidepressant fluoxetine did not show any further augmentation of the behavioural effects in these mice (Koponen et al 2005) (Fig. 2), thus suggesting that the elevated TrkB activity mimics the behavioural effects of antidepressants and occludes the effects of drug treatment.

Finally, it must be stressed that increased TrkB signalling is not associated with an antidepressant-like response in all brain areas. Whereas stress reduces BDNF mRNA levels in the hippocampus, the opposite is observed in the hypothalamus and amygdala (Berton & Nestler 2006, Duman & Monteggia 2006). Moreover, BDNF overexpression in the hippocampus produces an antidepressant-like behav-ioural response, but in the ventral tegmental area produces depression-like behav-iour (Berton & Nestler 2006). A depression-like behavioural response is also observed when TrkB signalling is blocked in the nucleus accumbens (Berton & Nestler 2006).

Neurotrophins, antidepressants and networks

The observations reviewed above strongly link BDNF and TrkB signalling with antidepressant drug effects in the hippocampus and cortex. But what does this information tell us about the pathophysiology of depression and the mechanism by which antidepressant treatments bring about mood recovery? The critical role of BDNF as a 'selector factor' in neuronal plasticity at the synaptic level suggests that neuronal plasticity and the stability of neuronal networks are critical components of mood disorders and antidepressant drug action. Indeed, a number of observations suggest that antidepressants, at least in some cases acting through BDNF signalling, regulate neuronal plasticity at several levels. As noted above, antidepressants regulate the proliferation and survival of neurons in the hippocampus (Dranovsky & Hen 2006, Sairanen et al 2005). ECT increases axon outgrowth in the mossy fibre pathway between the dentate gyrus and the CA3 area in a BDNF-dependent manner (Vaidya et al 1999). Furthermore, chronic antidepressant treatment increases synapse formation and synaptic density in CA1 and CA3 regions of hippocampus (Hajszan et al 2005). Stress inhibits the induction of long-term potentiation in the monosynaptic connection between hippocampus and prefrontal cortex, and this inhibition can be counteracted by antidepressant drug treatment, suggesting that antidepressants play a role in the regulation of synaptic strength (Rocher et al 2004). Using marker proteins of neuronal plasticity as indicators, we have recently provided evidence that chronic antidepressant treatment may regulate neuronal plasticity specifically in the prefrontal cortex, hippocampus and in the piriform cortex, (Sairanen et al 2007). Interestingly, the prefrontal cortex and hippocampus are the brain areas most often associated with mood disorders in humans (Drevets 2001).

Very recently, Normann et al (2007) investigated the effects of depression and antidepressant drugs on visually-evoked potentials (VEPs) in the human visual cortex. They showed that the adult visual cortex displays 'LTP-like' plasticity to visual stimuli and that this plasticity is compromised in depressed patients. Interestingly, they found that chronic treatment with the antidepressant sertraline significantly promoted the VEP plasticity in the visual cortex of healthy controls (Normann et al 2007). This important study demonstrates that depression and antidepressant drugs produce bidirectional changes in neuronal plasticity in the adult cortex and suggests that the effects of antidepressants on neuronal plasticity may not be confined to networks involved in mood control but perhaps extend to all cortical areas.

In addition to depression and antidepressant action, BDNF and TrkB signalling are implicated in a variety of physiological and pathophysiologal conditions such as addiction, dementia, chronic pain, eating disorders and schizophrenia. Similarly, antidepressants show potency in a variety of neuropsychiatric disorders in addition to depression, including chronic pain, obsessive-compulsive disorder and eating disorders, which is consistent with the idea that BDNF-TrkB signalling participates in antidepressant action in humans. These data suggest a model where neuronal plasticity and stability of neuronal networks is a critical pathophysiological mechanism in a variety of neuropsychiatric disorders and that

BDNF, as a critical tool in the plasticity of neuronal connectivity, is a critical mediator in successful treatment strategies against mood disorders (Castrén 2005).

Acknowledgments

We thank Dr Olivia O'Leary for comments and language revision. The Sigrid Jusélius Foundation and the Academy of Finland have financially supported the original work done in our laboratory.

References

Berton O, Nestler EJ 2006 New approaches to antidepressant drug discovery: beyond monoamines. Nat Rev Neurosci 7:137–151

Cabelli RJ, Hohn A, Shatz CJ 1995 Inhibition of ocular dominance column formation by infusion of NT-4/5 or BDNF. Science 267:1662–1666

Caspi A, Moffitt TE 2006 Gene-environment interactions in psychiatry: joining forces with neuroscience. Nat Rev Neurosci 7:583–590

Castrén E 2005 Is mood chemistry? Nat Rev Neurosci 6:241–246

Castrén E, Võikar V, Rantamäki T 2006 Role of neurotrophic factors in depression. Curr Opin Pharmacol 7:18–21

Chen B, Dowlatshahi D, MacQueen GM, Wang JF, Young LT 2001 Increased hippocampal BDNF immunoreactivity in subjects treated with antidepressant medication. Biol Psychiatry 50:260–265

Cohen-Cory S 2002 The developing synapse: construction and modulation of synaptic structures and circuits. Science 298:770–776

Dranovsky A, Hen R 2006 Hippocampal neurogenesis: regulation by stress and antidepressants. Biol Psychiatry 59:1136–1143

Drevets WC 2001 Neuroimaging and neuropathological studies of depression: implications for the cognitive-emotional features of mood disorders. Curr Opin Neurobiol 11:240–249

Duman RS, Monteggia LM 2006 A neurotrophic model for stress-related mood disorders. Biol Psychiatry 59:1116–1127

Egan MF, Kojima M, Callicott JH et al 2003 The BDNF val66met polymorphism affects activity-dependent secretion of BDNF and human memory and hippocampal function. Cell 112:257–269

Gervasoni N, Aubry JM, Bondolfi G et al 2005 Partial normalization of serum brain-derived neurotrophic factor in remitted patients after a major depressive episode. Neuropsychobiology 51:234–238

Hajszan T, MacLusky NJ, Leranth C 2005 Short-term treatment with the antidepressant fluoxetine triggers pyramidal dendritic spine synapse formation in rat hippocampus. Eur J Neurosci 21:1299–1303

Huang EJ, Reichardt LF 2001 Neurotrophins: roles in neuronal development and function. Annu Rev Neurosci 24:677–736

Karege F, Vaudan G, Schwald M, Perroud N, La Harpe R 2005 Neurotrophin levels in postmortem brains of suicide victims and the effects of antemortem diagnosis and psychotropic drugs. Brain Res Mol Brain Res 136:29–37

Koponen E, Rantamäki T, Voikar V, Saarelainen T, MacDonald E, Castrén E 2005 Enhanced BDNF signaling is associated with an antidepressant-like behavioral response and changes in brain monoamines. Cell Mol Neurobiol 25:973–980

Kuma H, Miki T, Matsumoto Y et al 2004 Early maternal deprivation induces alterations in brain-derived neurotrophic factor expression in the developing rat hippocampus. Neurosci Lett 372:68–73

Levi-Montalcini R 1987 The nerve growth factor: thirty-five years later. EMBO J 6:1145–1154

Liu D, Diorio J, Day JC, Francis DD, Meaney MJ 2000 Maternal care, hippocampal synaptogenesis and cognitive development in rats. Nat Neurosci 3:799–806

Lu B 2003 BDNF and activity-dependent synaptic modulation. Learn Mem 10:86–98

Lu B, Pang PT, Woo NH 2005 The yin and yang of neurotrophin action. Nat Rev Neurosci 6:603–614

Nibuya M, Morinobu S, Duman RS 1995 Regulation of BDNF and TrkB mRNA in rat brain by chronic electroconvulsive seizure and antidepressant drug treatments. J Neurosci 15:7539–7547

Normann C, Schmitz D, Furmaier A, Doing C, Bach M 2007 Long-term plasticity of visually evoked potentials in humans is altered in major depression. Biol Psychiatry 62:373–380

Post RM 2007 Role of BDNF in bipolar and unipolar disorder: clinical and theoretical implications. J Psychiatr Res 41:979–990

Rantamäki T, Knuuttila JE, Hokkanen ME, Castrén E 2006 The effects of acute and long-term lithium treatments on TrkB neurotrophin receptor activation in the mouse hippocampus and anterior cingulate cortex. Neuropharmacology 50:421–427

Rantamäki T, Hendolin P, Kankaanpää A et al 2007 Pharmacologically diverse antidepressants rapidly activate brain-derived neurotrophic factor (BDNF) receptor TrkB and induce phospholipase-Cγ signaling pathways in mouse brain. Neuropsychopharmacology 32:2152–2162

Roceri M, Hendriks W, Racagni G, Ellenbroek BA, Riva MA 2002 Early maternal deprivation reduces the expression of BDNF and NMDA receptor subunits in rat hippocampus. Mol Psychiatry 7:609–616

Rocher C, Spedding M, Munoz C, Jay TM 2004 Acute stress-induced changes in hippocampal/prefrontal circuits in rats: effects of antidepressants. Cereb Cortex 14:224–229

Saarelainen T, Hendolin P, Lucas G et al 2003 Activation of the TrkB neurotrophin receptor is induced by antidepressant drugs and is required for antidepressant-induced behavioral effects. J Neurosci 23:349–357

Sairanen M, Lucas G, Ernfors P, Castren M, Castren E 2005 Brain-derived neurotrophic factor and antidepressant drugs have different but coordinated effects on neuronal turnover, proliferation, and survival in the adult dentate gyrus. J Neurosci 25: 1089–1094

Sairanen M, O'Leary OF, Knuuttila JE, Castren E 2007 Chronic antidepressant treatment selectively increases expression of plasticity-related proteins in the hippocampus and medial prefrontal cortex of the rat. Neuroscience 144:368–374

Shimizu E, Hashimoto K, Okamura N et al 2003 Alterations of serum levels of brain-derived neurotrophic factor (BDNF) in depressed patients with or without antidepressants. Biol Psychiatry 54:70–75

Smith MA, Makino S, Kvetnansky R, Post RM 1995 Stress and glucocorticoids affect the expression of brain-derived neurotrophic factor and neurotrophin-3 mRNAs in the hippocampus. J Neurosci 15:1768–1777

Tsankova NM, Berton O, Renthal W, Kumar A, Neve RL, Nestler EJ 2006 Sustained hippocampal chromatin regulation in a mouse model of depression and antidepressant action. Nat Neurosci 9:519–525

Vaidya VA, Siuciak JA, Du F, Duman RS 1999 Hippocampal mossy fiber sprouting induced by chronic electroconvulsive seizures. Neuroscience 89:157–166

DISCUSSION

McAllister: How many classes of drugs have you looked at? I'm thinking of broad therapeutic classes as well as pharmacological mechanisms.

Castrén: We have looked at monoamine oxidase inhibitors. We have two different serotonin selectives, one noradrenaline selective and then two tricyclics. We also looked at electroconvulsive therapy (ECV) as a positive control. We were sure that this would increase TrkB phosphorylation, but it didn't. We dissected the time course. We looked as closely as we can and never found any evidence of increased TrkB phosphorylation after ECV shock treatment. After 30 min it goes down, so we thought there must be a quick peak somewhere, but we have never found it.

Lu: ECV could promote TrkB transcription rather than TrkB phosphorylation.

Castrén: We also looked at this. We treated them and after two weeks gave them another shock. We looked again half an hour after and still couldn't see anything.

McAllister: Did you test any antipsychotics, antianxiety drugs or psychomotor stimulants?

Castrén: No. These are live animal studies and take quite a lot of animals. We have a small animal house. I admit that there might be drugs that are not classically considered antidepressants that might produce the same effects.

Giedd: Is there much known about the developmental course of BDNF release? Could this help explain the age of onset of depression? Is there something in the system that changes in late adolescence or early adulthood when depression tends to manifest?

Castrén: There is evidence from animals that the BDNF expression picks up from postnatal life up to about 3 weeks. I don't know whether this coincides with synapse formation.

Barde: There is a tenfold increase in BDNF levels in the cerebral cortex or the hippocampus in the first three weeks after birth.

Sendtner: You showed multiple pieces of evidence that TrkB is necessary and sufficient for mediating the antidepressant effect, but didn't show evidence about BDNF. Is there also a dysfunction at the level of BDNF? Or could it be that disturbed transactivation of the TrkB receptor from other types of receptors such as dopaminergic receptors is responsible for the disease mechanism?

Castrén: We have seen the same behavioural effects in mice that have half BDNF or have reduced TrkB signalling. This indicates that the pair are required for the behavioural effect. The autophosphorylation response that we see after half an hour is another bit of evidence. Initially we thought they must be the same thing: since the behavioural effect requires BDNF then this is a reflection of the same thing. We can't rule out the possibility that there would be a transactivation event.

It might be completely through a transactivation event. We have done a study in which we injected BDNF heterozygotes with antidepressant. We looked at the phosphorylation response of TrkB. We found no difference. Even the baseline phosphorylation is the same, and gets increased in both cases. This system may be more complicated than we initially thought. We have very little molecular evidence of how these things are happening.

Chao: So is there any information about the steps that go from antidepressant action to the release of BDNF?

Lu: Antidepressants could activate TrkB through *trans*-activation (i.e. independent of BDNF). To answer the question whether BDNF mediates the antidepressant effects, there's an experiment by Ron Duman who made a stress-induced depression model. Then he infused BDNF into the hippocampus and rescued depressive behaviour (Shirayama et al 2002). This is probably direct evidence implicating BDNF, and not just TrkB, in antidepressant effects.

Castrén: This is in line with a genetic study I showed you. If you then increase TrkB signalling you get the same behavioural effect. In the behavioural domain it is clear that activation of the TrkB receptor through BDNF is what is important. But biochemical responses might be more complicated.

Raff: So is it the idea that the time course of the delay in the behavioural response, or the reversal of depression, is the time it takes for newly formed neurons to move into CA3 or other regions of the CNS and to differentiate?

Castrén: As far as I understand, that is what René Hen will suggest tomorrow. We have spent some time looking at the prefrontal cortex area where there is no evidence of neurogenesis. It may be one thing that takes time, but my working hypothesis is that there are other things happening at the same time, perhaps at a more subtle level, such as formation of new synapses and pruning of these. This also takes time but it may not require the birth of completely new neurons. Birth of neurons could be part of this response, though.

Raff: Is there reason to think that a hippocampal response is required for antidepressants to work in a mouse?

Castrén: We haven't gone into this.

Spedding: There are solid data showing stress-induced reductions in hippocampal dendritic arborisation changes with stress, which are reversed by some antidepressants (I will discuss these in my paper). These take 1–3 weeks. I have always thought that this is an important issue, and is probably why we will never get a rapid onset antidepressant that isn't also a psychostimulant.

Lu: I want to bring a slightly different issue into this. So far, your model of forced swim test addresses just one aspect of depression: behavioural despair. In clinical settings a more common issue for diagnosis is what is called anhedonia, which is a lack of interest in pleasurable behaviours. This involves a completely different brain system: the nucleus accumbens, VTA and the dopamine reward system. Have you looked at antidepressant effects there? We know BDNF function in this system is completely opposite to the system in the hippocampus. Have you looked at TrkB phosphorylation or other signal transduction machinery to see how they respond to antidepressants in the nucleus accumbens and VTA?

Castrén: No we haven't. We got into this work by studying dominant negative TrkB overexpressing animals. The promoter we have used doesn't work in nucleus accumbens or the striatum. You are right: it would have been relatively easy to dissect the accumbens to look for phosphorylation.

Lu: You could inject antidepressants into wild-type animals to see what happens.

Castrén: We haven't done that. In the initial study when we looked at different cortical areas, we found that the only cortical area where we see a significant difference is prefrontal cortex. However, in every cortical area there was a small increase. It wasn't significant, but we had a feeling that if we added a couple more mice we might have seen this. We do this all at the Western level; it is possible that there is a subset of cells responding and if we looked at these more directly we might understand better what is occurring.

Lu: Your animals—T1, conditional knockout or BDNF knockout mice—don't behave as if they are depressed. Perhaps BDNF itself (or more precisely, lack of it) is not involved in causing depression. It could be a parallel phenomenon. BDNF could be a target for antidepressants, because every time you treat the BDNF knockout animals with antidepressant they don't respond any more. BDNF may therefore be a target for antidepressants rather than an actual underlying mechanism for depression. If BDNF is simply a target of antidepressants, we should be able to use antidepressants to treat anxiety and all the other mood disorders in which impairments in BDNF signalling have been implicated.

Castrén: I would not like to say that BDNF is the mechanism. Neural plasticity is the mechanism involved in the drug action. In this mechanism BDNF is a tool. It is needed, and if this tool is not working properly then the function is not completely lost. It can be replaced with some other tools, but not quite as well.

Lee: In the realm of anxiety-related behaviours, if BDNF is reduced the mouse becomes more anxious (Rios et al 2001, Chan et al 2006, Monteggia et al 2007). Anxiety is a symptom of depression.

Akil: Not in rats. Fluoxetine would induce anxiety, and in the same acute time window it will look like an antidepressant. The time courses may be different and eventually with long-term treatment perhaps depression and anxiety will go together. But acutely you have to be careful about not equating them.

Lee: I was referring to two to three week treatments with antidepressants in animals, which have an anti-anxiety effect.

Lu: Let's say you do forced swim or other tests such as learned hopelessness, these tests are used to measure the ability of animals to respond to antidepressants, not depression or anxiety per se.

Lee: All the drug responses are within a day in those tests.

Lu: What I'm saying is that if we down-regulate BDNF or TrkB, you don't see the animal going into depression, when tested by available behavioural tests. When you challenge the BDNF knockouts or TrkB mutants with stress and they do get depressed, and when you treat them with antidepressants the drugs don't work any more. Thus, it seems to me that BDNF is more of a target of antidepressants than a molecular mechanism underlying depression itself.

Akil: I understand completely that in humans the comorbidity of anxiety and depression are very high. It's common to think of anxiety as a component or predisposing factor to depression. The problem is with some of the measures in animals. I don't think a lot of the measures of spontaneous anxiety tap the same thing as human anxiety. The elevated plus maze, the open field and the light/dark box correlate very highly with novelty seeking behaviours and measures of disinhibition. They are very hippocampal in nature. This is quite a different animal from associative anxiety and fear conditioning models. We have to be careful in the way we use the animal models or what you see with chronic social defeat or chronic stress.

McAllister: Many of the anti-anxiety models are based on the fact that they display responses to benzodiazepines. They have lent themselves preclinically for looking at drug effects compared with benzodiazepines. It has been great for the drug industry but takes us down the wrong road for a lot of the mechanisms.

Bothwell: At this point it seems compelling that some form of neuroplasticity is involved in depression and antidepressant drug action. But the term plasticity is used so broadly it is almost impossible to be wrong with that assertion. The cruel joke is that BDNF seems to be important for anything anyone has ever called plasticity in the cortex. So I guess one could argue that it would be amazing if BDNF and TrkB were not involved. Can we use what we know about BDNF and TrkB to somehow home in on what kind of plasticity is important here. Is it neurogenesis, dendritic arborisation or synapse by synapse competition?

Castrén: This is a construction problem. If you have to mount something on a wall you use a screwdriver. In this system, if some change is needed based on experience, you take the screwdriver, BDNF. From this perspective I would say that it isn't a surprise that anything involving neuroplasticity also involves BDNF. It is one of the major tools. What is it actually used for? It is not designing the construction; it is just a tool used in the process. This is a different story. By looking at whether BDNF and TrkB are involved I don't think we can work out the difference between anxiety and depression, for example. We should think of antidepressants in this context as being more permissive than instructive. They give people the opportunity to get better.

Flint: Do we know how antidepressants lead to the production of BDNF? Which cells produce it?

Tongiorgi: It depends. Different antidepressant drugs have differential effects in different neurons. This can be measured by *in situ* hybridization, looking at the up-regulation and down-regulation of BDNF. Once again, there is a nice parallel between the up and down of BDNF regulation and the behavioural effect. With short-lasting treatments there can be down-regulation of BDNF and then an up-regulation after a certain time. It is not always in the same brain areas.

Flint: Which cells secrete BDNF?

Tongiorgi: Mainly glutamatergic neurons but other neuronal types can secrete it also (Conner et al 1997). In addition, there is recent work from Canossa showing that although astrocytes cannot produce BDNF themselves they can nevertheless take up BDNF from extracellular spaces and then secrete it.

Castrén: If we wanted to play devil's advocate we could say that the causation is reversed. Long term treatment uses hippocampus more effectively. All those genes that are regulated by neural activity would go up. It could be that this is also a passive reaction to the increased activity within certain brain areas, which is then leading to the increase of those genes that are needed for the activity-dependent plasticity. It is difficult, especially in these long-term studies, to say what is the chicken and what is the egg. It could be that BDNF is working from both the chicken and egg side.

Tongiorgi: You can do exactly the same game as we discussed here concerning the genetic studies. You can do a meta-analysis comparing the different effects of fluoxetine in different papers. It can range from down-regulation to slight up-regulation to no effect. I would expect that the final outcome of this meta-analysis is that certain antidepressant drugs have no effect on BDNF mRNA levels. However, the real issue is that BDNF is a protein and we need to go through the entire biology of the protein, because it is not the same as the production of the mRNA. I have another question, which is about the idea of looking at the entire biology of the story. Do we have information about what really happens in terms of dendritic and axonal sprouting, and synapse formation in that system? If we know that, can we reproduce the effect by using a different molecule?

Castrén: We don't know. A lot of this is happening *in vivo*. The problem is that these are dynamic effects. We found not only an increase in production but also an increase in turnover. If you started to count the hippocampal neurons you wouldn't see any difference because one is taken away and one is added. You can label the newborn neurons at one point with BrdU and then follow up the same neuron, but the same can't be done with synapses. Histological sections are snap-shots that fail to capture the dynamics.

Raff: To what extent do we know that antidepressants work mainly through their effects on serotonin or noradrenaline?

Castrén: It is difficult to get into this. It is my feeling that their role is at least partially because at the time they were discovered to be involved it wasn't possible to measure anything else. This was in the 1960s. There are drugs that may be antidepressants that don't fit into this model.

Raff: I was thinking of the drugs that clearly have an effect on serotonin. Is this effect required to see BDNF changes?

Walsh: It has to be because these are drugs that have a single binding site in the CNS and that site is the transporter. The bit I'm struggling with is the rapidity of the effect. In my model there would be binding to serotonergic and noradrenaline transporter. As a consequence of that there will be increasing levels of serotonin. Everything you see is a consequence of that.

Lu: Only TrkB phosphorylation is rapid.

Walsh: When an antidepressant is given the first thing it does is bind to the transporter.

Raff: This isn't all they do, however. As my colleague Anne Mudge has found (unpublished observations) they can have effects on neurons that don't have serotonin transporters.

Walsh: That is controversial and unlikely to be physiologically important.

Talmage: Are there other examples where BDNF selectively stimulates autophosphorylation of subsets of sites?

Castrén: We have looked at the effect of morphine. It has a reduced nociceptive effect in NT4 knockout mice, and also in the TrkB dominant-negative overexpressing mice. When we looked at the brainstem region in morphine-treated mice, we found an increased phosphorylation of TrkB which is dependent on NT4. This phosphorylation is not seen in the Shc binding site but only in the PLCγ site, similarly to that seen after antidepressant treatment (Lucas et al 2003).

Talmage: So you are postulating that this may be an NT4-mediated, site-selective functional effect.

Castrén: We also did a small study where we looked at NT4 knockout mice in the antidepressant context. They seem to be normal in phosphorylation.

Talmage: This seems to speak to the possibility of an intermediate tyrosine kinase, other than TrkB, that is mediating the effect.

Chao: Yes, there is the possibility of selective phosphorylation of receptors by other non-receptor tyrosine kinases, such as Fyn.

Lu: It could be possible that whatever the antidepressant is doing, it is not inducing BDNF secretion but inducing a *trans*-activation of TrkB, either directly or through other small molecules (e.g. peptides). There are other molecules whose secretion could be induced by antidepressants, leading to TrkB phosphorylation.

Castrén: This is quite possible, but at the same time if we start to look more carefully at different phosphorylation sites the picture might not turn out to be so simple. It might also be more complex for EGF and FGF. Different phosphorylation sites may be preferentially used.

References

Chan JP, Unger TJ, Byrnes J, Rios M 2006 Examination of behavioral deficits triggered by targeting BDNF in fetal or postnatal brains of mice. Neuroscience 142:49–58

Conner JM, Lauterborn JC, Yan Q, Gall CM, Varon S 1997 Distribution of brain-derived neurotrophic factor (BDNF) protein and mRNA in the normal adult rat CNS: evidence for anterograde axonal transport. J Neurosci 17:2295–2313

Lucas G, Hendolin P, Harkany T et al 2003 Neurotrophin-4 mediated TrkB activation reinforces morphine-induced analgesia. Nat Neurosci 6:221–222

Monteggia LM, Luikart B, Barrot M et al 2007 Brain-derived neurotrophic factor conditional knockouts show gender differences in depression-related behaviors. Biol Psychiatry 61:187–197

Rios M, Fan G, Fekete C et al 2001 Conditional deletion of brain-derived neurotrophic factor in the postnatal brain leads to obesity and hyperactivity. Mol Endocrinol 15:1748–1757

Shirayama Y, Chen AC, Nakagawa S, Russell DS, Duman RS 2002 Brain-derived neurotrophic factor produces antidepressant effects in behavioral models of depression. J Neurosci 22:3251–3261

Genetics of bipolar disorder: focus on BDNF Val66Met polymorphism

Jinbo Fan*‡ and Pamela Sklar*†‡[1]

*Psychiatric and Neurodevelopmental Genetics Unit, Center for Human Genetics Research, Massachusetts General Hospital, 185 Cambridge Street, Boston, MA 02114, USA, †Department of Psychiatry, Harvard Medical School, Boston, Massachusetts, USA and ‡Program in Medical and Population Genetics, Broad Institute of MIT and Harvard, Seven Cambridge Center, Cambridge, Massachusetts 02139, USA

Abstract. Bipolar disorder is a chronic severe mood disorder that has been consistently demonstrated to have a strong inherited component. Traditional approaches to gene discovery have produced conflicting results regarding the association between genes and bipolar disorder. Numerous genes have been proposed as associated with bipolar disorder. This paper will focus on one of these, brain-derived neurotrophic factor (BDNF). BDNF is an interesting candidate gene for bipolar disorder because of its important role in the neurodevelopment of the CNS. Previous genetic work has identified a potential association between a Val66Met polymorphism in the BDNF gene and bipolar disorder. Meta-analysis based on all original published association studies between the Val66Met polymorphism and bipolar disorder up to May 2007 shows modest but statistically significant evidence for the association between the Val66Met polymorphism and bipolar disorder (random-effects pooled odds ratio [OR] = 1.13, 95% Confidence Interval [CI] = 1.04–1.23, Z = 2.85, $P = 0.004$) from 14 studies consisting of 4248 cases, 7080 control subjects and 858 nuclear families. Further large-scale studies are warranted to elucidate the relevant BDNF gene variation(s) that act as risk factors for bipolar disorder susceptibility.

2008 Growth factors and psychiatric disorders. Wiley, Chichester (Novartis Foundation Symposium 289) p 60–73

Bipolar disorder (BD) is a common, chronic, and often disabling mood disorder with a lifetime prevalence of approximately 0.5–1.5%. The diagnosis of bipolar I disorder includes one or more episodes of mania, whereas bipolar II disorder involves milder hypomanic episodes with recurrent depressive episodes. BD is an extremely disruptive illness, estimated to be the world's eighth largest cause of medical disability (Murray & Lopez 1996). The lack of understanding about the

---

[1] This paper was presented at the symposium by Pamela Sklar to whom correspondence should be addressed.

pathophysiology of BD severely handicaps the development of novel treatment strategies. Although there is intense interest in determining the aetiology of BD, with the goal of developing more effective treatment and prevention strategies, the biological basis for BD is still obscure.

Over a century of genetic epidemiological research shows that BD is a highly heritable disease (Tsuang & Faraone 1990). Family and epidemiological studies unequivocally demonstrate a strong contribution of inherited genetic variation to the risk for BD (Smoller & Finn 2003). The recurrence risk ratio for monozygotic twins is approximately 60, about four- to sixfold higher than for dizygotic twins, and the heritability of BD is estimated to be approximately 60% (Craddock et al 1995, Marneros & Angst 2000). Despite this, traditional linkage mapping strategies have failed to identify loci or genes that convincingly increase risk of BD. Less stringent or suggestive evidence for linkage has been obtained for essentially all chromosomes.

Traditional linkage methods for detection of susceptibility genes are not well powered to detect alleles that confer odds ratios less than 2. Effect sizes smaller than this are more efficiently detected by association studies (Risch & Merikangas 1996). New technical methods for assessing association across the entire genome simultaneously are now in active use. For many complex genetic disorders such as age-related macular degeneration, type 2 diabetes, breast cancer and others, these methods have led to identification of many new and compelling risk genes (WTCCC 2007, Dewan et al 2006, Easton et al 2007, Saxena et al 2007). A new generation of whole-genome studies in BD is underway and interpretation of their results is eagerly awaited.

To date, most association studies between genes and BD have focused on those candidate genes that contribute to pathways traditionally thought to be involved in biogenic amine modulation or lithium signalling, including genes encoding monoamine oxidase A (MAOA), catechol-O-methyltransferase (COMT), the serotonin transporter (SLC6A4), the serotonin 2A receptor (HTR2A), tryptophan hydroxylase 1 (TPH1) and brain-derived neurotrophic factor (BDNF), but consistent direction of effects and alleles have not been established for any of them (Hayden & Nurnberger 2006). The general pattern seen in bipolar association studies, as in many diseases of complex genetic structure, is that there is an initial positive study followed by many replication reports, some reporting positive findings and some reporting negative findings. These inconsistent results may be related to variation in ascertainment, phenotype definition and control selection, limited power (studies have typically included fewer than 200 cases or families) and possible confounding by population substructure. In almost all cases the limited sample sizes in the individual studies do not have the power to rule out or confirm an association, where the expected effect size of potential risk locus is less than 1.5-fold (Hirschhorn et al 2002).

BDNF is a member of the neurotrophin superfamily, which mediates neuronal differentiation and survival, modifies synaptic connections, and plays an important role in the neurodevelopment of the CNS (Poo 2001). Several converging lines of biological, pharmacological and genetic evidence suggest that the BDNF gene is an attractive candidate gene for BD susceptibility (Green & Craddock 2003, Hashimoto et al 2004). First, the chromosome 11p14.1 region, where the BDNF gene is located, has been implicated in BD by previous linkage studies (Craddock et al 1999). Second, reduced BDNF protein level has been observed in postmortem hippocampus from brain of BD patients compared with control subjects (Knable et al 2004). Third, direct evidence implicating the role of BDNF in susceptibility of BD has come from genetic studies (Geller et al 2004, Green et al 2006, Kremeyer et al 2006, Lohoff et al 2005, Muller et al 2006, Neves-Pereira et al 2002, Sklar et al 2002).

Position 196 in exon 5 of the BDNF gene contains a G to A transition (dbSNP: rs6265) that results in an amino acid substitution (valine to methionine) at codon 66 in the precursor BDNF peptide sequence (Cargill et al 1999). In a previous family-based association study, our group reported a significant excess transmission of the valine allele of the non-synonymous mutation (Val66Met) from parents to affected offspring ($P = 0.04$) in a screening sample of 136 parent-proband trios. Excess transmission of the same allele of Val66Met was observed in two independent samples totalling 334 parent-proband trios ($P = 0.066$). Genotyping of additional single nucleotide polymorphisms (SNPs) identified three SNPs associated with BD (Sklar et al 2002). An independent study also reported association between the same allele of Val66Met polymorphism and a complex repeat polymorphism located in regulatory region of the BDNF gene in their sample of 283 nuclear families (Neves-Pereira et al 2002). Following these two reports, a large number of association studies between BDNF gene polymorphisms and BD have been published. Most of them have specifically focused on the non-synonymous mutation (Val66Met) and have yielded conflicting results. Among them, three independent family-based studies and one case-control study have reported association with the Val allele (Geller et al 2004, Kremeyer et al 2006, Lohoff et al 2005, Muller et al 2006, Neves-Pereira et al 2002, Sklar et al 2002), while other studies failed to detect any association (Green et al 2006, Hong et al 2003, Kunugi et al 2004, Nakata et al 2003, Neves-Pereira et al 2005, Oswald et al 2004, Schumacher et al 2005, Skibinska et al 2004).

In view of the conflicting results, a meta-analysis was performed based on all original case-control and family-based association studies published up to May 2007, to comprehensively determine the overall strength of associations between BD and the non-synonymous (Val66Met) mutation. Furthermore, the linkage disequilibrium (LD) patterns of the BDNF gene locus were examined using the genotype data from the international HapMap project database (Altshuler et al 2005).

Methods

The identification, evaluation and processing of relevant studies for meta-analysis were performed as previously described (Fan & Sklar 2005, Faraone et al 2001, Glatt et al 2003). The pooled odds ratios (ORs) were calculated according to the DerSimonian-Laird random-effects model (DerSimonian & Laird 1986, Mantel & Haenszel 1959). In our study, pooled ORs are virtually identical for the fixed-effects and random-effects approaches. We choose to report only results from the random-effects model as the confidence intervals are more conservative. The combined effect from both case-control and family-based association studies was calculated as previously described (Lohmueller et al 2003). All P values were two-tailed, and the significance level was set at $P < 0.05$, unless stated otherwise.

The LD structure of a 200 kb region on chromosome 11p13 including the human BDNF gene was constructed using 110 single nucleotide polymorphisms (SNPs) from the international HapMap project database (*www.hapmap.org*), as previously described (Altshuler et al 2005, Barrett et al 2005, Fan & Sklar 2005). Only SNPs with minor allele frequencies (MAF) greater than 1% in all four populations (African, Asian and European ancestry) were included in the LD analysis. The BDNF Val66Met SNP (rs6265) was included despite being monomorphic in YRI population.

Results

Meta-analysis

Nine case-control and five family-based association studies met our criteria for inclusion in the meta-analysis. Table 1 shows the characteristics of the 14 studies. Data from four studies were not excluded due to non-independence from studies that were already included in the meta-analysis (Green et al 2006, Neves-Pereira et al 2002, Rybakowski et al 2006, Skibinska et al 2004). Additionally, the BD patients of NIMH trios families in the study of Sklar et al (2002) were partly overlapping with the patients in a case-control study with larger sample size (Lohoff et al 2005), thus, the NIMH families sample of the former study was excluded from current meta-analysis.

Case-control studies: Only one individual study found statistically significant differences in allele frequencies between patients and control subjects for this polymorphism (Table 1). The homogeneity analysis yielded a X^2 value of 4.42 (df = 8; $P = 0. 82$), which suggests there was no evidence for heterogeneity of the ORs among this group of studies. The pooled OR derived from nine case-control studies, including 4248 cases and 7080 control subjects, is nominally significant (random-effects pooled $OR_{cc} = 1.07$, 95% Confidence Interval [CI] = 1.00–1.15, $Z = 2.06$, $P = 0.04$). Sensitivity analysis generated a series of pooled ORs ranging from 1.05 to 1.08 with P values around 0.05 thresholds, except two studies

TABLE 1 Descriptive characteristics and meta-analysis of nine population-based and five family-based association studies between *BDNF* gene Val66Met polymorphism and bipolar disorder

CC study	Year	Number of cases/controls	Diagnostic criteria	Patients' phenotype	Ethnicity	HWE in controls*	Odds ratio	95% CI	P value
Hong CJ	2003	108/392	DSM-IV	BPD	Chinese	N.S.	1.12	0.83–1.52	0.46
Nakata K	2003	130/190	DSM-IV	102BPI + 30BPII	Japanese	N.S.	1.02	0.74–1.41	0.89
Kunugi H	2004	519/588	DSM-IV	347BPI + 172BPII	Japanese	N.S.	0.98	0.83–1.16	0.83
Oswald P	2004	108/158	DSM-IV	BPAD	Belgian	N.S.	0.89	0.59–1.35	0.59
Skibinska M	2004	352/375	DSM-IV	300BPI + 52BPII	Caucasian	N.S.	1.13	0.86–1.49	0.37
Lohoff FW	2005	621/998	DSM-IV	BPI	European	N.S.	1.22	1.02–1.47	0.03
Neves-Pereira M	2005	263/350	DSM-IV	BPAD	Caucasian	N.S.	1.07	0.81–1.41	0.63
Schumacher J	2005	281/1097	DSM-IV	BPAD	German	N.S.	1.01	0.80–1.28	0.94
WTCCC	2007	1866/2932	DSM-IV	BPAD[a]	British	N.S.	1.08	0.97–1.20	0.17
Pooled OR		4248/7080					1.07	1.00–1.15	0.04

TDT study	Year	Number of families	Diagnostic criteria	Patients' phenotype	Ethnicity	HWE in parents	Odds ratio	95% CI	P value
Sklar P	2002	136	RDC	106BPI + 26BPII + 4SAM	Caucasian/Hopkins	N/A	1.56	1.01–2.40	0.04
Sklar P	2002	145	DSM-IV	BPI	Caucasian/UK	N/A	1.19	0.74–1.90	0.47
Geller B	2004	53	DSM-IV	BPI (early onset)	Mixed/USA[b]	N/A	2.33	1.07–5.09	0.03
Kremeyer B	2006	212	RDC	BPI	Isolated South American	N.S.	1.40	0.79–2.49	0.25
Muller DJ	2006	312	DSM-IV	234BPI + 96BPII + 1NOS + 19SAD	Mixed[c]	N.S.	1.63	1.21–2.19	0.0013
Pooled OR		858					1.54	1.26–1.87	0.000019

Combined CC&TDT	Number of cases/controls or families						Odds ratio	95% CI	P value
Pooled OR	4248/7080 858						1.13	1.04–1.23	0.004

*N.S. means not significant in Hardy–Weinberg Equilibrium test.

[a]BPI (71%), schizoaffective disorder bipolar type (15%), BPII (9%) and manic disorder (5%).

[b]The probands were mainly Caucasians (88.7%), with others (11.3%).

[c]Participants were mainly White and of European origin (n = 332, 95%), with 12 Asians (3.4%), 3 Native Americans (0.8%), and 3 African–Americans (0.8%).

(WTCCC 2007, Lohoff et al 2005), suggesting that the P value of pooled OR was overly affected by these two studies (data not shown). For the nine case-control studies, the regression approach of Egger et al (1997) did not find significant evidence (a = –0.32, 95% CI = –1.83–1.20; t = 0.50, df = 7, P = 0.64) for small-study effects within this group of studies.

Family-based studies: Three individual studies found statistically significant over-transmission of the Val allele in their nuclear families. The homogeneity analysis yielded a X^2 value of 2.51 (df = 4; P = 0.64), which suggests there was no evidence for heterogeneity of the ORs among this group of studies. In five family-based studies with a total of 858 families, we found evidence for over-transmission of the Val allele of the Val/Met polymorphism from heterozygous parents to their affected offspring (254 transmitted vs. 165 not transmitted, Pooled OR_{tdt} = 1.54, 95% CI = 1.26–1.87, Z = 4.27, P = 0.000019, Table 1). Sensitivity analysis generated a series of pooled ORs ranging from 1.47 to 1.62 with 95% CIs that always excluded 1.0, suggesting that the pooled OR was not overly affected by any single study (data not shown). For the five family-based studies, the regression approach of Egger et al (1997) did not find evidence (a = 0.28, 95% CI = –3.95–4.50; t = 0.21, df = 3, P = 0.85) for small-study effects within this group of studies.

Combined case-control and family-based studies: The combined analysis of case-control and family-based association studies found moderate nominal association between the Val allele and BD (random-effects pooled OR_{all} = 1.13, 95% CI = 1.04–1.23, Z = 2.85, P = 0.004; Table 1). The homogeneity analysis yielded a X^2 value of 14.2 (df = 13; P = 0.36), which suggests there was no evidence for heterogeneity of the ORs among this group of studies. Sensitivity analysis generated a series of pooled ORs ranging from 1.09 to 1.16 with 95% CIs that always excluded 1.0, suggesting that the pooled OR was not overly affected by the inclusion of any single study (data not shown). For the fifteen studies, the regression approach of Egger et al (1997) found no evidence (a = 1.08, 95% CI = –0.25–2.41; t = 1.77, df = 12, P = 0.10) for small-study effects within this group of studies.

Structure of LD

The LD structure of the 200 kb region including the BDNF gene in four HapMap populations (European, Chinese, Japanese and Yoruban populations) are shown in Fig. 1. Using a block definition of 'strong LD' where the one-sided upper 95% confidence bound on D' > 0.98 as in Gabriel et al (2002), similar LD patterns were observed in the European (Fig. 1A), Chinese (Fig. 1C) and Japanese populations (Fig. 1D), while lower LD was observed in the Yoruban population (Fig. 1B).

In the European descent population, a large LD block (block 3, from left to right) contains the majority of the BDNF gene. Similar LD patterns were observed in the Chinese, Japanese, and Yoruba populations, while the BDNF coding region

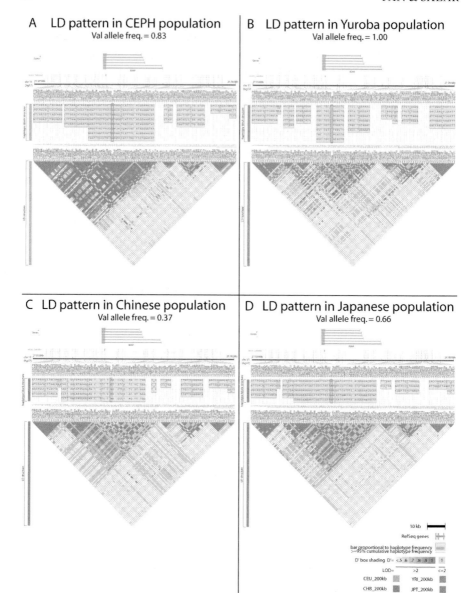

A LD pattern in CEPH population
Val allele freq. = 0.83

B LD pattern in Yuroba population
Val allele freq. = 1.00

C LD pattern in Chinese population
Val allele freq. = 0.37

D LD pattern in Japanese population
Val allele freq. = 0.66

was divided into two or three short regions of strong LD. Although the conservative block definition we have used separates these blocks, there is little evidence for recombination between blocks, with multi-allelic D' above than 0.90. The widely studied Val66Met polymorphism (rs6265) of BDNF gene was located in a region of strong LD in the European, Chinese and Japanese populations, while it is mono-morphic in HapMap Yoruba population. The Met allele predicts a unique haplotype in HapMap European and Japanese populations (frequency: 18% and 37% respectively), but not in Chinese and Yoruba populations.

Discussion

The functional Val66Met polymorphism in BDNF represents a strong biological candidate locus for various psychiatric disorders including BD. On the basis of 15 association studies that include 4248 cases, 7080 control subjects and 858 nuclear families, our meta-analysis revealed a moderate but nominally significant association between the Val allele and BD (random-effects pooled $OR_{all} = 1.13$, $P = 0.004$). This finding is not entirely unexpected since most of the individual studies (12 of 14 individual studies) showed over-representation or over-transmission of the Val allele in BD patients (OR > 1.0), although only four of them demonstrated statistically significant association (Geller et al 2004, Lohoff et al 2005, Muller et al 2006, Sklar et al 2002). Thus, many previous non-significant results likely resulted from the relatively low statistical power of the individual studies each of which comprised only a small number of subjects. The power to detect an association is dependent on sample size, risk allele frequency, and effect size of the risk allele. Using the Genetic Power Calculator (Purcell et al 2003), we determined that a sample of approximately 2500 cases and 2500 controls would be necessary to

◀──

FIG. 1.   Linkage disequilibrium (LD) structure of BDNF gene locus on chromosome 11p14.1 in four populations from the international HapMap project database. Graphical representation of the LD structure produced by Haploview and Locusview software (Barrett et al 2005; Petryshen, Kirby and Ainscow, unpublished software). The BDNF gene is shown by horizontal lines, exons are marked with vertical lines. The location of the Val66Met polymorphism (rs6265) is shown (box). SNP names and genotype data are those from dbSNP (*www.ncbi.nlm.nih.gov/SNP*) and the international HapMap project website (*www.hapmap.org*) (Altshuler et al 2005), vertical tick marks above each SNP name indicate the relative genomic position. The LD structure represents the pairwise calculation of D' for all possible combination of SNPs. D' of less than 0.5 is shown in white, D' = 1.0 in dark grey, with increasing shades of grey between representing increasing D' between the SNPs. D' was calculated using the program Haploview (Barrett et al 2005). Maximum likelihood haplotype blocks were calculated using an EM algorithm as in the study by Gabriel et al (2002). LD patterns were shown in the European (Fig. 1A), Yoruba (Fig. 1B), Han Chinese (Fig. 1C), and Japanese (Fig. 1D) populations, respectively.

achieve P value of 0.05 with 80% power to detect an effect size such as that we have observed in the combined analysis of case-control and family-based studies.

It has been suggested that the first significant study tends to overestimate the genetic effects (Ioannidis et al 2001). However, it is notable that the Val allele remained associated with BD (Pooled OR = 1.12, P = 0.013) even after removing the first significant report (Sklar et al 2002). Furthermore, we find no evidence that the overall findings resulted from any single study or small-study effects in the combined analysis of both case-control and family-based studies. A recent meta-analysis found no evidence for association between the Val66Met polymorphism and BD among eleven case-control association studies (Kanazawa et al 2007). The inclusion of different studies from the literature may explain the discrepancy between the current study and the recent report. First, Kanazawa et al (2007) included case-controls studies exclusively. Second, we have replaced the study of Green & Craddock (2003) with a recent study that presumably includes many individuals from the earlier study, but has a larger sample size (WTCCC 2007). Third, we excluded a single case-control study (Strauss et al 2004) from current meta-analysis because the patients were affected with childhood onset mood disorder rather than a more specific diagnosis of BD (inclusion of this study generated a pooled OR = 1.12, P = 0.009).

The allele frequencies of the BDNF gene Val66Met polymorphisms across individual studies and four HapMap populations showed significant global variation (as shown in Fig. 1) raising concerns of possible population stratification among case-control studies. However, all the case-control studies included in the current meta-analysis utilized case and control subjects from the same geographic region and ethnic origin, which should help to reduce the potential effects of stratification (Ardlie et al 2002), but formal assessments such as genomic control were not performed. Furthermore, the combined result from six family-based studies, which are robust to population stratification, also showed that the same Val allele of the Val66Met polymorphism was significantly over-transmitted (random-effects pooled OR_{TDT} = 1.54, P = 0.000019) from heterozygous parents to BD offspring. However, further analyses revealed significant discrepancy (Z = 3.39, P = 0.00035) between the pooled ORs from case-control studies (Pooled OR_{tdt} = 1.07) and family-based studies (Pooled OR_{tdt} = 1.54) (Cappelleri et al 1996), raising a concern regarding a more generalized transmission distortion at this locus that is not disease related. However, the observation of no excess transmission of the Val allele in non-BD trios families suggests this is not a likely explanation (Sklar et al 2002). Overall, the association observed in the current meta-analyses should be interpreted with caution and requires more replication studies for validation.

Evidence exists for functional effects of the Val66Met polymorphism, however, it is not possible to determine if this variant (or some variant in LD with it) is causally associated with increased risk of BD. The Met allele has been associated with relatively poorer human hippocampal functions (*in vivo*), and impaired intracellular trafficking and secretion of BDNF protein (*in vitro*) (Egan et al 2003); Met carriers had smaller hippocampus volumes in both schizophrenia patients and control subjects, and decreased hippocampal engagement during encoding and retrieval of information compared to Val/Val homozygotes (Hariri et al 2003, Szeszko et al 2005). These observations imply that the rarer Met allele is deleterious. Thus, it remains unknown why the more common Val allele was associated with increased risk of BD (or patients with rapid-cycling sub-phenotype).

One explanation for this observation is that the Val66Met polymorphism may be in strong LD with some other 'true' causal polymorphism, either in BDNF or even nearby gene(s). The haplotype block structure of the BDNF region in four HapMap populations shows that most of the BDNF gene coding region was located in a large block of strong LD (Fig. 1), whereas the Val66Met polymorphism localized in the middle of the LD block. The Met allele exclusively predicts a common haplotype uniquely found in HapMap European and Japanese populations, but not in Chinese and Yoruba populations. The strong LD between Val-66Met and nearby polymorphisms at the BDNF locus suggests the association in our meta-analysis may be due to nearby causal variation(s) in strong LD with the Val66Met polymorphism. This observation also suggests that testing the Val66Met polymorphism is inadequate to test comprehensively for association to BDNF and highlights the value of evaluating patterns of LD across a candidate gene, rather than relying on one or a few randomly selected markers.

The current status of BDNF genetics as viewed through meta-analysis revealed some evidence that the BDNF gene Val66Met variation is a risk factor for BD susceptibility. However, further large-scale studies are still warranted to elucidate the relevant BDNF gene variation(s) that act as risk factor for BD susceptibility.

Acknowledgements

We would like to thank Dr Tracey Petryshen for critical reviews and helpful discussion of the manuscript, and Andrew Kirby and Tracey Petryshen for Locusview software. This work was supported by grant MH062137 to PS, and a postdoctoral fellowship from the Charles A. King Trust, Bank of America, Co-Trustee to JBF. We thank the International HapMap Consortium and the International HapMap project, and Dr Falk W. Lohoff, Dr Barbara Geller, Dr Barbara Kremeyer and Dr Andres Ruiz-Linares for generous sharing of genotype data or for answering specific questions regarding their studies.

References

Altshuler D, Brooks LD, Chakravarti A et al 2005 A haplotype map of the human genome. Nature 437:1299–1320

Ardlie KG, Lunetta KL, Seielstad M 2002 Testing for population subdivision and association in four case-control studies. Am J Hum Genet 71:304–311

Barrett JC, Fry B, Maller J, Daly MJ 2005 Haploview: analysis and visualization of LD and haplotype maps. Bioinformatics 21:263–265

Cappelleri JC, Ioannidis JP, Schmid CH et al 1996 Large trials vs. meta-analysis of smaller trials: how do their results compare? JAMA 276:1332–1338

Cargill M, Altshuler D, Ireland J et al 1999 Characterization of single-nucleotide polymorphisms in coding regions of human genes. Nat Genet 22:231–238

Craddock N, Khodel V, Van Eerdewegh P, Reich T 1995 Mathematical limits of multilocus models: the genetic transmission of bipolar disorder. Am J Hum Genet 57:690–702

Craddock N, Lendon C, Cichon S et al 1999 Chromosome Workshop: Chromosomes 11, 14, and 15. Am J Med Genet 88:244–254

DerSimonian R, Laird N 1986 Meta-analysis in clinical trials. Control Clin Trials 7:177–188

Dewan A, Liu M, Hartman S et al 2006 HTRA1 promoter polymorphism in wet age-related macular degeneration. Science 314:989–992

Easton DF, Pooley KA, Dunning AM et al 2007 Genome-wide association study identifies novel breast cancer susceptibility loci. Nature 447:1087–1093

Egan MF, Kojima M, Callicott JH et al 2003 The BDNF Val66Met polymorphism affects activity-dependent secretion of BDNF and human memory and hippocampal function. Cell 112:257–269

Egger M, Davey Smith G, Schneider M, Minder C 1997 Bias in meta-analysis detected by a simple, graphical test. BMJ 315:629–634

Fan JB, Sklar P 2005 Meta-analysis reveals association between serotonin transporter gene STin2 VNTR polymorphism and schizophrenia. Mol Psychiatry 10:928–938, 891

Faraone SV, Doyle AE, Mick E, Biederman J 2001 Meta-analysis of the association between the 7-repeat allele of the dopamine D(4) receptor gene and attention deficit hyperactivity disorder. Am J Psychiatry 158:1052–1057

Gabriel SB, Schaffner SF, Nguyen H et al 2002 The structure of haplotype blocks in the human genome. Science 296:2225–2229

Geller B, Badner JA, Tillman R, Christian SL, Bolhofner K, Cook EH Jr 2004 Linkage disequilibrium of the brain-derived neurotrophic factor Val66Met polymorphism in children with a prepubertal and early adolescent bipolar disorder phenotype. Am J Psychiatry 161:1698–1700

Glatt SJ, Faraone SV, Tsuang MT 2003 Association between a functional catechol O-methyltransferase gene polymorphism and schizophrenia: meta-analysis of case-control and family-based studies. Am J Psychiatry 160:469–476

Green E, Craddock N 2003 Brain-derived neurotrophic factor as a potential risk locus for bipolar disorder: evidence, limitations, and implications. Curr Psychiatry Rep 5:469–476

Green EK, Raybould R, Macgregor S et al 2006 Genetic variation of brain-derived neurotrophic factor (BDNF) in bipolar disorder: case-control study of over 3000 individuals from the UK. Br J Psychiatry 188:21–25

Hariri AR, Goldberg TE, Mattay VS et al 2003 Brain-derived neurotrophic factor Val66Met polymorphism affects human memory-related hippocampal activity and predicts memory performance. J Neurosci 23:6690–6694

Hashimoto K, Shimizu E, Iyo M 2004 Critical role of brain-derived neurotrophic factor in mood disorders. Brain Res Brain Res Rev 45:104–114

Hayden EP, Nurnberger JI Jr 2006 Molecular genetics of bipolar disorder. Genes Brain Behav 5:85–95

Hirschhorn JN, Lohmueller K, Byrne E, Hirschhorn K 2002 A comprehensive review of genetic association studies. Genet Med 4:45–61

Hong CJ, Huo SJ, Yen FC, Tung CL, Pan GM, Tsai SJ 2003 Association study of a brain-derived neurotrophic-factor genetic polymorphism and mood disorders, age of onset and suicidal behavior. Neuropsychobiology 48:186–189

Ioannidis JP, Ntzani EE, Trikalinos TA, Contopoulos-Ioannidis DG 2001 Replication validity of genetic association studies. Nat Genet 29:306–309

Kanazawa T, Glatt SJ, Kia-Keating B, Yoneda H, Tsuang MT 2007 Meta-analysis reveals no association of the Val66Met polymorphism of brain-derived neurotrophic factor with either schizophrenia or bipolar disorder. Psychiatr Genet 17:165–170

Knable MB, Barci BM, Webster MJ, Meador-Woodruff J, Torrey EF 2004 Molecular abnormalities of the hippocampus in severe psychiatric illness: postmortem findings from the Stanley Neuropathology Consortium. Mol Psychiatry 9:609–620, 544

Kremeyer B, Herzberg I, Garcia J et al 2006 Transmission distortion of BDNF variants to bipolar disorder type I patients from a South American population isolate. Am J Med Genet B Neuropsychiatr Genet 141:435–439

Kunugi H, Iijima Y, Tatsumi M et al 2004 No association between the Val66Met polymorphism of the brain-derived neurotrophic factor gene and bipolar disorder in a Japanese population: a multicenter study. Biol Psychiatry 56:376–378

Lohmueller KE, Pearce CL, Pike M, Lander ES, Hirschhorn JN 2003 Meta-analysis of genetic association studies supports a contribution of common variants to susceptibility to common disease. Nat Genet 33:177–182

Lohoff FW, Sander T, Ferraro TN, Dahl JP, Gallinat J, Berrettini WH 2005 Confirmation of association between the Val66Met polymorphism in the brain-derived neurotrophic factor (BDNF) gene and bipolar I disorder. Am J Med Genet B Neuropsychiatr Genet 139:51–53

Mantel N, Haenszel W 1959 Statistical aspects of the analysis of data from retrospective studies of disease. J Natl Cancer Inst 22:719–748

Marneros A, Angst J 2000 Bipolar disorders: 100 years after manic-depressive insanity. Kluwer Academic Publishers

Muller DJ, de Luca V, Sicard T, King N, Strauss J, Kennedy JL 2006 Brain-derived neurotrophic factor (BDNF) gene and rapid-cycling bipolar disorder: family-based association study. Br J Psychiatry 189:317–323

Murray CJL, Lopez AD 1996 Evidence-based health policy—lessons from the global burden of disease study. Science 274:740–743

Nakata K, Ujike H, Sakai A et al 2003 Association study of the brain-derived neurotrophic factor (BDNF) gene with bipolar disorder. Neurosci Lett 337:17–20

Neves-Pereira M, Mundo E, Muglia P, King N, Macciardi F, Kennedy JL 2002 The brain-derived neurotrophic factor gene confers susceptibility to bipolar disorder: evidence from a family-based association study. Am J Hum Genet 71:651–655

Neves-Pereira M, Cheung JK, Pasdar A et al 2005 BDNF gene is a risk factor for schizophrenia in a Scottish population. Mol Psychiatry 10:208–212

Oswald P, Del-Favero J, Massat I et al 2004 Non-replication of the brain-derived neurotrophic factor (BDNF) association in bipolar affective disorder: a Belgian patient-control study. Am J Med Genet B Neuropsychiatr Genet 129:34–35

Poo MM 2001 Neurotrophins as synaptic modulators. Nat Rev Neurosci 2:24–32

Purcell S, Cherny SS, Sham PC 2003 Genetic Power Calculator: design of linkage and association genetic mapping studies of complex traits. Bioinformatics 19:149–150

Risch N, Merikangas K 1996 The future of genetic studies of complex human diseases. Science 273:1516–1517

Rybakowski JK, Borkowska A, Skibinska M, Hauser J 2006 Illness-specific association of Val-66Met BDNF polymorphism with performance on Wisconsin Card Sorting Test in bipolar mood disorder. Mol Psychiatry 11:122–124

Saxena R, Voight BF, Lyssenko V et al 2007 Genome-wide association analysis identifies loci for type 2 diabetes and triglyceride levels. Science 316:1331–1336

Schumacher J, Jamra RA, Becker T et al 2005 Evidence for a relationship between genetic variants at the brain-derived neurotrophic factor (BDNF) locus and major depression. Biol Psychiatry 58:307–314

Skibinska M, Hauser J, Czerski PM et al 2004 Association analysis of brain-derived neurotrophic factor (BDNF) gene Val66Met polymorphism in schizophrenia and bipolar affective disorder. World J Biol Psychiatry 5:215–220

Sklar P, Gabriel SB, McInnis MG et al 2002 Family-based association study of 76 candidate
    genes in bipolar disorder: BDNF is a potential risk locus. Brain-derived neutrophic factor.
    Mol Psychiatry 7:579–593
Smoller JW, Finn CT 2003 Family, twin, and adoption studies of bipolar disorder. Am J Med
    Genet C Semin Med Genet 123C:48–58
Strauss J, Barr CL, George CJ et al 2004 Association study of brain-derived neurotrophic factor
    in adults with a history of childhood onset mood disorder. Am J Med Genet B Neuropsy-
    chiatr Genet 131:16–19
Szeszko PR, Lipsky R, Mentschel C et al 2005 Brain-derived neurotrophic factor Val66Met
    polymorphism and volume of the hippocampal formation. Mol Psychiatry 10:631–636
Tsuang MT, Faraone SV 1990 The genetics of mood disorders. Johns Hopkins University Press
WTCCC (The Wellcome Trust Case Control Consortium) 2007 Genome-wide association study
    of 14,000 cases of seven common diseases and 3,000 shared controls. Nature 447:661–678

DISCUSSION

Chao: Could you compare the study you are doing with the Wellcome Trust study? How similar are they?

Sklar: The Wellcome Trust Case Control Consortium has completed the study of seven diseases, for which they looked at about 2000 cases of each, and they have 3000 controls from two different sources. The only psychiatric disease that was included was bipolar disorder, and this primarily focused on a collection of patients that Nick Craddock has at Cardiff University. The diagnoses of the patients are relatively similar. Both sets of patients were genotyped on the same Affymetrix chips that we are using, so the genotype data are directly comparable. These two studies are the largest, directly comparable studies. There was a smaller study that Huda Akil was involved in that used Illumina technology. The NIH has sponsored what is called the GAIN project, which involves four whole-genome scans for psychiatric disease: major depression, ADHD, bipolar disorder and schizophrenia.

Akil: We have done phase 1a and are doing phase 1b. We will have 1000 bipolars and 1000 controls done this month.

Sklar: Will you be sharing these data?

Akil: I hope so. This is a Foundation-based project and we need to clear matters with their lawyers. We want to share data. We know our sample is too small for us to reach conclusions: the more we can put the data together the better. For your information, these are the NIMH samples and Pablo Gejman controls that we did stratification on to match them as well as possible. The quality of the genotyping is fantastic. We are working hard and hopefully this will add to the information available.

Owen: The Wellcome Trust data are going to be made publicly available. The control data are already available and the case genotype data will be available in a few months' time.

Sklar: That is true for our data also. Our control data are already in the database.

Chao: You mentioned that there was a weak genetic association with the potential candidate risk gene dysbindin. What would you tell those working on dysbindin about the significance of this association?

Sklar: Substantial genetic work needs to be done for us to understand whether there is a genetic association with this gene. People working on dysbindin should work on it because they think it is an interesting gene. The genetic studies are at present inconclusive. Researchers in the field need to get together and come up with a common set of markers. These markers need to be genotyped in one lab under controlled conditions to assess whether there is a real association. Whole-genome scan data should be informative because many more DNA samples will be genotyped across that locus. One explanation often offered for the apparent inconsistency between findings is that there is epistasis. This is formally possible, but has yet to be demonstrated. If one proposes the hypothesis that there is epistasis one needs to measure it and conclusively demonstrate epistasis. Similarly, if epigenetics is proposed. If one has a hypothesis about why this gene is involved in a non-standard way, then the onus is to demonstrate those things rather than simply assert them.

Brandon: Have you looked at any other genes which have this same locus heterogeneity, such as *DISC1* and neuregulin?

Sklar: Yes. We are almost finished with dysbindin 1. Dysbindin was a small gene, as they go. The genes just get bigger and more complicated. The next one we have broached is *DISC1*. First we construct a framework map so we can put all of the association data on that map. This is done by joining up genotyping of markers from the HapMap with previously reported associations in the literature by genotyping all SNPs on the HapMap Caucasian sample. *DISC1* is a much more complex locus, and I do not think it will be as simple. My current interpretation of the data for *DISC1* is that there is very little consistency in the genetic association data at present.

Flint: I want to comment on the family-based versus population data association studies. One explanation for the differences is the presence in the families of rare variants.

Sklar: Yes. We have done a fair amount of sequencing, for example of *BDNF*, and have not come up with rare variants that are sticking out. For *BDNF*, the promoter structure is quite complicated. There is some evidence for the *BDNF* locus being under selection, which probably makes some sense given how important it is. Recently we have been focusing on trying to understand what is going on in the promoter region, looking at whether there is evidence for selection.

Flint: Did the whole-genome association study hit anything that people have looked at before?

Sklar: There is a threshold issue. We looked at a few of the prior candidate genes. I do not know how to define properly what a hit would look like, given the fact that for a gene such as neuregulin there are 261 SNPs on the chip. What threshold do I set, even though there is a prior theory?

Mechanisms of neuregulin action

David A Talmage[1]

Institute of Human Nutrition and Department of Pediatrics, Columbia University Medical Center, 630 West 168th Street, New York, NY 10024, USA

Abstract. Neuregulin 1 (Nrg1) and ErbB receptor tyrosine kinase signalling is essential for the formation and proper functioning of multiple organ systems and inappropriate Nrg1/ErbB signalling severely compromises health, contributing to such diverse pathologies as cancer and neuropsychiatric disorders. Numerous genetic modelling studies in mice demonstrate that Nrg1 signalling is important in the development of normal neuronal connectivity. Recent studies have identified novel signalling mechanisms and revealed unexpected roles of Nrg1 isoforms in both the developing and adult nervous system. Of particular interest to this discussion are findings linking deficits in Nrg1–ErbB4 signalling to perturbations of synaptic transmission, myelination, and the survival of particular sets of neurons and glia.

2008 Growth factors and psychiatric disorders. Wiley, Chichester (Novartis Foundation Symposium 289) p 74–86

Genetic association of neuregulin 1 and schizophrenia

The Nrg1 gene is a schizophrenia susceptibility gene. This was initially reported by deCODE in 2002 in a study in which a seven-marker haplotype (five single nucleotide polymorphisms [SNPs] and two microsatellites) at the extreme 5' end was identified as significantly associated with disease diagnosis in an Icelandic population (Stefansson et al 2002). The association of these, and/or additional sequence polymorphisms in the Nrg1 gene with disease has been reproduced in numerous studies in multiple populations. A recent count of the literature indicates that there have been at least 30 studies of which about two-thirds show association between Nrg1 and schizophrenia and the rest do not. Both positive and negative findings have been reported in case-control and family based studies and in numerous geographically distinct populations (for recent update, see: *http://www. schizophreniaforum.org/res/sczgene/geneoverview.asp?geneid=311*). Several recent studies have extended the Nrg1 connection beyond schizophrenia raising the possibility

---

[1] Current Address: Department of Pharmacology, State University of New York, Stony Brook, USA.

that dysregulation of Nrg1–ErbB signalling contributes to other disorders such as bipolar (Thomson et al 2007) and Alzheimer's disease with psychosis (Go et al 2005). In addition there are data emerging that support additional links between ErbB4 and schizophrenia susceptibility (Silberberg et al 2006, Law et al 2007).

Over 80 SNPs have been described in the association studies between the Nrg1 gene and risk of schizophrenia and disease associated SNPs are grouped into several 'at risk' haplotypes that span much of the 1–1.5 million base pairs encoding Nrg1 proteins. Of these 80, only four result in changes in the predicted coding sequence of the protein. The significance of these changes is not known but the most recent, a valine to leucine substitution in the transmembrane domain, will be discussed below (Walss-Bass et al 2006). The absence of clear mutations in protein coding sequences that are associated with disease risk, are consistent with the conclusion that changes in the level of expression of one or more isoforms of Nrg1 contribute to the aetiology of this disorder (Law et al 2006).

Neuregulin 1 functions: why are there so many isoforms, and does this diversity provide insight into pathology?

We face two major challenges to bridging the gap between results of human genetic studies and understanding how Nrg1–ErbB signalling contributes to psychiatric disease. First, we need to identify the relevant DNA sequence polymorphisms and gain insight into how these polymorphisms affect expression of the Nrg1 gene. Second, we need to acquire a deep enough understanding of how Nrg1 functions in the CNS to allow us to make the leap from DNA sequences to changes in function that might explain the cell and neuronal circuit based changes that contribute to disease.

In the following sections I will (1) review the functional importance of different exons/isoforms and (2) present data supporting the use of genetically modified mice to better understand the role of Nrg1 in establishing and maintaining important (with respect to this disease) circuits in the mouse brain.

Neuregulin 1 is one of about 20 vertebrate genes encoding ligands for the four ErbB receptors (Stein & Staros 2006). In general, ErbB1 (=EGFR) and ErbB4 are the key targets—seven genes encode ligands for ErbB1 and nine encode ligands for ErbB4 (with three, HB-EGF, epiregulin and betacellulin, shared). ErbB3 is more selective; to date only Nrg1 and Nrg2 and neuroglycan have been shown to bind directly to ErbB3. ErbB2 (also called Her2/neu) is a co-receptor that does not bind ligand on its own, but forms heterodimers with the other ErbBs altering their signalling properties.

Nrg1 is a large and complex gene that encodes 15–20 different proteins. These isoforms are generated following transcription from six promoters coupled with a significant degree of alternative splicing of primary transcripts (Fig. 1). Aspects of

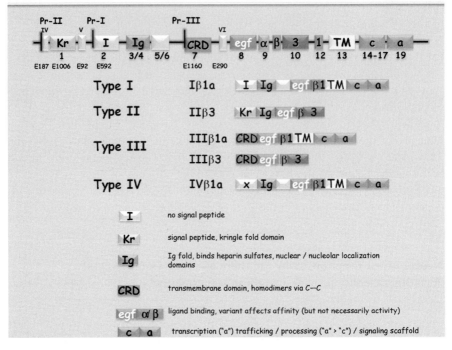

FIG. 1.   The Neuregulin 1 (Nrg1) gene encodes an abundance of related but functionally distinct proteins. The Nrg1 gene is schematized at the top. Boxes represent coding exons drawn approximately to scale. Introns are not shown to scale. In primates, six families of Nrg1 isoforms have been described and are thought to all be transcribed from distinct core promoters (I–VI) (Steinthorsdottir et al 2004). Only types I–III appear to be present in non-primates. Each of the six families of isoforms has a unique N-terminal sequence that is encoded by 6 different 5' exons (I = E592, II= E1006, III = E1160, IV = E187, V = E92 and VI = E290). No clear signal sequence is present in E592, E187, E92 or E290. E1006 encodes a classic signal peptide and E1160 enocodes a transmembrane domain that anchors the type III isoforms in the membrane. Other domains of interest include the Ig domain (encoded by exons 3 and 4), the EGF domain encoded by exon 8, the C-terminal EGF-like domain encoded by combinations of exons 9–12, the common transmembrane domain encoded by exon 13 and the intracellular domain, encoded by exons 14–19. The functions associated with these domains are described in the text. What is clear from this diagram is that combinations of differential promoter usage with differential splicing gives rise to families of proteins with distinct signalling strategies.

both promoter usage and splicing appear to be developmentally regulated and occur in tissue and cell type specific patterns. Until recently little attention has been paid to the factors that regulate the choice of these promoters and/or splice sites. This lack of data on the function of non-coding sequences in neurons and glia limit the ability to generate informed hypotheses linking disease associated polymorphisms with potential functional consequences. A very recent report from A. Law and colleagues provides the first experimental demonstration that a disease associated polymorphism alters promoter strength, a result that should pave the way for a more systematic assessment of the biological significance of non-coding SNPs in the Nrg1 gene (Tan et al 2007).

To date Nrg1 isoforms have been divided into three major families (types I, II and III) present in all vertebrates examined and three minor families (types IV, V and VI) which appear to be restricted to primates. Although post-mortem studies have focused attention on type I Nrg1 and type IV Nrg1 (Law et al 2006), the fact that SNPs and haplotypes spanning nearly the entire 1.5 Mbp have been linked to disease risk, reinforces the need to understand the functional contribution of all of the isoforms to the development and maintenance of the CNS.

In contrast to what we know about non-coding regions, we know a lot more about the functions of discrete regions of the encoded proteins, both those that are common to all known functional isoforms and those that are isoform or family specific. In sum: the unique N-termini associated with types I, II and III all have functional implications. The N-terminus of the type I isoforms (and presumably types IV–VI) is notable for what it lacks: a signal sequence or alternative mechanism for entering the secretory pathway. Type I Nrg1 isoforms depend on the central transmembrane domain and portions of the intracellular domain to enter the secretory pathway, reach the cell surface and then undergo proteolytic release of the growth factor domain (Liu et al 1998, Montero et al 2000, Wang et al 2001). Without a transmembrane domain, type 1 Nrg1 does not reach the cell surface, and experimentally, are expressed as soluble, cytosolic proteins that are targeted to the nucleolus (Golding et al 2004).

The type II isoforms contain N-terminal domains blessed with both a classic signal peptide and a Kringle-like domain. These isoforms readily enter the secretory pathway and are released from cells. Kringle domains in other proteins mediate protein–protein interactions, but no partners for type II Nrg1 have been reported.

Types I, II, IV and V contain an immunoglobulin-like domain near their N-termini. In peripheral nerves and tissues outside of the nervous system, this Ig-domain is thought to contribute to specific interactions with extracellular matrix components and modify (a) the distance over which these growth factors act and (b) the local concentration of growth factor (Li & Loeb 2001).

Type III Nrg1 is unique in a number of ways. First, type III expression is mostly limited to neurons; no other isoform displays this degree of restricted expression (Yang et al 1998, Wolpowitz et al 2000). Second, the cysteine-rich domain encoded by the type III-specific N-terminal exon forms a transmembrane domain (Wang et al 2001). As a result, type III Nrg1 proteins have cytosolic N-termini, and have membrane-tethered EGF-like domains. This topology (a) restricts type III Nrg1 signalling to cell–cell interactions (i.e. juxtacrine signalling) and (b) allows type III Nrg1 to act as a receptor. Indeed we have demonstrated that type III Nrg1 is a bidirectional signalling protein that functions as both a ligand that activates ErbB receptors and as a receptor that modulates the behaviour of type III Nrg1-expressing neurons (Bao et al 2003).

All known functional variants of Nrg1 contain an EGF-like domain essential for interaction with ErbB receptors. The EGF-like domain consists of three regions; the N-terminal part of the EGF domain is constant for all Nrg1 isoforms. This is followed by either an α type or a β type exon and a variable 'stalk' region (the stalk is the extracellular juxtamembrane segment separating the EGF-like domain from the transmembrane domain). The variability in the EGF-like domain has functional implications. Variations in this region affect the affinity of the Nrg1 ligand for receptors with the β isoforms having significantly greater affinity than α isoforms. The relatively subtle variations in the stalk region affect the efficiency by which the transmembrane precursors are processed by metalloproteases (which for non-type III Nrg1 isoforms is necessary for release of active growth factor), with longer 'stalks' being better substrates than shorter ones (Montero et al 2000). These relatively subtle differences have not been explored in depth *in vitro* or *in vivo*.

The C-terminal intracellular domain (ICD) has important functions. As noted above, in the case of the type I Nrg1 isoforms, the intracellular domain is required for intra-cellular trafficking of the protein (Liu et al 1998). In addition, the longest variant of the intracellular domain (the 'a' form) functions as an inducible transcription factor (Bao et al 2003, 2004). Both ErbB binding and depolarization stimulate a γ-secretase catalysed intramembranous cleavage that releases the C-terminal ICD. Subsequent to cleavage, the ICD translocates to the nucleus where it contributes to the transcriptional regulation of genes involved in neuronal survival and in synaptic maturation and maintenance. In more recent studies we have uncovered additional signalling mechanisms that are engaged by Nrg1-ICD, and find that these signalling events regulate growth cone dynamics and trafficking of neurotransmitter receptors. The latter responses, in which Nrg1 behaves like a receptor, require that the full length form of Nrg1 is presented at the cell surface. In our hands, only type III Nrg1 isoforms elicit responses consistent with this receptor-like function, but in the systems we have studied, type I/II isoforms are rapidly released from the cell surface and therefore are unlikely to contribute to bidirectional signalling. In addition, in recent studies we have found a number of amino acid residues within the transmembrane domain that are necessary for γ-secretase cleavage. The recent finding of a Val/Leu substitution within the transmembrane domain that is associated with risk of schizophrenia in some populations (Walss-Bass et al 2006) raises the possibility that alterations in bidirectional signalling could contribute to disease pathology.

Although the complexity of the Nrg1 gene has been known for 15 years, there is still relatively little information available about how the functional diversity of the Nrg1 isoforms influences the biology of the CNS. What information we do have comes from two general types of experimental approaches; addition of recombinant neuregulin to neurons followed by measurements of various responses, and studies on the effect of genetic disruption of one or more Nrg1 isoforms in mice. The results of these studies provide compelling evidence for the biological plausibility of Nrg1 as a schizophrenia susceptibility gene. In particular, these studies demonstrate that Nrg1 is critical for neuronal development (including neurogenesis, migration, axonal targeting, and neurotransmitter expression and targeting), the survival of neurons and the maintenance of circuit plasticity.

Using mouse genetic models to probe Nrg1 function in brain circuitry

In order to study aspects of the biological changes that underlie psychiatric diseases, one would ideally like to introduce disease associated mutations into model systems. Unfortunately most of the DNA sequence changes that link Nrg1 with schizophrenia occur in regions of the gene that do not encode protein and are believed to have subtle effects on levels and/or patterns of expression. As a starting point, we and others have examined the effects of reducing Nrg1 expression by half on the behaviour of adult mice (homozygous mutations in Nrg1 result in embryonic or perinatal lethality) (Meyer & Birchmeier 1995, Wolpowitz et al 2000). Mutations that have been examined include those that eliminate all Nrg1 expression as well as ones that eliminate Ig-Nrg1 expression (types I and II) (Gerlai et al 2000, Bjarnadottir et al 2007), type III Nrg1 expression or all Nrg1 isoforms that contain the common transmembrane domain (all type I and subsets of types II and III) (Stefansson et al 2002, O'Tuathaigh et al 2006, Bjarnadottir et al 2007, Boucher et al 2007, Karl et al 2007). Not surprisingly, the results are complicated. Some behaviours are altered in all mutants examined whereas others are associated with the disruption of specific Nrg1 isoforms. In addition, behaviours affected include those that are thought to correspond to endophenotypes associated with schizophrenia as well as behaviours that do not model schizophrenia phenotypes. For example, Nrg1 mutant mice show elevated levels of activity in a novel open environment (with the exception of the type III Nrg1 mutants), have deficits in pre-pulse inhibition of an acoustic startle reflex (a model of sensorimotor gating), alterations in anxiety related behaviours, and altered responses to drugs including THC (tetrahydrocannabinol) and nicotine (Boucher et al 2007). Similar results have been noted in mice bearing mutations in ErbB receptors, although the effect of mutation tends to be less pronounced in ErbB mutant mice than in Nrg1 mutant mice (Gerlai et al 2000, Stefansson et al 2002). We are tempted to speculate that the picture will clarify once more precise mutations are generated, both in terms of specific brain regions affected as well as studying more 'schizophrenia-like' alterations in Nrg1.

Neuregulin 1 signalling in synaptic development and maintenance: building the case for biological plausibility

The pathology of schizophrenia has been associated with underlying deficits in a number of cellular and molecular systems in the brain, including those involving oligodendrocytes, prefrontal and striatal dopamine signalling, cortical GABAergic interneurons and diffuse NMDA mediated glutamatergic transmission (Lewis 2000, Hof et al 2002, Coyle & Tsai 2004, Harrison & Weinberger 2005). *In vivo* studies in rodents, as well as *in vitro* studies using tissue from a variety of species including human post-mortem samples, have provided evidence that Nrg1–ErbB signalling can affect each of these targets. For example, Nrg1 is essential for direct-ing myelination of peripheral nerves (Michailov et al 2004, Taveggia et al 2005) and disruption of oligodendroglial ErbB signalling alters myelination of central axons and widely dysregulates dopamine signalling (Roy et al 2007). Nrg1–ErbB signalling is an essential regulator of tangential migration of cortical GABAergic interneurons during early brain development and adult mice lacking neuronal ErbB4 expression or heterozygous for disruption of type III Nrg1 expression have deficits in subpopulations of these cortical interneurons (Flames et al 2004). *In vitro* studies show that short-term responses of cerebellar and cortical neurons to the application of recombinant Nrg1 include transcriptional regulation of GABA-A receptor expression (Rieff et al 1999, Okada & Corfas 2004) and presynaptic modulation of GABA release (Woo et al 2007). Thus, Nrg1–ErbB signalling con-tributes to the migration, differentiation and modulation of a population of cortical interneurons that are affected in individuals with schizophrenia.

Nrg1–ErbB signalling also affects glutamatergic transmission, again at multiple levels. Early in development Nrg1–ErbB signalling is important for radial migra-tion of differentiating pyramidal neurons and for targeting of glutamatergic projec-tions from the dorsal thalamus to the neocortex (Anton et al 1997, Lopez-Bendito et al 2006). We have found that heterozygous type III Nrg1 mutant mice have alterations in the formation and function of glutamatergic ventral hippocampal synapses on striatal medium spiny neurons (unpublished observations). Altering Nrg1–ErbB signalling has complex effects on activity dependent synaptic plasticity in hippocampal and cortical slice cultures, altering both NMDA receptor levels and phosphorylation and AMPA receptor trafficking. Although these studies point to complex, and sometimes contradictory effects of Nrg1–ErbB signalling at glu-tamatergic synapses, in sum they point to the need for a fine balance of Nrg1–ErbB signalling with both deficient and excessive signalling interfering with synaptic plasticity (Gu et al 2005, Kwon et al 2005, Hahn et al 2006, Bjarnadottir et al 2007,

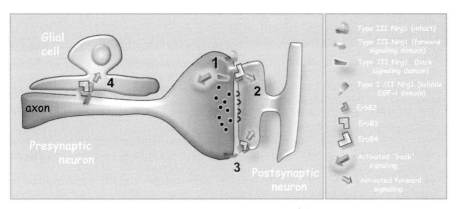

FIG. 2.   Differential axonal expression of Neuregulin 1 isoforms affects synaptic Nrg1-ErbB
signalling strategies. On the left is a cartoon depicting an axon terminal segment interacting
with a postsynaptic spine and a glial cell (1). At the synapse, presynaptic type III Nrg1 interacts
with post-synaptic ErbB4 dimers (shown as an ErbB4:ErbB2 heterodimer, but could also be
an ErbB4 homodimer). This interaction activates ErbB tyrosine kinase activity eliciting both
local changes in the spine and transcriptional responses in the post-synaptic neuron (2). At
glutamatergic synapses responses include regulation of NMDA receptor expression and regulation of both NMDA and AMPA receptor trafficking; responses that modulate synaptic plasticity. Type III Nrg1–ErbB interactions can also result in signalling by the type III Nrg1 in the
presynaptic cell. One type of signalling that we have described (Bao et al 2003) involves the γ-
secretase dependent cleavage of type III Nrg1 releasing the C-terminal intracellular domain
which has transcriptional regulatory activity. 'Back-signalling' contributes to the survival of
presynaptic neurons during development and regulates the targeting of neurotransmitter receptors to presynaptic sites where these receptors modulate synaptic activity. Non-type III Nrg1
isoforms also signal at synapses, but are likely to do so in a predominantly unidirectional
manner (3). Altering the ratio of type III Nrg1 to non-type III Nrg1 levels is predicted to
change the balance of unidirectional vs. bidirectional signalling. Axonal Nrg1 also interacts
with ErbB3:ErbB2 heterodimers on glia (4), a signalling partnership that is essential for proper
myelination.

Li et al 2007, Role & Talmage 2007). It is likely that there is a similar requirement
for balanced signalling at other synapses and at extrasynaptic sites (Fig. 2). Given
the apparent sensitivity of the Nrg–ErbB signalling network to perturbations, it
is becoming clearer how subtle changes in the levels and types of Nrg1–ErbB
interactions could alter the ability of key brain circuits to withstand additional
genetic and environmental insults and contribute to disease.

Acknowledgements

All work, published and unpublished, from the Talmage lab has been carried out in collaboration with Dr Lorna W. Role and was funded by NS29071.

References

Anton ES, Marchionni MA, Lee KF, Rakic P 1997 Role of GGF/neuregulin signaling in interactions between migrating neurons and radial glia in the developing cerebral cortex. Development 124:3501–3510

Bao J, Wolpowitz D, Role LW, Talmage DA 2003 Back signaling by the Nrg-1 intracellular domain. J Cell Biol 161:1133–1141

Bao J, Lin H, Ouyang Y et al 2004 Activity-dependent transcription regulation of PSD-95 by neuregulin-1 and Eos. Nat Neurosci 7:1250–1258

Bjarnadottir M, Misner DL, Haverfield-Gross S et al 2007 Neuregulin 1 (NRG1) signaling through Fyn modulates NMDA receptor phosphorylation: differential synaptic function in NRG1+/– knock-outs compared with wild-type mice. J Neurosci 27:4519–4529

Boucher AA, Arnold JC, Duffy L, Schofield PR, Micheau J, Karl T 2007 Heterozygous neuregulin 1 mice are more sensitive to the behavioural effects of Delta9-tetrahydrocannabinol. Psychopharmacology (Berl) 192:325–336

Coyle JT, Tsai G 2004 NMDA receptor function, neuroplasticity, and the pathophysiology of schizophrenia. Int Rev Neurobiol 59:491–515

Flames N, Long JE, Garratt AN et al 2004 Short- and long-range attraction of cortical GABAergic interneurons by neuregulin-1. Neuron 44:251–261

Gerlai R, Pisacane P, Erickson S 2000 Heregulin, but not ErbB2 or ErbB3, heterozygous mutant mice exhibit hyperactivity in multiple behavioral tasks. Behav Brain Res 109:219–227

Go RC, Perry RT, Wiener H et al 2005 Neuregulin-1 polymorphism in late onset Alzheimer's disease families with psychoses. Am J Med Genet B Neuropsychiatr Genet 139:28–32

Golding M, Ruhrberg C, Sandle J, Gullick WJ 2004 Mapping nucleolar and spliceosome localization sequences of neuregulin1-beta3. Exp Cell Res 299:110–118

Gu Z, Jiang Q, Fu AK, Ip NY, Yan Z 2005 Regulation of NMDA receptors by neuregulin signaling in prefrontal cortex. J Neurosci 25:4974–4984

Hahn CG, Wang HY, Cho DS et al 2006 Altered neuregulin 1-ErbB4 signaling contributes to NMDA receptor hypofunction in schizophrenia. Nat Med 12:824–828

Harrison PJ, Weinberger DR 2005 Schizophrenia genes, gene expression, and neuropathology: on the matter of their convergence. Mol Psychiatry 10:40–68

Hof PR, Haroutunian V, Copland C, Davis KL, Buxbaum JD 2002 Molecular and cellular evidence for an oligodendrocyte abnormality in schizophrenia. Neurochem Res 27:1193–1200

Karl T, Duffy L, Scimone A, Harvey RP, Schofield PR 2007 Altered motor activity, exploration and anxiety in heterozygous neuregulin 1 mutant mice: implications for understanding schizophrenia. Genes Brain Behav 6:667–687

Kwon OB, Longart M, Vullhorst D, Hoffman DA, Buonanno A 2005 Neuregulin-1 reverses long-term potentiation at CA1 hippocampal synapses. J Neurosci 25:9378–9383

Law AJ, Lipska BK, Weickert CS et al 2006 Neuregulin 1 transcripts are differentially expressed in schizophrenia and regulated by 5' SNPs associated with the disease. Proc Natl Acad Sci USA 103:6747–6752

Law AJ, Kleinman JE, Weinberger DR, Weickert CS 2007 Disease-associated intronic variants in the ErbB4 gene are related to altered ErbB4 splice-variant expression in the brain in schizophrenia. Hum Mol Genet 16:129–141

Lewis DA 2000 GABAergic local circuit neurons and prefrontal cortical dysfunction in schizophrenia. Brain Res Brain Res Rev 31:270–276

Li Q, Loeb JA 2001 Neuregulin-heparan-sulfate proteoglycan interactions produce sustained erbB receptor activation required for the induction of acetylcholine receptors in muscle. J Biol Chem 276:38068–38075

Li B, Woo RS, Malinow R 2007 The neuregulin-1 receptor ErbB4 controls glutamatergic synapse maturation and plasticity. Neuron 54:583–597

Liu X, Hwang H, Cao L et al 1998 Domain-specific gene disruption reveals critical regulation of neuregulin signaling by its cytoplasmic tail. Proc Natl Acad Sci USA 95:13024–13029

Lopez-Bendito G, Cautinat A, Sánchez JA et al 2006 Tangential neuronal migration controls axon guidance: a role for neuregulin-1 in thalamocortical axon navigation. Cell 125:127–142

Meyer D, Birchmeier C 1995 Multiple essential functions of neuregulin in development. Nature 378:386–390

Michailov GV, Sereda MW, Brinkmann BG et al 2004 Axonal neuregulin-1 regulates myelin sheath thickness. Science 304:700–703

Montero JC, Yuste L, Diaz-Rodriguez E, Esparis-Ogando A, Pandiella A 2000 Differential shedding of transmembrane neuregulin isoforms by the tumor necrosis factor-alpha-converting enzyme. Mol Cell Neurosci 16:631–648

Okada M, Corfas G 2004 Neuregulin 1 downregulates postsynaptic GABAA receptors at the hippocampal inhibitory synapse. Hippocampus 14:337–344

O'Tuathaigh CM, O'Sullivan GJ, Kinsella A et al 2006 Sexually dimorphic changes in the exploratory and habituation profiles of heterozygous neuregulin-1 knockout mice. Neuroreport 17:79–83

Rieff HI, Raetzman LT, Sapp DW, Yeh HH, Siegel RE, Corfas G 1999 Neuregulin induces GABA(A) receptor subunit expression and neurite outgrowth in cerebellar granule cells. J Neurosci 19:10757–10766

Role LW, Talmage DA 2007 Neurobiology: new order for thought disorders. Nature 448:263–265

Roy K, Murtie JC, El-Khodor BF et al 2007 Loss of ErbB signaling in oligodendrocytes alters myelin and dopaminergic function, a potential mechanism for neuropsychiatric disorders. Proc Natl Acad Sci USA 104:8131–8136

Silberberg G, Darvasi A, Pinkas-Kramarski R, Navon R 2006 The involvement of ErbB4 with schizophrenia: association and expression studies. Am J Med Genet B Neuropsychiatr Genet 141:142–148

Stefansson H, Sigurdsson E, Steinthorsdottir V et al 2002 Neuregulin 1 and susceptibility to schizophrenia. Am J Hum Genet 71:877–892

Stein RA, Staros JV 2006 Insights into the evolution of the ErbB receptor family and their ligands from sequence analysis. BMC Evol Biol 6:79

Steinthorsdottir V, Stefansson H, Ghosh S et al 2004 Multiple novel transcription initiation sites for NRG1. Gene 342:97–105

Tan W, Wang Y, Gold B et al 2007 Molecular cloning of a brain-specific, developmentally regulated Neuregulin 1 (NRG1) isoform and identification of a functional promoter variant associated with schizophrenia. J Biol Chem 282:24343–24351

Taveggia C, Zanazzi G, Petrylak A et al 2005 Neuregulin-1 type III determines the ensheathment fate of axons. Neuron 47:681–694

Thomson PA, Christoforou A, Morris SW et al 2007 Association of Neuregulin 1 with schizophrenia and bipolar disorder in a second cohort from the Scottish population. Mol Psychiatry 12:94–104

Walss-Bass C, Liu W, Lew DF et al 2006 A novel missense mutation in the transmembrane domain of neuregulin 1 is associated with schizophrenia. Biol Psychiatry 60:548–553

Wang JY, Miller SJ, Falls DL 2001 The N-terminal region of neuregulin isoforms determines the accumulation of cell surface and released neuregulin ectodomain. J Biol Chem 276:2841–2851

Wolpowitz D, Mason TB, Dietrich P, Mendelsohn M, Talmage DA, Role LW 2000 Cysteine-rich domain isoforms of the neuregulin-1 gene are required for maintenance of peripheral synapses. Neuron 25:79–91

Woo RS, Li XM, Tao Y et al 2007 Neuregulin-1 enhances depolarization-induced GABA
    release. Neuron 54:599–610
Yang X, Kuo Y, Devay P, Yu C, Role L 1998 A cysteine-rich isoform of neuregulin controls
    the level of expression of neuronal nicotinic receptor channels during synaptogenesis.
    Neuron 20:255–270

DISCUSSION

Chao: In the heterozygotes for neuregulin, what is the level of the type III
proteins?

Talmage: It is close to 50% of wild-type levels in systems where we can get clean
tissue and good clean blots.

Chao: Are the other isoforms of neuregulin affected?

Talmage: They are unaffected at the RNA level. There aren't good antibody
probes to look at protein expression levels, but we have done RNase protection
assays for various isoforms, and they are unaffected by the full type III
knockout.

Akil: Do you have any inducibles?

Talmage: Not at this point.

Akil: I am basing my comment on my thinking on fibroblast growth factor
(FGF). There is one programme during development, and quite a different programme during adulthood. It might be worth sorting out which one we are talking
about when we are thinking about animal models.

Talmage: We want to do those experiments. As an example, the interneuron
migration story involves neuregulins. The migrating interneurons don't express
neuregulin, but they express ErbB4. At that point in development in the mouse,
the E12/E14 window, there is very little neuregulin and type III is not expressed
in the neocortex. It is expressed in regions of the developing striatum where
it interacts with the migrating neurons and the axons that have been targeted.
By E18 there is type III expression in the cortex. In adults there is clear
expression in both pyramidal and non-pyramidal cortical neurons. There is
a window where it is important in setting up the structure of the neocortex
but it is not expressed in the cells that get there. Yet it is turned on later. One
would expect it would then have another function distinct from its role in early
development. We think there are probably both embryonic and adult
phenotypes.

Lu: The functional studies you did were in cultures of extracellular domain
(ECD) of the ErbB4 receptor. Let's think about the physiological context: how
would the ECD be generated and is it regulated? Is it regulated at the synapse?

Talmage: One possibility is that the ErbB4 ECD is released from cells in a regulated fashion.

Lu: Has that been demonstrated?

Talmage: In vitro, yes. There are splice variants of ErbB4 that undergo ecto-domain shedding and γ-secretase-mediated processing (e.g. Rio et al 2000, Ni et al 2000). We think there is direct interaction between type III neuregulin and ErbB4 (or ErbB3). Neuregulin is shipped to axons that go to target fields where ErbB4 is expressed. Everyone is in the right place, but we don't know at the electron microscopy (EM) level if they are really in the right place. Conceptually, both proteins are where they need to be to do what we think they are doing. The γ-secretase processing of type III neuregulin can be stimulated by activity as well.

Lu: I have another question about the acute versus long-term effects. The long-term regulation is a nuclear event. How long does it take for the intracellular fragment to go into the nucleus, and do you know about the targets?

Talmage: It takes 12–15 minutes to appear in the nucleus after stimulus. It physically interacts with Eos, a member of the Ikaros transcription family (Bao et al 2004). We have genes whose transcription is regulated up and down as a consequence of stimulating the back signalling event. We get slightly different transcriptional profiles if we stimulate with Erb4 than we do following depolarization. There may be additional subtleties. We haven't shown binding to promoter for those target genes yet.

Bothwell: What do Alzheimer disease mutations of amyloid precursor protein (APP) or presenilins do to neuregulin signalling?

Talmage: I don't know. Processing of type III neuregulin does not occur in cells from presenilin knockout mice

Buonanno: Is the back signalling of type I neuregulin also included in this? Are type I and ErbB4 in those axons that you were talking about?

Talmage: We don't detect ErbB4 in those axons. If we inhibit ErbB4 kinase activity it affects nothing. If we add soluble neuregulin we don't get any of the same responses. Type I and type II neuregulin isoforms are probably expressed but in these neurons type I (or type II) seems to be constitutively released from the cell surface, so we can't ask whether it participates in back-signalling. There are other cells where type I neuregulin stays on the surface much longer and its release is regulated by other events. It probably can function as a receptor in those contexts.

Buonanno: So if you use an antibody that is specific for type III and run this on a western blot, do you see that the proportion of unprocessed type III is large compared with type I?

Talmage: Yes, and we are also collecting type I from the conditioning medium, showing that it is there. We have stained neurons from type III knockout animals with the ErbB4 extracellular domain so we can look where it is binding. Without type III expression we don't detect any ErbB4 binding.

References

Bao J, Lin H, Ouyang Y et al 2004 Activity-dependent transcription regulation of PSD-95 by neuregulin-1 and Eos. Nat Neurosci 7:1250–1258

Ni CY, Murphy MP, Golde TE, Carpenter G 2000 γ-Secretase cleavage and nuclear localization of ErbB-4 receptor tyrosine kinase. Science 294:2179–2181

Rio C, Buxbaum JD, Peschon JJ, Corfas G 2000 Tumor necrosis factor-alpha-converting enzyme is required for cleavage of ErbB4/HER4. J Biol Chem 275:10379–10387

General discussion I

Chao: For this general discussion there are three topics I'd like to raise. First, we have covered a number of different assays and models, but I haven't heard anything about simple organisms such as *Drosophila* and *Caenorhabditis elegans*. Is there any utility in these models? Second, we have brought up the influence of white matter myelination. How important is this issue in psychiatric disorders? Third, there's the interesting proposal of the push for whole-genome association analysis. If there were unlimited money and resources, what would we choose to do? I'm amazed at the level of 'big science' projects that has occurred. Related to that, I understand that some genetic analyses has uncovered similarities and overlap between bipolar disorder and schizophrenia. Is there any substance to this?

Flint: I'll pick up your first point about the model organisms. I've had this discussion with various people. People working on model organisms like to promulgate their particular organism, and I have heard claims about anxious worms and psychotic flies. There are some mechanisms that these models could probably deal with. Prepulse inhibition seen in the mouse could be done in the fly. You can startle a fly, make it respond and measure that startle response. You can also give it a prepulse stimulus and see how much that reduces. There is no reason why we couldn't set up a screen to look for that. What this will produce is unknown. There is another issue: we work in a paradigm that says if we look at a synapse in sea slugs, it will be the same synapse in *Drosophila*, mice and humans. I've heard some suggestions that this isn't true. The idea that evolutionary change from invertebrates to our own species is simply growth in the nervous system may be a reflection of changes at a synapse that allow that growth to take place. The fundamental unit may not be the neuron; rather, the fundamental unit may be the synapse, and this has changed with evolution. This suggests that there is a qualitative, not simply a quantitative difference in neural development through evolution.

Talmage: To add to that from my perspective, worms don't have neuregulin. They have an epidermal growth factor (EGF)-like gene and an EGF receptor. Flies do have a neuregulin-like gene, with one receptor and three ligand genes. But its structure is different. So an increase in complexity with the genes tracks an increase in complexity with the organisms. If the complexity is important for function in mammalian and human brains then simple model organisms won't help a great deal.

Bothwell: I would suggest that behavioural screens in zebrafish are every bit as easy to do as in *Drosophila* and *C. elegans*, and have a better chance of leading somewhere.

Buonanno: If you are interested in uncovering the biology of a pathway that is relevant to higher organisms, I would take the other side and suggest that invertebrate studies are useful. One of the surprises I had in writing a review was that if we look in *Drosophila* at the processing of the single EGF receptor and its ligand, we could make predictions about the process used to regulate the EGF receptor and its ligand before any of this was published (Buonanno & Fischbach 2001).

Lu: The fly model has been successfully used in Parkinson's disease research. In genetic screens, people haven't looked at behaviour, but rather at what is called inclusion bodies in the pathology of the neurons. This gets back to the idea of an intermediate phenotype, and using simpler assays to identify genes involved. Take working memory as an example: the ability to hold information for a short period of time is reflected in the delayed, sustained neuronal firing. If working memory is used as an assay, perhaps we can find some genes involved in maintaining sustained firing. This might be helpful for schizophrenia research, for example. The advantage of using a simple organism is getting at the genes through screening, and coming up with unexpected genes.

Akil: A lot depends on how you think about these psychiatric disorders, and whether you take a top–down or bottom–up approach. In Western cultures we always start with the forebrain, and think it is about thought and cognition. This is true for mood and schizophrenia. But in fact there are differences in sensory feedback and processing, and so on. For controlling affect, Buddhism suggests that you need to control your breathing. In Western cultures we say we need to think differently. This seems silly, but it colours how we model these disorders and what we consider relevant for measurement. There is a lot of projecting going on from our idea of the illness to what model systems we use. This is why I favour a somewhat more agnostic approach. If the genetics were to work broadly enough that you could then go back and look at the traits, clusters and measures that map on to the genes, this would open the door to all kinds of levels of analysis. Currently we are trapped: we can't imagine an animal model of schizophrenia, and certainly not in a worm.

Malaspina: We have spoken about schizophrenia and its age of onset. There is a premorbid deterioration in many cases, but there is also a large proportion of cases with normal childhood and early adolescent function. Huda Akil mentioned that there might be different programmes for early life gene expression. It seems that some understanding of how these programmes shift, and in which alleles, might be helpful in understanding these diseases. They are not present by and large from early life.

Raff: Most people think that schizophrenia involves a strong genetic predisposition as well as some *in utero* stress or insult. We haven't discussed this. What is going on *in utero* and why the delay in the onset of the disease? This seems to be a critical question for autism, as well as for schizophrenia. There is a related question: are the depressive psychoses also developmental brain disorders?

Flint: As far as we know, major depression is not a developmental issue.

Raff: What has been done to address the question?

Flint: As far as I know, no one has looked at the neuropathology in development.

Malaspina: Many of the adult-onset chronic diseases that have no pathology before they present are the results of fetal programming. There is no reason to presume that fetal programming doesn't play a very important role in depression.

Raff: The cognitive impairment in schizophrenia can apparently be detected in children, well before the onset of psychosis. What about affective disorders? Are children that go on to develop bipolar disorder normal, for example?

Flint: We need to separate bipolar disorder from major depression.

Castrén: Isn't there a study that looked at the effect of early maltreatment, and found that hippocampus size was affected only in those individuals who had experienced early life maltreatment (Vythilingam et al 2002)?

Flint: There is lots of evidence that there is an effect of stress on the hippocampus mediated by glucocorticoids. That is pretty well established. It is not as if that is internally generated.

Akil: I don't know that this has been fully tested. We have bred animals based on drug-seeking behaviour. It turns out that one of the biggest differences between them is hippocampal morphology. The difference between them is subtle differences in hippocampal morphology and neurogenesis, but the laminae around the dentate gyrus, which are hard to study in human, are clearly different in these different lines of animals. These are established early in life during a window in development that would be equivalent to third trimester in humans. This persists in adulthood and affects a range of behaviours, including stress responsiveness. Our view of the hippocampus as a monitor of salience in the environment would be consistent with some nuances in the changes in that structure really changing how the environment impacts on the individual. I am struck by this finding on post-traumatic stress disorder (PTSD) from a Harvard study. They looked at Vietnam veterans who had a non-combatant twin. The brain size of the unaffected twin predicted the magnitude of PTSD in the one that went to war. The size of the hippocampus is a predictor and not a consequence of the stress response.

Flint: It seems to me that this is different from the model that Martin Raff was proposing of what has gone wrong in schizophrenia, which is some sort of qualitative difference in the brain. What we see in major depression is different.

Akil: It is a continuum. It is not broken in the same sense. But I wouldn't say that it is not developmentally mediated.

Flint: What you are saying is that there are some basic triggers that have happened, perhaps prenatally, that will determine a later outcome. For schizophrenia this may be the case, but not for major depression.

Malaspina: A portion of cases of schizophrenia are also well until onset, so perhaps it is just as much a mystery that schizophrenia has developmental underpinnings. Serious depression can be degenerative as well.

Raff: Another way of asking the question is the following: in those mouse models where the fetus is exposed to a drug or a toxin *in utero* to induce a behavioural phenotype in the adult, does one ever see what you define as a depressive phenotype?

Javitt: One of the major disconnects in the field is that from the schizophrenia pathology perspective we are going towards a 10 or 15 hit model of schizophrenia, where the genetic liability helps, but there needs to be perhaps perinatal hypoxia, head trauma during childhood and a bad environment, whereas all the models are unifactorial. In order to get a phenotype as severe as is seen in schizophrenia from an environmental intervention, it has to be a whopping environmental intervention that in turn produces brain changes that are much larger than would be seen in schizophrenia itself.

Raff: You could test whether an infection in a pregnant mouse carrying a predisposition gene for a psychiatric disorder increases the risk of a behavioural phenotype in the adult.

Javitt: This is being done now. Ina Weinerin (Tel Aviv) is doing perinatal poly-IC models. She gets latent inhibition deficits that look a lot like what is seen in schizophrenia, but the brain pathology she gets is much more severe than one would ever see. The striking thing about the schizophrenia brain is that you can't easily see the difference. All the deficits are statistical deficits: changes of 5–10%. With single interventions there are huge changes in brain structure.

Raff: With the Patterson mouse polyI-polyC model (Shi et al 2003), perhaps the dose of polyI-polyC could be reduced in mice with a genetic predisposition.

Javitt: That's what we need to do. The pharmacologists need to interact more with the geneticists.

Chao: One process that may be involved is myelination, which occurs postnatally. Some believe it occurs throughout adult life. How important is white matter dysfunction?

Javitt: In terms of signals coming from schizophrenia that could be translated, the changes in white matter that we get are very robust and seem to occur relatively early in the illness, perhaps even before the onset of symptoms. Whatever is breaking down on the diffusion tensor imaging (DTI) level is happening early. It is hard to know what is driving this on the pathological level. We assume myelin is involved, but some of the demyelination studies suggest that myelin is not driving the DTI signal quite as much as you would expect. It may have more to do with water transport across the membrane rather than the myelin itself. We now have to go back to the animal models to try to figure out what is driving the DTI changes. To do this we need to try to collaborate with groups that have potentially informative mice that we can then go back and do the DTI with to see whether these mutations or behavioural interventions are affecting DTIs.

Talmage: There is not a consistent story in post-mortem tissue about myelination defects. There are groups who think it is the cause, but the neuropathologists I talk to don't see these defects in histology.

Javitt: It is a white matter change; it is not necessarily myelin. There is something going on in the white matter and we hope it is myelin.

Buonanno: The myelin that has been described with neuregulin is peripheral myelin, not central myelin.

Javitt: We are trying to look at central myelin. We are doing this *in vitro*, or at least in anaesthetized mice. There is some suggestion that there may be functional aspects to DTI. Neuronal axonal transmission may have dynamic changes, which could be driving the DTI signal also. For example, diffusivity measures are altered during seizures, suggesting that there may be a functional component. DTI is evidently less affected than diffusivity (Diehl et al 2005), but it raises the issue that factors that affect water diffusion across the axonal membrane may also affect DTI.

Buonanno: My understanding from speaking with Judith Rappoport about her retrospective studies with children with early onset schizophrenia, is that one of the early behavioural hallmarks is the age children begin to walk. Children who eventually will develop schizophrenia walk later. Have people looked at peripheral myelin in schizophrenia?

Javitt: I don't know of any. Nerve conduction studies have not shown very much.

Buonanno: How severe would demyelination have to be to have an effect on conduction velocity?

Javitt: I don't know.

Buonanno: For the effects of neuregulin, the heterozygote mice were 50% down and the effects on the myelin were not severe.

Talmage: There is a 50% reduction in neuregulin and there is a 30% reduction in conduction velocity in the mice.

Malaspina: Is it measurable as processing speed?

Talmage: It has been calculated from the latency between compound action potential using the tail (Michailov et al 2004).

Akil: Perhaps the change is in gene expression within glial cells as opposed to number or amount, and we see that in gene expression profiling studies in lots of disorders. Even in classical neurotransmitter systems you are just mining after the fact. One of the more reliable changes is in transporters for GABA and glutamate in glia. There is likely to be a cross-talk between neurons and glia, and the production of GABA and glutamate in the cortex that is modulated by glial function.

Raff: I am trying to think of how we can make progress in figuring out what is developmental and what isn't, and when pathology or dysfunction really starts. In high density families, one would want to study the children as early as possible. Some will get schizophrenia and some will get depression, and it would helpful to know what the earliest differences are.

Malaspina: People have done high risk studies which show early deficits in attention, measurable on a CBT test, are good predictors of later onset (Cornblatt & Malhotra 2001). In early childhood verbal memory is a good predictor of who will later have onset.

Raff: Are you talking about schizophrenia?

Malaspina: Yes, these are offspring of mothers with schizophrenia.

Javitt: The complication is that you don't know that some of these families will be multiply affected until the older siblings start coming down with the illness. By then the other children are into the age of risk already. This is where the genetics could be useful.

Owen: I am aware of more studies on high-risk families in schizophrenia than bipolar disorder. Eve Johnstone has been doing a high-risk study in schizophrenia on people with strong family histories. She has some interesting data on prodromal symptoms, structural brain abnormalities and even genetics that predict who will make the transition. But the numbers are still small (Hall et al 2006).

Raff: Are there international websites for patients and their families, which would make it much easier to collect data?

Owen: There would be ethical objections to doing this for identifiable families such as the DISC1 family.

Malaspina: NIMH has a group called Naples. It is a movement by NIMH to take all the different prodromal studies that meet a certain criteria and are funded by NIMH. They have adopted common diagnostic interviews and longitudinal forms so these studies can be pooled. Some of the people with the worst outcome may not necessarily develop schizophrenia but have other types of severe impairment.

Giedd: I am doing longitudinal imaging studies which include typically developing children and adolescents from non-high risk families. Participants are between four and 20 years when they enter the study and are scanned at approximately two-year intervals. Out of 300 people who had no evidence of psychopathology when they began the study 17 have now developed depression and four have developed bipolar disorder. None have developed schizophrenia. Our seventeen before and after depression scans do not provide enough power to make meaningful statements but as the study progresses and participants go through ages of increased prevalence for depression we should be able to address this question. It will take enormous sample sizes to get enough prospective data for before illness and after illness comparisons for rarer conditions

Javitt: If you nationalize your health service these studies are good to do retrospectively. Enough people will have magnetic resonance imaging (MRI) scans somewhere along the line, so if they later develop illness you can compare their current scan with the one they had before symptoms appeared.

Sklar: There are some specific issues related to bipolar disorder that have to do with the lack of agreement about what the phenotype looks like in children, and whether it exists in children. It is frequently overlaid with attention deficit hyperactivity disorder (ADHD). The current diagnosis of paediatric bipolar disorder includes many of the same criteria: using the standard Diagnostic and Statistical Manual (DSM-IV) in use, in the US children diagnosed with paediatric bipolar disorder will meet criteria for paediatric ADHD. There also appears to be a genetic overlap.

References

Cornblatt BA, Malhotra AK 2001 Impaired attention as an endophenotype for molecular genetic studies of schizophrenia. Am J Med Genet B Neuropsychiatr Genet 105:11–15

Buonanno A, Fischbach GD 2001 Neuregulin and ErbB receptor signaling pathways in the nervous system. Curr Opin Neurobiol 11:287–296

Diehl B, Symms MR, Boulby PA et al 2005 Postictal diffusion tensor imaging. Epilepsy Res 65:137–146

Hall J, Whalley HC, Job DE et al 2006 A neuregulin 1 variant associated with abnormal cortical function and psychotic symptoms. Nat Neurosci 9:1477–1478

Michailov GV, Sereda MW, Brinkmannet BG al 2004 Axonal neuregulin-1 regulates myelin sheath thickness. Science 304:700–703

Shi L, Fatemi SH, Sidwell RW, Patterson PH 2003 Maternal influenza infection causes marked behavioral and pharmacological changes in the offspring. J Neurosci 23:297–302

Vythilingam M, Heim C, Newport J et al 2002 Childhood trauma associated with smaller hippocampal volume in women with major depression. Am J Psychiatry 159:2072–2080

The fibroblast growth factor family and mood disorders

H. Akil, S. J. Evans, C. A. Turner, J. Perez, R. M. Myers*, W. E. Bunney†, E. G. Jones‡, S. J. Watson and other members of the Pritzker Consortium

*University of Michigan, Ann Arbor, USA, *Stanford University, California, USA, †University of California, Irvine, USA and ‡University of California, Davis, USA*

Abstract. While there has been a great deal of interest in the role of brain-derived neurotrophic factor (BDNF) in mood disorders and/or the mode of action of anti-depressants, less is known about the role of other growth factors. This paper is focused on a group of growth factors, the fibroblast growth factor (FGF) family and their potential role in mood disorders.

2008 Growth factors and psychiatric disorders. Wiley, Chichester (Novartis Foundation Symposium 289) p 94–100

Our focus on the fibroblast growth factor (FGF) family arose as a result of an unbiased search aimed at describing the 'neural phenotype' or molecular signature of mood disorders in postmortem human brains. This was carried out by a collaborative group of investigators, the Pritzker Consortium for Severe Psychiatric Disorders, which includes scientists from the University of Michigan, Stanford University, the University of California at Irvine, the University of California at Davis and Cornell University. Using microarray technology, consortium scientists carried out gene expression profiling on several limbic and cortical brain regions from carefully selected and well-characterized human brains. Various types of gene ontology analyses all pointed to factors such as neurodevelopment, neurogenesis, neural growth and cell signalling as being significantly altered. The FGF family as a whole was the most dramatically altered, with some transcripts being significantly elevated and other transcripts, especially two of the FGF receptors (FGFR2 and FGFR3) being significantly down-regulated (Evans et al 2004, Turner et al 2006). While the original findings were in two regions of the cortex (anterior cingulate and dorsolateral prefrontal cortex), additional unpublished studies from the consortium have revealed dysregulation in numerous limbic and brain stem regions. Evidence from the human studies suggested that the decrease in several FGF transcripts seen in major depression was not secondary to treatment with selective serotonin reuptake inhibitor (SSRI) antidepressants (Evans et al 2004). The general finding of dysregulation of the FGF system in mood disorders has recently been independently confirmed in the human hippocampus (Gaughran et al 2006)

These results in human, while novel and provocative, could not be fully interpreted in isolation. Thus, changes in the FGF family may be primary or secondary to the illness and they may or may not have functional consequences. We therefore undertook a series of rodent studies to assess the role of the FGF family in emotional behaviour. While the FGFs had been implicated in brain development, there was little information about their relevance to affective behaviour. Therefore our studies addressed the following questions:

(1) Are there *basal differences* in the expression of FGF transcripts in animals that are selectively bred for differences in their level of anxiety?
(2) Are members of the FGF family altered by manipulations that *decrease* anxiety-like behaviour in the rodent?
(3) Are members of the FGF family altered by manipulations that *increase* anxiety-like behaviour in the rodent?
(4) Are members of the FGF family altered following *stress and animal models of depression?*
(5) What is the impact of acute and chronic administration of *exogenous FGF2 on anxiety behaviour?*
(6) Are these effects different as a function of the animal's genotype—e.g. high versus low anxiety animals?
(7) What is the impact of acute and chronic administration of exogenous FGF2 on an animal *model of depression?*
(8) What are the consequences of chronic administration of FGF2 on hippocampal neurogenesis?
(9) Do experimental alterations of the FGF system induced in early life produce lifelong changes in emotional behaviour?
(10) Do experimental alterations of the FGF system induced in early life produce lifelong changes in neurogenesis and/or hippocampal morphology?

The talk presented the results of this series of studies in the rat, focusing on FGF2 (or basic FGF), which is the best-studied member of the FGF family in the brain. Taken together, the outcome of this work demonstrated that FGF2 and the FGF receptors are clearly involved in the control of emotionality. Thus, animals that have high levels of spontaneous anxiety have lower resting levels of FGF2 in various hippocampal fields. A manipulation that decreases spontaneous anxiety, environmental complexity, also induces FGF2 mRNA levels and the impact is greatest in the high anxiety animals. These findings are mirrored by the impact of exogenous FGF2. Thus, chronic administration of FGF2 was anxiolytic, and the impact was most profound in the high anxiety animals. Moreover, the same treatment produces alterations in hippocampal neurogenesis. It was apparent that high chronic levels of FGF2, whether endogenous or exogenous, were related to decreasing anxiety behaviour.

Similarly, we were able to implicate FGF2 in depression-like behaviour in the rat, using the Porsolt Forced Swim Test. Thus, two animal models of depression, chronic social defeat and chronic unpredictable stress, led to decreased levels of FGF2 mRNA in the hippocampus. Interestingly, chronic stress also altered both the levels and the alternative splicing pattern of two of the FGF receptors, favouring a splice form which is typically less efficacious in *in vitro* assays. Moreover, administration of exogenous FGF2 acted as an antidepressant in the Porsolt Forced Swim Test.

It therefore appears that the observed changes in gene expression that emerged from the human postmortem studies point to an important new set of molecular players that play a key role in the pathophysiology and/or trajectory of mood disorders. Alterations in the FGF system expression and function may well contribute to the negative mood and increased anxiety seen in many severely depressed patients. It will be important to ascertain whether some of these alterations are part of the initial pathophysiology of the illness, or whether they are secondary to the expression of the illness, as we have shown that chronic stress and anxiety can themselves lead to dysregulation of this system. Genetic studies, for example, will help determine whether allelic variations in members of the FGF family are associated with severe mood disorders. Whether these molecules represent vulnerability genes, or whether their alterations result from environmental changes during development and in adulthood, it is clear that they are important molecular actors in the manifestation of the illness. Therefore, we hypothesize that the re-setting of the FGF system may be a critical step that is required for neural remodelling that mediates the action of effective antidepressants, and indeed there is already some evidence to this effect from the work of other groups (Maragnoli et al 2004). Moreover, analogues of the FGF molecules may themselves prove to be interesting targets for the treatment of mood disorders.

References

Evans SJ, Choudary PV, Neal CR et al 2004 Dysregulation of the fibroblast growth factor system in major depression. Proc Natl Acad Sci USA 101:15506–15511
Gaughran F, Payne J, Sedgwick PM, Cotter D, Berry M 2006 Hippocampal FGF-2 and FGFR1 mRNA expression in major depression, schizophrenia and bipolar disorder. Brain Res Bull 70:221–227
Maragnoli ME, Fumagalli F, Gennarelli M, Racagni G, Riva MA 2004 Fluoxetine and olanzapine have synergistic effects in the modulation of fibroblast growth factor 2 expression within the rat brain. Biol Psychiatry 55:1095–1102
Turner CA, Akil H, Watson SJ, Evans SJ 2006 The fibroblast growth factor system and mood disorders. Biol Psychiatry 59:1128–1135

DISCUSSION

Bothwell: I am sure that you are aware that there a lot of FGF receptor mutations in humans that cause disease. They are mainly skeletal disorders. Astonishingly, most of these mutations have almost no recorded phenotype in brain. A few have mild mental retardation; I'm wondering whether anyone has looked for psychiatric disorders in those patients.

Akil: I don't know that they have. We have thought about this in the other direction: we have asked whether any of the FGFs might be good candidate genes. We are doing genome-wide studies. In the course of doing some candidate gene work we chose 100 genes to look at and only at a small number of patients. Our biggest hit was highly significant, but this was not FGF. Our second hit was FGFR3. It is not at a level of significance that makes us want to write home about it. It might fall apart when we look at larger populations.

Bothwell: One of the reasons one might speculate that these diseases that cause skeletal abnormalities are so skeletal specific, is that many mutations occur in domain Ig3. This is the osteoblast-specific Ig3, not the one that is primarily expressed in the brain. You showed that with stress you are up-regulating the exon that contains these mutations. If you stress a person with Crouzon syndrome, you are up-regulating a mutant receptor.

Malaspina: The data that the FGFRs are involved in mediating stress are convincing. Having highly stressed mothers increases their expression and participation. But it seems that an epigenetic understanding of these might be just as likely as the idea that these are candidate genes, and the idea that the enriched environment rescues sounds like high maternal nurture.

Akil: I am agnostic about whether this has anything to do with an initial genetic difference. We went into the gene expression profiling with the notion that while it would be interesting to know what the genes are, downstream changes are important and changes induced by the environment are important. They can not only become drug targets but also a means of thinking about the disease process or the protection from diseases.

Walsh: I'd like to commend you for your heroic effort in dealing with the pathological material. My colleagues and I have often thought about doing these types of experiments but haven't been able to see past the real problems. I am concerned about the extent of variability in the disease state, and getting reproducible data. But more important is the drug history of individuals. Even small amounts of drugs can change gene transcriptional profiling. I guess you have come to the conclusion that you can overcome these very obvious limitations and problems.

Akil: I think we miss a lot of real effects because they get drowned in the noise that comes from exactly these variables. These are small numbers of samples relative to what we would like to have. They have varied histories that we can't control. We have tried to measure lithium levels in their brains and other drug levels. We do the best we can, but we know that there is a lot of variance. When we first started on this, I kept worrying that the noise would obscure all the results. So I was stunned that we can actually see a difference. This is the low hanging fruit of what really drives feeling horrible when you are depressed or whatever happens when you are bipolar. But I am sure there are a lot of varied, unique changes that we can't pick up in this way.

Walsh: I am interested in your logic in terms of moving to the FGF family. The output shows that lots of things are changing. There are so many things changing it is hard to know what is important. The way Gene Logic data are displayed by the computer is slightly misleading. What it shows are potential interacting partners rather than real ones.

Akil: We didn't rely on Ingenuity analyses for our selection. It was gene ontology analysis.

Walsh: Have you any evidence of the FGF receptor pathway changing? I've never seen this in pathological materials.

Akil: The main driver was the number of FGF molecules that was changed given the number of FGF molecules that were detectable on the chip. This was highly significant, and more significant than any other family that we have looked at. We have also looked at GABA and glutamate and mitochondrial genes. We focused on FGF initially because of the BDNF story.

Brandon: I have been involved in a lot of these sorts of studies and their follow-up. Are any of the transcript changes you see shown at the protein level?

Akil: We are doing proteomics on some of these samples, but I don't yet have enough data to report. We are also using specific antibodies to phosphoproteins. As you know, human post-mortem tissue presents challenges. We are also doing DNA analysis on the same tissue to look for promoter and splice variance, and how these relate to gene expression.

Brandon: My experience is that you can get transcript changes but the protein changes might not be there. Where does this lead you?

Akil: I agree: it would be nice to show the changes in protein.

Spedding: 20 years ago in the first round of enthusiasm about administering growth factors, my group was involved with Frank Collins and Rusty Gage in terms of looking at the effects of growth factors directly. We found that FGF2 given intravenously was the most powerful agent in terms of having a beneficial effect in stroke models. The effects were remarkable. Therefore you are looking at an agent that is very powerful in terms of changes in plasticity in animal models. FGF2 was then taken through toxicology assessment and some phase I studies were done. Chronic dosing with toxicological doses of FGF2 has marked effects on animals including making the choroid plexus grow quite remarkably. This means we have to be careful about the chronic dosing effects of the growth factors themselves.

Akil: I'm not recommending it as a clinical treatment as such. It would be important to make sure it is targeted in a particular way because it is so powerful. Conceptually, it is helpful to think about.

Talmage: The anxiety behaviour in your two rat groups shows remarkable similarity to recent results from T. Karl's group in Australia on one of the neuregulin heterozygous animals (Karl et al 2007). In their work, the heterozygote had greater levels of activity and exhibited less anxiety behaviour. It is a parallel example of decreasing signalling through a receptor tyrosine kinase pathway. This raises two possibilities. First, the speculation that neuregulin is negatively regulating FGF in the hippocampus. Second, underlining the points of looking at downstream signalling at the protein level; FGF receptors and ErbB receptors share many of the same signalling targets yet the genetic phenotypes are quite distinct, so it will be interesting to see what mechanisms are used *in vivo*.

Akil: In the rat we are raring to go on the protein side. Both *in vitro* cell biological studies and *in vivo* protein and phosphorylation studies are the next step.

Chao: The FGFs are ubiquitous. Is there a preferential cellular source of FGFs?

Akil: They are not in every neuron or every glia, by any stretch. In the hippocampus, for example, its expression is clearly delineated. But some of them are in glia, some are in neurons, for some the ligand is in the neuron and the receptor is in the glia depending on the brain region. There is a lot of neuron–glia cross talk in this system, plus the FGF experts will tell you that they cross-regulate each other in complicated ways.

Lu: There is an old literature by Professor Yutaka Oomura who identified the hypothalamus as the satiety centre. According to him, in his papers published in the 1980s, food intake and an increase in blood glucose concentration dramatically stimulates the hypothalamus to produce/secrete FGF, which somehow passes through the hippocampus and regulates hippocampal synaptic plasticity (Oomura 1988). Along these lines, if you can't identify the source of FGF, identification of FGF receptor-expressing cells would be helpful. We recently did some work on the FGF receptor that supports your ideas about the role of FGF in neurogenesis and plasticity (Zhao et al 2007). We generated a line of mutant mice in which the FGFR1 gene is specifically deleted in the CNS. Some of the effects are expected: we see an effect on the production of new neurons but no effect on their differentiation. One of the surprising findings was that when we looked at long-term potentiation (LTP) in the dentate, there are two pathways for the granule cell apical dendrites, and the LTP deficit was only in the medial perforant path (MPP). This was the biggest effect I've ever seen on all the studies of growth factor regulation of LTP.

Akil: In the conditionals, when did you knock FGFR1 out?

Lu: We crossed Nestin-Cre mice with FGFR1 floxed mice, to delete FGFR1 gene during early development. Behaviourally, when these animals were tested in the conventional Morris water maze we saw normal spatial learning. However, more dramatic effects were seen in a four-episode training water maze study where each day the location was changed (moving platform). It turns out their ability to acquire new information is the same as for wild-type, but their ability to retain older information is lost. There is a neurogenesis problem which only involves the survival or proliferation of new neurons, and the LTP deficit that contributes to the retention of old memory.

Kahn: We have just completed a study of 300 schizophrenia patients. We looked at brain imaging in about 100 of them, comparing them with 100 controls. FGF2 and FGFR1 were significantly related to brain volume and especially grey matter volume. The FGF system came out highly significant, much more than the others. This fits with the social deficit and stress hypothesis.

References

Karl T, Duffy L, Scimone A, Harvey RP, Schofield PR 2007 Altered motor activity, exploration and anxiety in heterozygous neuregulin 1 mutant mice: implications for understanding schizophrenia. Genes Brain Behav 6:677–687

Plata-Salaman CR, Yamamoto T, Oomura Y, Shimizu N, Sakata T 1988 Food intake suppression in rats by a substance isolated from human feces. Physiol Behav 43:365–369

Zhao M, Li D, Shimazu K, Zhou YX, Deng CX, Lu B 2007 Fibroblast growth factor receptor-1 is required for long-term potentiation, memory consolidation, and neurogenesis. Biol Psychiatry 62:381–390

Trajectories of anatomic brain development as a phenotype

Jay N. Giedd, Rhoshel K. Lenroot, Philip Shaw, Francois Lalonde, Mark Celano, Samantha White, Julia Tossell, Anjene Addington and Nitin Gogtay

Brain Imaging Unit, Child Psychiatry Branch NIMH, 10 Center Drive, MSC 1367 Bethesda, MD 20892, USA

Abstract. Many cognitive, emotional and behavioural traits, as well as psychiatric disorders are highly heritable. However, identifying the specific genes and mechanisms by which this heritability manifests has been elusive. One approach to make this problem more tractable has been to attempt to identify and quantify biological markers that are intermediate steps along the gene-to-behaviour path. The field of neuroimaging offers several anatomic and physiologic possibilities to quantify. Stability over time has been proposed as a desired feature for these intermediate phenotypes. However, in this paper we discuss the value of looking at trajectories of anatomic brain development (i.e. morphometric changes over time), as opposed to static measures, as a phenotype. Examples drawn from longitudinal anatomic magnetic resonance imaging studies of typical development, attention deficit/hyperactivity disorder, and childhood-onset schizophrenia are used to demonstrate the utility of trajectories of brain development as a phenotypic bridge between genes and behaviour in health and in illness.

2008 Growth factors and psychiatric disorders. Wiley, Chichester (Novartis Foundation Symposium 289) p 101–118

The path from genes to behaviour is an elaborate and tortuous journey coursing through the most complex biological structure known, the human brain. One approach to elucidate this path has been to study biological measures at various stages along the way, sometimes referred to as intermediate phenotypes.

The rationale for this approach is that the intermediate phenotypes are more fundamental constituents of the behavioural phenomenon and are 'closer' to the gene effects, thereby more likely to demonstrate higher penetrance (Gottesman & Gould 2003). As sensible as this approach is, the benefits of utilizing intermediate phenotypes have not proved to be a panacea for simplifying the staggeringly complicated relationship between genes, brain and behaviour (Flint & Munafò 2007).

The field of imaging genetics encompasses various types of investigations linking neuroimaging outcome measures to genetic variation (Meyer-Lindenberg

& Weinberger 2006). 'Reverse genetics' approaches attempt to identify the neural circuitry influence by a given gene variant by finding genetic associations with a clinical diagnosis and then exploring neuroimaging outcome measures thought to differ between the clinical group and controls within the normative population to determine if allelic variation occurring outside the presence of the disorder is associated with a similar phenotypic signature (Meyer-Lindenberg & Zink 2007). This allows the much greater pool of information from healthy control populations to be used to determine specific effects of particular polymorphisms and thus inform mechanisms underlying neuropsychiatric disorders.

In this paper we discuss a subset of imaging genetics targeting the trajectories of anatomic brain development (i.e. changes in the size/shape of brain structures with time) as the measures to link to genetic variation. Examples of the merits of trajectories as a phenotype are discussed in the context of typical development, attention deficit hyperactivity disorder (ADHD), and childhood-onset schizophrenia (COS).

Project design

Since 1989, the Child Psychiatry Branch of the National Institute of Mental Health has been conducting a longitudinal study in which participants return at approximately two-year intervals for brain imaging, psychological and behavioural testing, and genetics. Currently, the data set consists of approximately 4000 scans from 2000 subjects, about half of them typically developing and the other half from various clinical populations.

Trajectories of brain development in healthy children and adolescents

Singleton subjects for the typical development component of the project are recruited from the local community and twin subjects are recruited nationally. Subjects are screened via an initial telephone interview, mailed questionnaires, and subsequent in-person assessment which includes a clinical evaluation and neuropsychological testing. Exclusion criteria include having a psychiatric diagnosis or first-degree relatives with psychiatric diagnoses, head injury, or any known learning, developmental, or medical conditions likely to have affected brain development. Exclusion criteria related to pregnancy and birth events included gestational age of <30 weeks; very low birth weight (<3 lbs 4 oz), any known exposure to psychotropic medications during pregnancy, and significant perinatal complications.

The merit of using trajectories, as opposed to static 'final' morphometry, has been demonstrated in a previous study by our group that examined the relationship between IQ and cortical thickness (Shaw et al 2006a). In this study of 307 unrelated children and adolescents the developmental trajectory of cortical thickness in the right superior frontal gyrus (and other brain regions), but not the cortical thickness itself, was different amongst groups with average intelligence (IQ range 83–108), high intelligence (IQ range 109–120), and superior intelligence (IQ range 121–149).

Trajectories have also been shown to be superior to static measures in discriminating male and female brains in our cohort (Lenroot et al 2007). In a study of 829 scans from 287 subjects aged 3 to 27 years, total cerebral volume peaked at age 10.5 in females and 14.5 in males (see Fig. 1). White matter increased across this age span in both males and females but with a steeper rate of increase in males during adolescence. Cortical and subcortical grey matter trajectories follow an inverted U-shaped path with peak sizes 1 to 2 years earlier in females.

The inverted U shaped trajectories of grey matter volumes coinciding with improved cognitive abilities confound straightforward relationships between size and function. In a study of 13 subjects who had each been scanned 4 times at approximately 2 year intervals, the peak age of gray matter density along the inverted U-shaped trajectories of gray matter were used as a proxy for maturation on a voxel level of analysis throughout the cortex (Gogtay et al 2004). An animation of these changes is available at *http://www.loni.ucla.edu/~thompson/DEVEL/ dyanamic.html*. The peaks occurred earliest in the primary sensorimotor areas and latest in heteromodal association areas of the dorsolateral prefrontal cortex (DLPFC), inferior parietal and superior temporal gyrus. Implications of ongoing maturation throughout adolescence of the DLPFC (which is a key component of circuitry subserving control of impulses, judgment, organization, and long range planning) have prominently entered clinical, social, educational and judicial realms.

These examples from the typical development literature support the contention that trajectories of anatomic brain changes are often more powerful predictors of cognition and behaviour than static measures.

Trajectories of brain development in ADHD

Subjects meeting criteria for ADHD as defined by the Diagnostic and Statistical Manual of Mental Disorders, Fourth Edition (DSM-IV) (American Psychiatric Association 1994) are recruited from the surrounding community. Inclusion criteria are hyperactive, inattentive, and impulsive behaviours that cause impairment in at least two settings and a Conners' Teacher Hyperactivity rating greater than 2 SD above age- and sex-specific means (Werry et al 1975)

In a study analysing 544 scans from 152 people with ADHD (age range, 5–18 years) and 139 age- and sex-matched controls (age range, 4.5–19 years) total

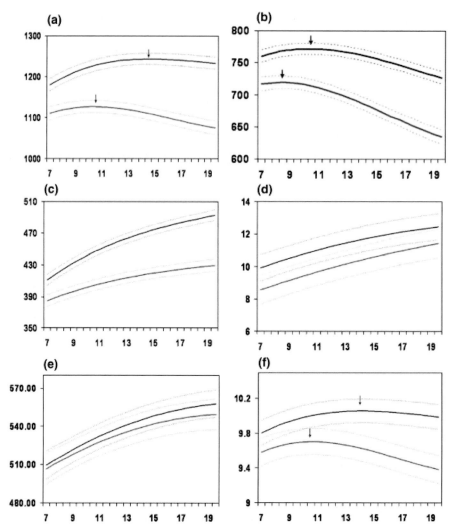

FIG. 1.   Mean volume by age in years for males (top lines, N = 475 scans) and females (bottom lines, N = 354 scans). Middle lines in each set of three lines represent mean values, and upper and lower lines represent upper and lower 95% confidence intervals. All curves differed significantly in height and shape with the exception of lateral ventricles, in which only height was different, and mid-sagittal area of the corpus callosum, in which neither height nor shape was different. (a) Total brain volume, (b) grey matter volume, (c) white matter volume, (d) lateral ventricle volume, (e) mid-sagittal area of the corpus callosum, and (f) caudate volume. (Adapted from Lenroot et al 2007.)

cerebral and cerebellar volumes were smaller in ADHD and the difference persisted across this age span (Castellanos et al 2002). However, caudate volume was smaller in ADHD during childhood but the difference became statistically nonsignificant as caudate volumes decreased for both patients and controls during adolescence.

The relationship between trajectories of brain morphometry and clinical outcome in ADHD was examined in three studies. In the first, volumes of six cerebellar hemispheric lobes, the central white matter, and three vermal subdivisions were quantified on 229 scans from 36 subjects with ADHD and 36 controls. A measure of global clinical outcome and DSM-IV criteria were used to split the 36 ADHD subjects into groups of better or worse outcome (Mackie et al 2007). The superior cerebellar vermis was smaller in ADHD but did not show progressive loss with age and did not relate to clinical outcome. However, in the worse outcome group inferior–posterior cerebellar lobes became progressively smaller during adolescence than in the better outcome or control groups. An implication of this work is that the cerebellar hemispheres may constitute a more plastic, state-specific marker that could be targeted for clinical intervention.

In the second study relating anatomic trajectories to outcome in ADHD, cortical thickness was quantified on 636 scans from 163 children with ADHD (mean age at entry, 8.9 years) and 166 controls (Shaw et al 2006b). The ADHD group had thinner cortex globally, most pronounced in medial and superior prefrontal and precentral regions, with the worse outcome group having thinner left medial prefrontal cortex at baseline than the better outcome and control groups. Trajectories of right parietal cortex thickness converged with the control group in the better outcome but not worse outcome group. This normalization in patients with a better outcome may represent compensatory cortical change (Fig. 2).

In a follow up of the previous study, information regarding the type of dopamine D4 receptor polymorphism was combined with cortical thickness measures quantified on 442 scans from 105 subjects with ADHD and 103 controls (Shaw et al 2007). The DRD4 seven-repeat allele is associated with greater risk for ADHD. The group with the risk allele had thinner right orbitofrontal/inferior prefrontal and posterior parietal cortex, regions that were generally thinner in subjects with ADHD. However, ADHD subjects with the risk allele had a better clinical outcome and only this group demonstrated the previously mentioned normalization of the right parietal cortical region.

As with the studies of typical development, assessment of trajectories in brain morphometric studies of ADHD yields information linking genes to behaviour not discerned with static measures.

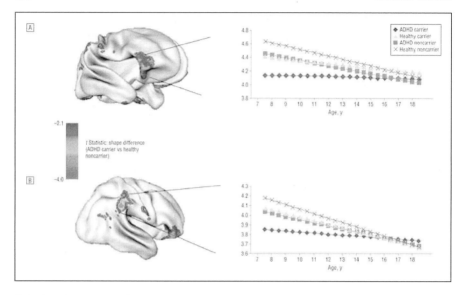

FIG. 2.   Brain maps of clusters where attention-deficit/hyperactivity disorder (ADHD) carriers of the seven-repeat allele of dopamine d4 receptor differ in trajectory of cortical growth and graphs illustrating trajectories for these clusters. (Adapted from Shaw et al 2007.)

Trajectories of brain development in childhood-onset schizophrenia (COS)

COS is defined as onset of psychosis by the age of 13 and occurs in approximately 1 in 40000 people (Nicolson & Rapoport 1999). Although neurobiologically continuous with the adult onset form of schizophrenia (Nicolson & Rapoport 1999, Rapoport et al 2005), COS subjects have more pronounced delays in social, motor and language function (Alaghband-Rad et al 1995, Hollis 1995), a 10% rate of chromosomal abnormalities (Sporn et al 2004), higher familial rates of schizophrenia spectrum disorders (Nicolson et al 2003), and smooth pursuit eye movement abnormalities (Sporn et al 2005). These features suggest that genetic influences may be more salient in COS (Rapoport et al 2005).

As of August 2007 the NIMH Child Psychiatry Branch has acquired a sample of 95 well characterized cases of COS. The participants were recruited nationwide in a process involving over 1400 chart reviews and 230 in person screenings. The diagnosis was established by two psychiatrists using clinical and structured interviews of the patient and family and in-hospital observation during a 1–3 week medication-free period.

Several studies have identified anomalous trajectories of brain anatomy in this cohort. As in typical development grey matter volumes reduce during adolescence, although in COS the rate of reduction of gray matter volumes is significantly more pronounced during adolescence (Sporn et al 2003, Thompson et al 2001b) and progresses in a parieto-frontal direction. Across ages 7 to 26 the cortex is thinner in the COS group. However, with increasing age posterior (parietal) regions normalize while anterior regions (frontal and temporal) remain thinner merging with the pattern reported in adult onset schizophrenia studies (Greenstein et al 2006). A study examining 113 scans from 52 healthy siblings of this cohort revealed significant child and adolescent gray matter reductions in left prefrontal and bilateral temporal cortices and smaller deficits in the right prefrontal and inferior parietal cortices compared with the controls (Gogtay et al 2007). These differences normalized by age 20 years at which time there were statistically significant differences and the GM thickness correlated positively with the overall functioning of the healthy siblings (GAS scores). Similarly, thicker cortical GM in prefrontal and superior temporal cortices also correlates positively with the remission status at discharge 3–4 months after the MRI scans, suggesting that there may be a direct correlation between cortical thickness and functional outcome.

Gene variants have also been shown to influence trajectories in this COS cohort. GAD1 (2q31.1) encodes glutamic acid decarboxylase (GAD67), which expression studies show is decreased in dorsolateral prefrontal cortex in schizophrenic patients relative to controls. The effects of variants of GAD1 on grey and white matter trajectories were investigated in a family-based TDT and haplotype association analysis (Addington et al 2005). Three adjacent SNPs in the 5′ upstream region of GAD1 showed a positive pairwise association with illness and quantitative trait TDT analyses indicated several SNPs were associated with an increased rate of frontal grey matter loss.

In a subsequent study of a slightly extended sample (78 COS patients and 165 healthy controls) 56 markers (54 single-nucleotide polymorphisms and two microsatellites) spanning the NRG1 locus were genotyped (Addington et al 2007). The risk allele was associated with poorer premorbid social functioning and diagnostically specific different trajectories of grey and white matter lobar volumes (see Fig. 3). In the typically developing group the risk allele affected only frontal and temporal gray matter, whereas in the COS group the risk allele was associated with greater initial total gray and white volume but with an accelerated decline into adolescence.

We have started to explore these findings further using finer cortical thickness measures. Our initial results show that both COS probands ($n = 61$, 149 scans) and their healthy siblings ($n = 24$, 50 scans) who have the risk allele for GAD1 have steeper slopes for GM loss in prefrontal and parietal cortices compared to their counterparts without the risk allele suggesting the influence of risk genes (e.g. GAD) in a regionally specific manner.

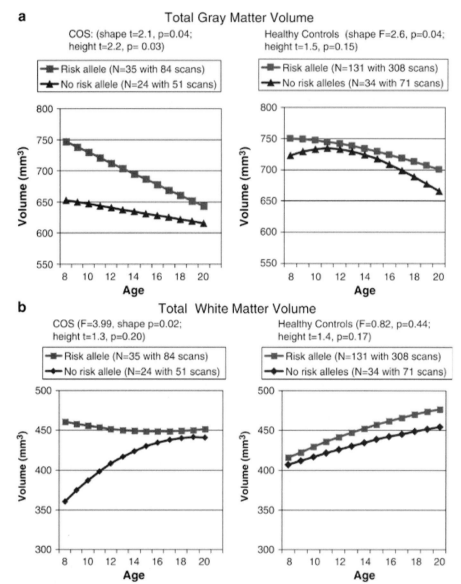

FIG. 3.   Effect of risk allele status at 420M9-1395 on brain MRI volume trajectories in COS and healthy controls for total (a) grey matter and (b) white matter. (Adapted from Addington et al 2005.)

Discussion

Development is the means by which genes express themselves in phenotypes, and there has been increasing recognition of the importance of understanding the factors regulating the developmental process itself in attempting to parse the factors associated with a healthy or pathological phenotype. Specific traits such as head circumference or height have characteristic patterns of healthy growth, and the detection of abnormalities in these patterns can be one of the first clues that development is going awry. The advent of non-invasive magnetic resonance imaging has made possible longitudinal measurements of the development of brain structure in children and adolescents and consequent characterization of the growth patterns of this previously elusive organ. The studies previously described have demonstrated the inverted U-shaped curves associated with normal brain development, the differences between male and female brain development, the relevance of trajectories as a measure of brain function such as IQ, and the specific impact of different neuropsychiatric disorders and associated genetic polymorphisms.

The sensitivity of growth patterns to such factors raises the question of whether the patterns themselves can serve as intermediate phenotypes in the search for specific genes associated with neurodevelopmental disorders such as schizophrenia. Such a goal presents significant challenges. The developmental course of a complex trait is the product of the interaction of multiple genetic and environmental factors over time. A fundamental step in assessing the usefulness of brain developmental trajectories as intermediate phenotypes is determining whether these trajectories are heritable (Gottesman & Gould 2003). Twin studies have shown that brain volumes are highly heritable (Baare et al 2001, Reveley et al 1984), and cortical thickness to be regionally so (Thompson et al 2001a). The potential interaction of age with heritability measures is supported by results from the large-scale paediatric twin study being carried out by our group, which has shown evidence of age-related changes in heritability of brain lobar volumes (Wallace et al 2006).

Evidence for the possibility that trajectories may prove to be heritable is supported by the well-documented findings of high heritability of growth patterns in other somatic traits such as height (Hauspie et al 1994). It has been observed in both humans and animal models that variance tends to decrease over development, which has been taken as evidence of the operation of canalization. Canalization refers to the frequently observed robustness of phenotypes against minor genetic or environmental perturbations, as in the example of compensatory growth (Flatt 2005, Schmalhausen 1949, Tanner 1963, Waddington 1942). Gene–environment interactions have been proposed as one path by which variance can be decreased over the course of development. Genetic determinants of plasticity in response to the environment may constrain structures to develop along a heritable trajectory from an undifferentiated beginning to a genetically determined mature state (Garlick 2002). Repetitive pattern of activity may also sculpt plastic developing structures. Zelditch and colleagues found that variance in murine skull morphometry decreased during early postnatal development. They hypothesized that high initial variance was due to the random stresses placed on skull tissues from relatively unorganized muscular activity early in life, and that variance decreased as patterns of activity took on the predictable characteristics of maturity (Zelditch et al 2004). Such a process could be relevant to activity-dependent changes in the cerebral cortex. The presence of canalization serves to stabilize developmental trajectories towards a specific heritable phenotypic target. Conversely, impairment of these buffering factors through pathology may be detectable as an increase in the variance seen in developing structures. Recent advances in statistical methodologies such as functional mapping (Wu & Lin 2006), which are designed to describe the genetic architecture of quantitative traits over development, show promise for disentangling these factors.

The ability to directly quantify aspects of brain structure and function has given us tools with which to form bridges between the genetic and environmental factors shaping biology and the resulting behaviours. Evidence from the first longitudinal structural brain imaging studies in children and adolescents who are developing normally or who have neurodevelopmental disorders has shown that trajectories can be sensitive to both genetic and functional factors. However, little is known about the heritability of other potential brain phenotypic measures such as the microstructural properties assessed with diffusion tensor imaging (DTI) or the functional BOLD responses that are the target of fMRI studies, and quantification of the heritability of the trajectories themselves awaits completion of longitudinal twin studies.

In contrast to the literature claiming stability over time as a desiderata (desired feature) for intermediate phenotypes (Almasy & Blangero 2001, Waldman 2005, Weinberger 1999), these examples illustrate the utility of trajectories of brain development as a phenotypic bridge between genes and behaviour in health and in illness.

References

Addington AM, Gornick M, Duckworth J et al 2005 GAD1 (2q31.1), which encodes glutamic acid decarboxylase (GAD67), is associated with childhood-onset schizophrenia and cortical gray matter volume loss. Mol Psychiatry 10:581–588

Addington AM, Gornick MC, Shaw P et al 2007 Neuregulin 1 (8p12) and childhood-onset schizophrenia: susceptibility haplotypes for diagnosis and brain developmental trajectories. Mol Psychiatry 12:195–205

Alaghband-Rad J, McKenna K, Gordon CT et al 1995 Childhood-onset schizophrenia: the severity of premorbid course. J Am Acad Child Adolesc Psychiatry 34:1273–1283

Almasy L, Blangero J 2001 Endophenotypes as quantitative risk factors for psychiatric disease: rationale and study design. Am J Med Genet 105:42–44

American Psychiatric Association 1994 Diagnostic and statistical manual of mental disorders. American Psychiatric Association, Washington, D.C.

Baare WF, Hulshoff Pol HE, Boomsma DI et al 2001 Quantitative genetic modeling of variation in human brain morphology. Cereb Cortex 11:816–824

Castellanos FX, Lee PP, Sharp W et al 2002 Developmental trajectories of brain volume abnormalities in children and adolescents with attention-deficit/hyperactivity disorder. JAMA 288:1740–1748

Flatt T 2005 The evolutionary genetics of canalization. Q Rev Biol 80:287–316

Flint J, Munafò MR 2007 The endophenotype concept in psychiatric genetics. Psychol Med 37:163–180

Garlick D 2002 Understanding the nature of the general factor of intelligence: the role of individual differences in neural plasticity as an explanatory mechanism. Psychol Rev 109:116–136

Gogtay N, Giedd JN, Lusk L et al 2004 Dynamic mapping of human cortical development during childhood through early adulthood. Proc Natl Acad Sci USA 101:8174–8179

Gogtay N, Greenstein D, Lenane M et al 2007 Cortical brain development in nonpsychotic siblings of patients with childhood-onset schizophrenia. Arch Gen Psychiatry 64:772–780

Gottesman I, Gould TD 2003 The endophenotype concept in psychiatry: etymology and strategic intentions. Am J Psychiatry 160:636–645

Greenstein D, Lerch J, Shaw P et al 2006 Childhood onset schizophrenia: cortical brain abnormalities as young adults. J Child Psychol Psychiatry 47:1003–1012

Hauspie RC, Bergman P, Bielicki T, Susanne C 1994 Genetic variance in the pattern of the growth curve for height: a longitudinal analysis of male twins. Ann Hum Biol 21:347–362

Hollis C 1995 Child and adolescent (juvenile onset) schizophrenia. A case control study of premorbid developmental impairments. Br J Psychiatry 166:489–495

Lenroot RK, Gogtay N, Greenstein DK et al 2007 Sexual dimorphism of brain developmental trajectories during childhood and adolescence. Neuroimage 36:1065–1073

Mackie S, Shaw P, Lenroot R et al 2007 Cerebellar development and clinical outcome in attention deficit hyperactivity disorder. Am J Psychiatry 164:647–655

Meyer-Lindenberg A, Weinberger DR 2006 Intermediate phenotypes and genetic mechanisms of psychiatric disorders. Nat Rev Neurosci 7:818–827

Meyer-Lindenberg A, Zink CF 2007 Imaging genetics for neuropsychiatric disorders. Child Adolesc Psychiatr Clin N Am 16:581–597

Nicolson R, Rapoport JL 1999 Childhood-onset schizophrenia: rare but worth studying. Biol Psychiatry 46:1418–1428

Nicolson R, Brookner FB, Lenane M et al 2003 Parental schizophrenia spectrum disorders in childhood-onset and adult-onset schizophrenia. Am J Psychiatry 160:490–495

Rapoport JL, Addington AM, Frangou S 2005 The neurodevelopmental model of schizophrenia: update 2005. Mol Psychiatry 10:434–449

Reveley AM, Reveley MA, Chitkara B, Clifford C 1984 The genetic basis of cerebral ventricular volume. Psychiatry Res 13:261–266

Schmalhausen II 1949 Factors of evolution. The theory of stabilising selection. The Blakiston Co., Philadelphia

Shaw P, Greenstein D, Lerch J et al 2006a Intellectual ability and cortical development in children and adolescents. Nature 440:676–679

Shaw P, Lerch J, Greenstein D et al 2006b Longitudinal mapping of cortical thickness and clinical outcome in children and adolescents with attention-deficit/hyperactivity disorder. Arch Gen Psychiatry 63:540–549

Shaw P, Gornick M, Lerch J et al 2007 Polymorphisms of the dopamine d4 receptor, clinical outcome, and cortical structure in attention-deficit/hyperactivity disorder. Arch Gen Psychiatry 64:921–931

Sporn AL, Greenstein DK, Gogtay N et al 2003 Progressive brain volume loss during adolescence in childhood-onset schizophrenia. Am J Psychiatry 160:2181–2189

Sporn A, Addington A, Reiss AL et al 2004 22q11 deletion syndrome in childhood onset schizophrenia: an update. Mol Psychiatry 9:225–226

Sporn A, Greenstein D, Gogtay N et al 2005 Childhood-onset schizophrenia: smooth pursuit eye-tracking dysfunction in family members. Schizophr Res 73:243–252

Tanner JM 1963 The regulation of human growth. Child Dev 34:817–847

Thompson PM, Cannon TD, Narr KL et al 2001a Genetic influences on brain structure. Nat Neurosci 4:1253–1258

Thompson PM, Vidal C, Giedd JN et al 2001b Mapping adolescent brain change reveals dynamic wave of accelerated gray matter loss in very early-onset schizophrenia. Proc Natl Acad Sci USA 98:11650–11655

Waddington CH 1942 Canalization of development and the inheritance of acquired characters. Nature 150:563–565

Waldman ID 2005 Statistical approaches to complex phenotypes: evaluating neuropsychological endophenotypes for attention-deficit/hyperactivity disorder. Biol Psychiatry 57:1347–1356

Wallace GL, Schmitt JE, Lenroot RK et al 2006 A pediatric twin study of brain morphometry. J Child Psychol Psychiatry 47:987–993

Weinberger DR 1999 Schizophrenia: new phenes and new genes. Biol Psychiatry 46:3–7

Werry JS, Sprague RL, Cohen MN 1975 Conners' Teacher Rating Scale for use in drug studies with children—an empirical study. J Abnorm Child Psychol 3:217–229

Wu R, Lin M 2006 Functional mapping—how to map and study the genetic architecture of dynamic complex traits. Nat Rev Genet 7:229–237

Zelditch ML, Lundrigan BL, Garland T Jr 2004 Developmental regulation of skull morphology. I. Ontogenetic dynamics of variance. Evol Dev 6:194–206

DISCUSSION

Raff: There is also a story about cortical thickness or brain-size trajectories in autism. There is thought to be an excessive enlargement, followed by an excessive decrease. People have been thinking in terms of abnormalities in the regressive processes that occur in normal neural development, such as neuronal culling and axonal pruning. Is this the same kind of thing you are seeing but with a different time course?

Giedd: That's a key question. Most autism researchers agree that the heads are bigger in the first few years. There is less consensus about the persistence of the larger head circumference but substantial evidence that by adolescence the heads are not bigger. The fundamental one-two punch of CNS development throughout the animal kingdom is overproduction followed by competitive or selective elimination. To use the musical chairs analogy of many people (i.e. synaptic connections) competing for a smaller number of chairs: in typical development it would be like 20 people for 12 chairs, but in autism like 200 people for the 12 chairs and it becomes chaos, with disruption of the regular checks and balances. Of course at this point this should be considered metaphorical and speculative as we really don't have any direct evidence that something like this is going on.

Another feature of autism is the prominence of short connections over long connections. There are white matter:grey matter ratio differences, for instance a proportionally smaller corpus callosum, that suggest greater local processing and less of a Gestalt picture. Behaviourally, people with autism tend not to do as well with certain visual illusions where the whole picture has to be taken in. As with much of the form/function speculation, I am unaware of any studies actually predicting Gestalt abilities from gray matter:white matter ratios in a given individual, but conceptually it seems consistent. In COS the typical adolescent decrease in frontal gray matter thickness is exaggerated: 28% COS versus 7% for typical development. Although this exaggerated thinning is not causal as it occurs after onset of symptoms it may in some way be related to disease progression. If so, might the prevention of over-pruning have positive clinical effects? Lithium is not a standard treatment for schizophrenia but it is on the list of augmenting agents and may prevent over-pruning through its effect on BDNF. Other agents that promote BDNF might also be considered. This is one speculative but possible clinical implication of focusing on the trajectories.

Flint: You have a developmental model and you argue that there is a lot happening in late adolescence. We see schizophrenia's peak incidence around that time. You then looked at a set of childhood-onset cases which presumably must differ because you don't have these processes occurring. How do these stories reconcile?

Giedd: Yes, you are correct. By the time I am seeing these grey matter changes they have had symptoms for a long time. It can't be causal: it can't be that the over-pruning leads to hallucinations or delusions. I have struggled with how best to interpret the gray matter trajectory differences. Is it a medication effect? Is it that the some as-yet-unknown process both leads to symptoms earlier and the trajectory changes later? Is it a compensatory process stemming from the brain's response to the illness?

Flint: Is it possible that there is a different mechanism for those childhood onset cases?

Giedd: I don't think so. We initially thought it was related to early-onset puberty. Several of our early cases had puberty at eight or nine, which technically isn't precocious these days but which seemed awfully early to us. Our current perspective is that COS looks very similar to severe adult-onset schizophrenia both clinically and by imaging.

Flint: So are there any clues from looking at this unusual group?

Giedd: No. I think the idea was sound: looking at an extreme. But we have been more struck by how similar they are. We haven't found anything different about the childhood group.

Talmage: I was struck by your childhood-onset group when you split out at-risk from not-at-risk alleles for neuregulin, and found that the pattern of developmental changes in gray and white matter volume were quite different. Is there anything symptomatic about those two populations that sets them apart?

Giedd: Not yet. We haven't found any outcome or medication-response differences. We have for ADHD: by looking at the early ADHD scans we are able to predict outcome 10 years later (Shaw et al 2006). I am not sure we are looking in the right places. There's nothing obvious.

Castrén: This trajectory business in brain development looks interesting. Different brain areas have their own timing. This is probably a developmental programme. It might be interesting to think about whether the environmental influences might change the shape of the trajectories. Early fibroblast growth factor (FGF) treatment might in certain brain areas prematurely force the maturation of certain brain areas, freezing it in place. Enriched environment might allow a more long-term trajectory. The genetic programme and environmental programme are intermingled differently in different time scales.

Giedd: Yes, this would be good to pursue. When I started this work I thought that it would be like children learning to walk at different ages, but the sequence of crawling and scooting and then walking isn't varying. So I was surprised that the sequence of which areas reach peak cortical thickness can vary from person to person. Some people may mature physically at one age but psychologically at a different age. There can be decoupling of maturation in different realms. What affects these rates of maturation for good or ill? We know very little about this.

Sendtner: It would be interesting to compare these changes of size of grey matter with other measurements such as changes in excitability or indirect measures of this, and then correlate this with the clinical symptoms. What is known about the time correlation of these changes in terms of disease onset or other alterations in excitability? Do you think that these morphological brain alterations are a consequence, or are they a reason for the mechanisms that underlie the clinical symptoms? How does this correlate on a time scale?

Giedd: Clinically, not very well. It is very hard to capture in individuals. One would want high frequency scans in individuals every three to six months. This hasn't been done as far as I know. We are constrained by our ethics board to 2 year intervals, which has more to do with convention than science or safety. The link may be better pursued in non-human primate studies where scans can be acquired more frequently.

Akil: In the animal models, the low-risk-taking and high-risk-taking have different hippocampal trajectories as measured by both gene expression profiling and rates of neurogenesis, both birth and survival. When they are adult they don't look quite as different. But there are subtle differences in morphology that are thought to be related to inhibitory circuitry. These relate to the behavioural inhibition that we see in the high anxiety low responder animals versus the others. When you give a small dose of FGF you change the time course. At 21 d there are high rates of neurogenesis in these FGF animals, with high rates of survival. But what happens is that in adults it slows down, there is more density and packing, there is no change in volume but there are more cells and they look normal, although they are twitchy and more prone to drug abuse. The trajectory is changed: it looks good early on but then it falls apart. So there must be feedback mechanisms that we need to understand at the cell biology level and which determine how big things grow and put the brakes on development.

Giedd: There may be biological constraints on size. An analogy would be a college that has room for 10 000 students: if there are 20 000 applicants then one set of GPAs is needed, but if there are 50 000 applicants everything goes up quality wise but there will still be 10 000 students.

Lee: As a model for early life stress, what has the adoption literature looked like for adoptees in terms of trajectories?

Giedd: Martin Teicher at Harvard looked at the effect of abuse on corpus callosum morphology (Teicher et al 2003). It's mostly bad news. If one affects early brain development, it looks like certain aspects of the neurobiology stay affected even with a corrected environment (Glaser 2000).

Spedding: You mean it is irreversible?

Giedd: Well, I am not sure if it is irreversible, but if it is reversible we don't yet know how to go about it. Earlier studies showing temporal lobe differences with positron emission tomography (PET) scans showed that even with loving families the impairments were still there (Chugani et al 2001). There's a good study going on by Charles Nelson at Harvard with Romanian orphans that may shed light on this important question (see *www.macbrain.org/beip.htm*). In this study it looks like attentive one-on-one care does improve physical growth, intelligence, and improved ability to express positive emotions.

It can be difficult to separate primary from 'downstream' effects. For instance, in autism the primary hit may be that you don't have a strong bias to attend to faces, but from then on, for the rest of your life, you will be having a different experience of the world. There may be a lot of secondary affects that are not obviously connected to the genetic hit and which are more impairing later. Any deviation from the path early on could have downstream effects.

Malaspina: Would you call those critical periods?

Giedd: A critical period for the visual system is pretty well established. There are times in development when the proper environmental input is essential for optimal organization of the networks. In that system the critical period is paralleled by particularly dynamic structural and physiological changes. If there are critical or sensitive periods for systems other than vision perhaps they are also related to times of particularly dynamic structural or physiological changes. That is something we can detect with neuroimaging. Perhaps we can work backwards from discerning the times of most dynamic structural changes to times when certain educational or therapeutic interventions might have their greatest impact. We are not there yet.

Malaspina: For social capacity, which underlies these diseases, it has been difficult to identify critical periods and the determinants for life-long social capacity. Without this many of these other things may follow.

Giedd: A trait that has been studied in ADHD is the ability to estimate time (Barkley et al 1997). At both millisecond and minute scales people with ADHD tend to be less accurate in estimating elapsed intervals. For example, you can present subjects with two tones at a certain time interval apart and then give them a third tone and have them push a thumb button at what they think is the same interval as the first two tones. People with ADHD are not as accurate—they do not miss consistently in either direction—they can estimate the interval either too long or too short. This may seem irrelevant for everyday life but many of our social interactions require exquisitely sensitive timing. A slightly longer pause in speech may indicate sarcasm, an eye gazing away for just a little too long may portray dishonesty. Much of this subtlety may blow right past the ADHD kids. They are in a group where people are joking around but they will say something that really hurts someone's feelings. They are not as good at detecting the subtle social boundaries. The genetics might be related primarily to the timing skills but the damaging effect is its impact on the social skills.

Malaspina: For what other things in life other than social communication and verbal language do we need such exquisite timing? So many of these things are elaborations of our interdependence on social cues. It is hard to say that the exquisite sense of timing and pitch is anything but a social capacity.

Giedd: Yes, as Robin Dunbar has illustrated social network size is the best predictor of brain size and may have been the most important driving force for creating the unique features of the human brain (Dunbar 1993).

Sklar: One of the reasons that you would try to select such an early-onset group, would be for the possibility of finding a Mendelian form of schizophrenia, which runs very strongly through families. 20 years ago no one knew whether there was a childhood form, and if so whether it was consistent with adult disease. You have shown clearly that what you identify in children is schizophrenia, at least phenomenologically. What do the genetics look like in these children? Is it a more genetically based form of the disease?

Giedd: In genetic studies of other illnesses such as rheumatoid arthritis very early onset cohorts are thought to be a more homogeneous subgroup with more 'pure' genetics (Childs 1996). So I anticipated that we would have found clearer genetic/familial links in our childhood onset schizophrenia group but it didn't really turn out that way.

Sklar: But what I'm asking is do they have a larger number of relatives, is the risk to siblings greater? If so one might want to sequence and look for mutations. The approach is different if you were convinced you had early onset families.

Giedd: Schizophrenia spectrum disorders were more common in parents of childhood onset schizophrenia than those with adult onset (Nicolson et al 2000). As far as I remember we haven't found the kind of clues you are talking about. COS is about 1/500th as common as the adult form. It could just be the tail end of the normal age distribution. We haven't found any unique features of the group that would explain the early onset.

Owen: Have you looked systematically for chromosomal abnormalities?

Giedd: Yes. We have a higher incidence of chromosomal abnormalities but quite a variety of them. Nine of our 96 COS patients have chromosomal abnormalities. Four are VCFS, three have X chromosome abnormalities, one is a 1:7 balanced translocation (inherited), and one is 5q32-ter segmental iUPD (Yan et al 2000, Nicolson et al 1999).

Owen: I know that there were 22q11 deletions in the early cases. But these cases are a high-risk group because a huge number of them go on to develop psychosis at some part of their life. Have you thought of doing prospective imaging in children with deletions, to compare the trajectories of those that go on to develop psychosis with those who don't?

Giedd: That would be a great idea. I think Alan Reiss at Stanford might be looking at this and perhaps some other investigators as well.

References

Barkley RA, Koplowitz S, Anderson T, McMurray MB 1997 Sense of time in children with ADHD: effects of duration, distraction, and stimulant medication. J Int Neuropsychol Soc 3:359–369

Childs B 1996 A logic of disease. Lipids 31:3–6

Chugani HT, Behen ME, Muzik O, Juhasz C, Nagy F, Chugani DC 2001 Local brain functional activity following early deprivation: a study of postinstitutionalized Romanian orphans. Neuroimage 14:1290–1301

Dunbar RIM 1993 Co-evolution of neocortex size, group size and language in humans. Behav Brain Sci 16:681–735

Glaser D 2000 Child abuse and neglect and the brain—a review. J Child Psychol Psychiatry 41:97–116

Nicolson R, Giedd JN, Lenane M et al 1999 Clinical and neurobiological correlates of cytogenetic abnormalities in childhood-onset schizophrenia. Am J Psychiatry 156:1575–1579

Nicolson R, Giedd JN, Blumenthal J et al 2000 A longitudinal MRI study of children and adolescents with atypical psychotic disorders. Biol Psychiatry 47:494–494

Shaw P, Lerch J, Greenstein D et al 2006 Longitudinal mapping of cortical thickness and clini-
    cal outcome in children and adolescents with attention-deficit/hyperactivity disorder. Arch
    Gen Psychiatry 63:540–549
Teicher MH, Polcari A, Anderson CM, Andersen SL, Lowen SB, Navalta CP 2003 Rate depen-
    dency revisited: understanding the effects of methylphenidate in children with attention
    deficit hyperactivity disorder. J Child Adolesc Psychopharmacol 13:41–51
Yan WL, Guan XY, Green ED et al 2000 Childhood-onset schizophrenia/autistic disorder and
    t(1;7) reciprocal translocation: identification of a BAC contig spanning the translocation
    breakpoint at 7q21. Am J Med Genet 96:749–753

Cell biology of BDNF and its relevance to schizophrenia

Bai Lu and Keri Martinowich

Genes, Cognition and Psychosis Program (GCAP), NIMH and Section on Neural Development & Plasticity, NICHD, National Institutes of Health, Bethesda, MD 20892-3714, USA

Abstract. BDNF is a key regulator of synaptic plasticity and hence is thought to be uniquely important for various cognitive functions. While correlations of schizophrenia with polymorphisms in the BDNF gene and changes in BDNF mRNA levels have been reported, specific links remain to be established. Cell biology studies may provide clues as to how BDNF signalling impacts schizophrenia aetiology and pathogenesis: (1) the Val-Met polymorphism in the pro-domain affects activity-dependent BDNF secretion and short-term, hippocampus-mediated episodic memory. (2) pro-BDNF and mBDNF, by interacting with their respective p75[NTR] and TrkB receptors, facilitate long-term depression (LTD) and long-term potentiation (LTP), two common forms of synaptic plasticity working in opposing directions. (3) BDNF transcription is controlled by four promoters, which drive expression of four BDNF-encoding transcripts in different brain regions, cell types and subcellular compartments (dendrites, cell body, etc.), and each is regulated by different genetic and environmental factors. A role for BDNF in early- and late-phase LTP and short- and long-term, hippocampal-dependent memory has been firmly established. Extending these studies to synaptic plasticity in other areas of the brain may help us to better understand how altered BDNF signalling could contribute to intermediate phenotypes associated with schizophrenia.

2008 Growth factors and psychiatric disorders. Wiley, Chichester (Novartis Foundation Symposium 289) p 119–135

BDNF is the most widely distributed neurotrophin in the CNS. BDNF was initially isolated and defined as a secretory molecule capable of promoting the survival of peripheral neurons through activation of its receptor TrkB. This has been shown in cultured CNS neurons including hippocampal and cortical, cholinergic, dopaminergic and serotonergic neurons. However, current thinking, derived largely from genetic and behavioural studies, posits that the primary function of BDNF in the adult brain is to regulate synaptic transmission and plasticity, rather than cell survival (Lu 2003). Hypotheses that BDNF may play a potential role in the pathophysiology of schizophrenia are based on the idea that BDNF is a key regulator of synaptic plasticity, and therefore various cognitive functions (Lewis et al 2005). Data from animal models of schizophrenia in which BDNF signalling is abnormally regulated lent initial support to these hypotheses (Angelucci et al 2004). In humans, genetic studies have further bolstered a link between BDNF and schizophrenia, as well as with brain dysfunction associated with the disorder (Szekeres et al 2003). In addition, changes in levels of BDNF and its receptor TrkB in the dorsal-lateral pre-frontal cortex (DF-PLC) (Hashimoto et al 2005, Weickert et al 2003) as well as in serum (Toyooka et al 2002) of patients with schizophrenia have been reported. However, complex interactions between BDNF and neuronal activity may be key components in the control of sophisticated cognitive functions in the mammalian brain that are impaired in schizophrenia. Recent progress in BDNF research revealed multiple levels at which BDNF signalling can be regulated or altered. Thus, when studying the role of BDNF in schizophrenia, it is necessary to take the full spectrum of BDNF cell biology into consideration as opposed to simply focusing on up- or down-regulation of BDNF mRNA or protein levels.

Cell biology of BDNF

The precursors of neurotrophins, proneurotrophins, were once considered functionally inactive. This view is no longer valid after the discovery that proneurotrophins can promote apoptosis via the p75 neurotrophin receptor (p75^{NTR}) (Lee et al 2001). Activation of pro-BDNF- p75^{NTR} and mature BDNF (mBDNF)-TrkB signalling pathways also elicit completely opposite effects on synaptic plasticity (Lu et al 2005). Considering the opposing roles of pro- and mature BDNF, cleavage of proneurotrophins may serve an important regulatory mechanism in the mammalian brain. A key characteristic of BDNF cell biology is its activity dependence (Lu 2003). For example, visual input and stimulation of the vibrissae control BDNF expression in the visual and barrel cortex, respectively. In addition to regulation of BDNF gene expression, neuronal activity can control cellular processes affecting BDNF, including intracellular trafficking, secretion, and perhaps cleavage.

Transcription

BDNF's complex genomic structure is ideal for regulation and control at multiple levels. In rodents, there are at least four promoters, each driving a short 5′ exon that is alternatively spliced onto a common 3′ exon (exon V) encoding the pre-pro-BDNF protein (Timmusk et al 1993). Recent studies indicate that there are as many as seven promoters and eight exons in human and mouse (Liu et al 2005). What is the purpose of multiple BDNF transcripts if they encode the same protein?

It has been shown that BDNF transcripts are distributed in different brain regions, different cell types, and even in different parts of the cell (e.g. soma versus dendrites). Importantly, a wide variety of physiological stimuli could elicit differential regulation of these transcripts.

Because it is regulated by neuronal activity in the amygdala, hippocampus and cortex, promoter III transcription has attracted much attention. Increases in promoter III-driven transcription have been associated with long-term potentiation (LTP) and learning and memory (Korte et al 1995, Minichiello et al 2002, Patterson et al 1996). BDNF gene expression relies on intracellular Ca^{2+}, which signals through three Ca^{2+}-dependent elements located in BDNF promoter III (West et al 2001). Tight regulation of BDNF exon III transcription by several mechanisms allows for the coupling of neuronal activity with gene transcription. Impairment in promoter III-driven BDNF transcription has been implicated in Rett Syndrome and depression. MeCP2, a methyl-CpG-dependent transcriptional repressor that is mutated in Rett Syndrome, binds methylated DNA in promoter III. Neuronal depolarization induces dissociation of MeCP2, resulting in derepression of exon III (Chen et al 2003, Martinowich et al 2003). Depressive-like behaviours in mice are associated with a decrease in BDNF promoter III-mediated transcription, an effect which can be counteracted by antidepressants via induction of histone acetylation (Tsankova et al 2006).

Processing and trafficking

Pro-BDNF, translated from BDNF mRNA in the endoplasmic reticulum (ER), is folded in the trans-Golgi network, packaged into secretory vesicles, and sorted into one of two principal pathways, the constitutive (i.e. spontaneous release) or regulated (i.e. release in response to stimuli) (Mowla et al 1999). BDNF-containing vesicles are trafficked to their appropriate sub-cellular compartments, including dendritic spines and axonal terminals, and secreted in response to extracellular and intracellular signals.

BDNF's pro-domain is important for dendritic trafficking and synaptic localization. A single-nucleotide polymorphism (SNP) in the pro-region of human BDNF produces a valine to methionine substitution at amino acid 66 (Val66Met). In cultured hippocampal neurons, Val-BDNF is localized to both the cell body and dendrites with a fraction localized to the synapse, whereas Met-BDNF is largely found in the cell body and proximal dendrites. Met-BDNF is largely absent from distal dendrites and the synapse (Egan et al 2003, Chen et al 2004).

It is possible that pro-BDNF is processed to mBDNF in the secretory granules by intracellular proteases. However, a large fraction of neuronal BDNF is actually secreted in the pro-form, which is converted to mBDNF by extracellular proteases including plasmin and the matrix metalloproteinases (Lee et al 2001, Teng et al 2005). Because pro-BDNF and mBDNF elicit distinct biological effects via different receptor systems, the proteolytic step is important in influencing BDNF's functional output. An interesting candidate that could be influential in this step is tissue plasminogen activator (tPA), an extracellular protease that converts the inactive zymogen plasminogen to plasmin. Conceivably, neuronal activity could control pro-BDNF→mBDNF conversion by triggering tPA secretion from axon terminals in response to activity (Pang et al 2004).

Secretion

Unlike other growth factors, BDNF is secreted primarily through the regulated, rather than the constitutive, pathway. BDNF secretion occurs at both pre- and postsynaptic sites. In general, tetanic stimulation is more effective in inducing BDNF secretion than low frequency stimulation. The effects of the Val66Met polymorphism have drawn attention to the pro-domain's role in activity-dependent BDNF secretion. In neurons expressing Met-BDNF, depolarization-induced secretion is selectively impaired while the integrity of constitutive secretion is preserved (Egan et al 2003). Recent studies have identified a new receptor for pro-BDNF called sortilin (Nykjaer et al 2004). Sortilin specifically interacts with the pro-domain in a region encompassing Val66Met. Inhibition of the pro-domain/sortilin interaction attenuates depolarization-induced secretion of BDNF (Chen et al 2005). However, since sortilin is likely to interact with the pro-domains of neurotrophins incapable of regulated secretion, the mechanism may not be specific. Interaction between the sorting motif on mBDNF and the well-known sorting receptor, carboxypeptidase E (CPE), allows for sorting of pro-BDNF into regulated pathway vesicles for activity-dependent secretion (Lou et al 2005).

BDNF and synaptic plasticity

Accumulated evidence supports the notion that BDNF is a key regulator of several forms of synaptic plasticity in the hippocampus and cortex. These studies have led to the idea that BDNF may be involved in various cognitive brain functions.

Early phase LTP

LTP can be divided into an early phase (E-LTP, lasting ~1–2 hours) and a later phase (L-LTP, lasting days). This distinction is based not only on the duration of LTP, but also its dependence on gene transcription and protein synthesis. Early work focused on the role of BDNF in E-LTP. In the neonatal hippocampus, where endogenous BDNF levels are low, application of high frequency stimulation (HFS) induced short-term potentiation but not LTP. In hippocampal slices treated with BDNF, LTP can be reliably induced (Figurov et al 1996). Conversely, in the adult hippocampus, where endogenous levels of BDNF are relatively high, inhibition of BDNF activity attenuates expression of E-LTP (Figurov et al 1996). Moreover, a subthreshold tetanus that normally induces only weak potentiation can elicit pronounced LTP (Figurov et al 1996). These findings are backed by studies using BDNF knockout mice. Heterozygous mice (BDNF$^{+/-}$) exhibit severe impairments in E-LTP (Korte et al 1995, Patterson et al 1996). The LTP deficit in BDNF mutant mice can be reversed by introducing BDNF back into the system (Korte et al 1995, Patterson et al 1996). TrkB knockout mice also exhibit deficits in E-LTP (Minichiello et al 2002).

The mechanisms by which BDNF regulates E-LTP have largely been worked out (Lu & Chow 1999). Genetic and biochemical studies support a model in which BDNF facilitates the docking of synaptic vesicles to presynaptic membranes through TrkB-mediated phosphorylation of synaptic proteins such as synapsin I and synaptobrevin. An actin motor complex containing Myo6 and a Myo6-binding protein, GIPC1, might be involved in the presynaptic function of BDNF (Yano et al 2006). An increase in the number of docked vesicles would enhance the ability of hippocampal synapses to respond to HFS, resulting in the facilitation of hippocampal E-LTP. Despite overwhelming evidence for BDNF regulation of presynaptic transmitter release at excitatory synapses, a postsynaptic role of BDNF cannot be excluded. Indeed, BDNF has been shown to regulate properties of NMDA channels (Levine et al 1998), and elicit both acute and long-term effects on dendritic spines (Ji et al 2005).

Late-phase LTP

A number of early studies proposed a role for BDNF in L-LTP. Expression of BDNF and TrkB mRNAs is selectively enhanced by tetanic stimulation that is capable of inducing L-LTP, and the time course of BDNF synthesis correlates well with that of L-LTP (Patterson et al 1992). This transcription is partially dependent on CREB, a transcription factor known to be necessary for L-LTP. In BDNF$^{+/-}$ mice, application of strong tetanic stimulation such as long theta burst stimulation (TBS) (e.g., 12 sets of TBS) or forskolin failed to induce L-LTP (Korte et al 1998, Patterson et al 2001). Moreover, in conditions in which only E-LTP could occur, such as delivering weak tetanus (three sets of TBS) or strong tetanus (12 TBS) in the presence of protein synthesis inhibitors, robust L-LTP can be induced after application of exogenous BDNF (Pang et al 2004). Several recent studies further reveal the importance of activity-dependent BDNF transcription, possibly through promoter III. When protein synthesis was completely blocked, perfusion of exogenous BDNF could restore L-LTP (Pang et al 2004). In VP16-CREB mice in which CREB-mediated BDNF transcription is elevated, a weak, E-LTP-inducing tetanus could induce L-LTP, and this could be reversed by application of BDNF scavenger TrkB-IgG (Barco et al 2005). Finally, we have recently generated a line of mutant mice in which activity-dependent, promoter III-mediated BDNF transcription is blocked. Remarkably, L-LTP was selectively impaired, but E-LTP remained intact (K. Sakata 2005 Society for Neuroscience, abstract). Thus, BDNF is a key protein synthesis product responsible for L-LTP expression.

In addition to activity-dependent transcription of BDNF, L-LTP is also dependent on conversion of pro-BDNF to mBDNF by extracellular proteases, particularly, the tissue plasminogen activator (tPA)/plasmin system. tPA is an enzyme that can cleave plasminogen (an inactive precursor) to plasmin. These proteases are expressed in the brain and secreted at hippocampal synapses. Plasmin has been shown to cleave pro-BDNF and generate mBDNF *in vitro* (Lee et al 2001). Mice lacking tPA exhibit selective impairments in L-LTP, but not E-LTP (Baranes et al 1998). These results have led us to hypothesize that L-LTP requires an enzymatic cascade in which tPA cleaves the inactive zymogen plasminogen to plasmin, which then cleaves pro-BDNF to mBDNF. Indeed, in both tPA and plasminogen mutant mice, pro-BDNF is elevated in the hippocampus. Moreover, application of mBDNF, but not uncleavable pro-BDNF, can rescue the L-LTP deficit seen in tPA and plasmin knockout mice (Pang et al 2004). These results provide a mechanistic link between these two seemingly independent molecular systems in L-LTP expression.

Long-term depression (LTD)

LTD is defined as a persistent reduction in synaptic strength, which is induced by prolonged low frequency stimulation (LFS). Several different forms of LTD exist, each sub-served by different glutamate receptors. NMDA-dependent LTD, the most well-known form of LTD, is robustly expressed in young, but not adult animals. Several recent studies have implicated pro-BDNF-p75[NTR] in the NMDAR-dependent form of LTD (Woo et al 2005, Zagrebelsky et al 2005). In p75[NTR] mutant mice, NMDAR-dependent LTD was absent while other forms of plasticity, including NMDAR-dependent LTP and NMDAR-independent LTD, remained intact. Furthermore, protein levels of NR2B, an NMDAR subunit implicated in LTD, as well as NR2B-mediated currents were significantly reduced in the p75[NTR] mutant hippocampus. Importantly, cleavage-resistant pro-BDNF was able to increase NR2B-mediated synaptic currents and enhance LTD in the wild type, but not the mutant, p75[NTR] hippocampus (Woo et al 2005). These results implicate pro-BDNF as an endogenous ligand of p75[NTR], which enhances expression of LTD via an NR2B-mediated mechanism.

BDNF, cognition and schizophrenia

The profound effects of BDNF on hippocampal plasticity, particularly LTP, strongly suggest a role for BDNF in hippocampal-dependent forms of memory. In rodents, disruption of BDNF or TrkB signalling markedly impairs two hippocampal-dependent forms of memory. In humans, studies of the BDNF Val66Met polymorphism, where the Met allele was shown to be associated with abnormal hippocampal structure and function, provided the first evidence for direct involvement of BDNF (Hariri et al 2003, Egan et al 2003, Pezawas et al 2004). Direct tests of memory function show that human subjects with two copies of the Met allele exhibit selective impairment in short-term episodic memory, but not in hippocampal-independent working memory or semantic memory tasks (Egan et al 2003). The high frequency of the BDNF Val66Met SNP in the population also facilitated the ability to run association analyses between this polymorphism and other cognitive tasks. In one report, elderly carriers of two BDNF Met alleles score higher in non-verbal reasoning, verbal fluency and logical memory (Harris et al 2006), whereas in another report, young Chinese that are homozygous for the Val allele score higher on IQ tests (Tsai et al 2004). In addition, the BDNF Met allele has been associated with decreased hippocampal volume (Pezawas et al 2004).

The BDNF gene is one of just a few genes that are prominently implicated in cognitive functions. This, coupled with the impairments in hippocampal structure and memory functions that have been associated with the BDNF Val66Met polymorphism, have generated a great deal of interest in linking deficits in BDNF signalling/function with schizophrenia and/or its intermediate phenotypes. It is believed that inappropriate or inadequate neurotrophic support during brain development could underlie structural and functional disorganization of neural and synaptic networks, leading to the decreased ability of the brain to make necessary adaptive changes seen in schizophrenia. The studies so far fall into three categories. (1) Numerous studies have reported association between BDNF Val66Met and other single nucleotide polymorphisms (SNPs) and schizophrenia (Craddock et al 2006). However, these associations have not been replicated in some recent studies (Craddock et al 2006). (2) A more consistent finding is the decrease in the serum (or plasma) BDNF levels in schizophrenic patients (Toyooka et al 2002). However, in drug-naïve first-episode schizophrenic patients, serum BDNF levels are increased (Jockers-Scherubl et al 2004). Thus, it is unclear whether the reduction in serum BDNF is truly associated with the illness or antipsychotic drug administration. (3) A more relevant study might be to examine BDNF expression levels in relevant brain regions from animal models of schizophrenia or postmortem schizophrenic brains. Neonatal lesion of rodent ventral hippocampus recapitulates many schizophrenia-like phenotypes. In this model, BDNF mRNA levels were reduced in the hippocampus, prefrontal cortex (PFC), and cingulate cortex

(Ashe et al 2002, Lipska et al 2001, Molteni et al 2001). In postmortem brains from schizophrenia patients, there is a significant decrease in BDNF mRNA in dorsal lateral PFC and hippocampus (Hashimoto et al 2005, Weickert et al 2003). In parallel, expression of TrkB and calbindin-D, a marker for GABAergic neurons, was significantly reduced in the hippocampus or PFC (Hashimoto et al 2005, Weickert et al 2003, Takahashi et al 2000). Again, it is unclear whether the changes in BDNF or TrkB expression are direct consequences of the illness or secondary to antipsychotic drug treatment. Rodents could be used to directly test the effect of antipsychotics. Chronic treatment of rodents with typical antipsychotic drugs generally suppresses BDNF expression in the brain, whereas atypical antipsychotics increase BDNF expression (Lipska et al 2001, Chlan-Fourney et al 2002).

When thinking about future research on the role of BDNF in schizophrenia, several points warrant further discussion. First, given BDNF's complex genomic structure, it may be helpful to examine expression of specific BDNF transcripts in the schizophrenic brain, particularly in relevant regions such as hippocampus and sub-regions of PFC. Second, BDNF gene expression is subject to strong epigenetic regulation. Thus, lack of genetic association does not automatically suggest that BDNF is not involved. A recent precedent was the demonstration that social defeat stress induced long-lasting down-regulation of BDNF transcripts III and IV, and chronic antidepressants reversed this down-regulation by increasing histone acetylation at these promoters (Tsankova et al 2006). Third, studies of the BDNF Val66Met polymorphism suggest that the mode of BDNF secretion (regulated versus constitutive), rather than the levels of BDNF per se, might be more important in cognitive functions and behaviours. Indeed, BDNF (Met/Met) knock-in mice, which exhibit increased anxiogenic behaviours, have normal BDNF levels in the brain, but show significantly impaired activity-dependent secretion of BDNF (Chen et al 2006). Third, all studies thus far have used methods that cannot distinguish pro-BDNF from mBDNF. Since pro-BDNF and mBDNF elicit opposing actions on synaptic plasticity, their distinction is paramount to determining the role of pro-BDNF and mBDNF in specific aspects of cognitive behaviours relevant to schizophrenia. Finally, given that the majority of negative symptoms in schizophrenia are associated with PFC deficits such as impairments in working memory and executive functions, future efforts should be directed towards studying the regulation of PFC function by BDNF. Since synchronized firings in the PFC last only a few seconds, LTP-like mechanisms may not be involved. It is more likely that BDNF controls the development of underlying cortical networks. A major target is the parvalbumin (PV)-positive GABAergic interneurons, which co-ordinate sustained firing of pyramidal neurons within a PFC network. Among all interneurons, TrkB is preferentially expressed in PV interneurons. Accumulated data suggest that TrkB signalling is disrupted in the PV interneurons in schizophrenic patients, leading to decreased expression of GABA-related genes (Lewis et al 2005). Multidisciplinary approaches, particularly network recording and behavioural assays relevant to PFC functions, should be used to study BDNF regulation of the development of GABAergic interneurons, and its functional consequences. How impairments in cortical network are linked to the pathophysiology of schizophrenia is a fascinating subject worthy of future studies.

References

Angelucci F, Mathe AA, Aloe L 2004 Neurotrophic factors and CNS disorders: findings in rodent models of depression and schizophrenia. Prog Brain Res 146:151–165

Ashe PC, Chlan-Fourney J, Juorio AV, Li XM 2002 Brain-derived neurotrophic factor (BDNF) mRNA in rats with neonatal ibotenic acid lesions of the ventral hippocampus. Brain Res 956:126–135

Baranes D, Lederfein D, Huang YY, Chen M, Bailey CH, Kandel ER 1998 Tissue plasminogen activator contributes to the late phase of LTP and to synaptic growth in the hippocampal mossy fiber pathway. Neuron 21:813–825

Barco A, Patterson S, Alarcon JM et al 2005 Gene expression profiling of facilitated L-LTP in VP16-CREB mice reveals that BDNF is critical for the maintenance of LTP and its synaptic capture. Neuron 48:123–137

Chen WG, Chang Q, Lin Y et al 2003 Derepression of BDNF transcription involves calcium-dependent phosphorylation of MeCP2. Science 302:885–889

Chen ZY, Patel PD, Sant G et al 2004 Variant brain-derived neurotrophic factor (BDNF) (Met66) alters the intracellular trafficking and activity-dependent secretion of wild-type BDNF in neurosecretory cells and cortical neurons. J Neurosci 24:4401–4411

Chen ZY, Ieraci A, Teng H et al 2005 Sortilin controls intracellular sorting of brain-derived neurotrophic factor to the regulated secretory pathway. J Neurosci 25:6156–6166

Chen ZY, Jing D, Bath KG et al 2006 Genetic variant BDNF (Val66Met) polymorphism alters anxiety-related behavior. Science 314:140–143

Chlan-Fourney J, Ashe P, Nylen K, Juorio AV, Li XM 2002 Differential regulation of hippocampal BDNF mRNA by typical and atypical antipsychotic administration. Brain Res 954:11–20

Craddock N, O'Donovan MC, Owen MJ 2006 Genes for schizophrenia and bipolar disorder? Implications for psychiatric nosology. Schizophr Bull 32:9–16

Egan MF, Kojima M, Callicott JH et al 2003 The BDNF Val66Met polymorphism affects activity-dependent secretion of BDNF and human memory and hippocampal function. Cell 112:257–269

Figurov A, Pozzo-Miller LD, Olafsson P, Wang T, Lu B 1996 Regulation of synaptic responses to high-frequency stimulation and LTP by neurotrophins in the hippocampus. Nature 381:706–709

Hariri AR, Goldberg TE, Mattay VS et al 2003 Brain-derived neurotrophic factor Val66Met polymorphism affects human memory-related hippocampal activity and predicts memory performance. J Neurosci 23:6690–6694

Harris SE, Fox H, Wright AF et al 2006 The brain-derived neurotrophic factor Val66Met polymorphism is associated with age-related change in reasoning skills. Mol Psychiatry 11:505–513

Hashimoto T, Bergen SE, Nguyen QL et al 2005 Relationship of brain-derived neurotrophic factor and its receptor TrkB to altered inhibitory prefrontal circuitry in schizophrenia. J Neurosci 25:372–383

Ji Y, Pang PT, Feng L, Lu B 2005 Cyclic AMP controls BDNF-induced TrkB phosphorylation and dendritic spine formation in mature hippocampal neurons. Nat Neurosci 8:164–172

Jockers-Scherubl MC, Danker-Hopfe H, Mahlberg R et al 2004 Brain-derived neurotrophic factor serum concentrations are increased in drug-naive schizophrenic patients with chronic cannabis abuse and multiple substance abuse. Neurosci Lett 371:79–83

Korte M, Carroll P, Wolf E, Brem G, Thoenen H, Bonhoeffer T 1995 Hippocampal long-term potentiation is impaired in mice lacking brain-derived neurotrophic factor. Proc Natl Acad Sci USA 92:8856–8860

Korte M, Kang H, Bonhoeffer T, Schuman E 1998 A role for BDNF in the late-phase of hippocampal long-term potentiation. Neuropharmacology 37:553–559

Lee R, Kermani P, Teng KK, Hempstead BL 2001 Regulation of cell survival by secreted proneurotrophins. Science 294:1945–1948

Levine ES, Crozier RA, Black IB, Plummer MR 1998 Brain-derived neurotrophic factor modulates hippocampal synaptic transmission by increasing N-methyl-D-aspartic acid receptor activity. Proc Natl Acad Sci USA 95:10235–10239

Lewis DA, Hashimoto T, Volk DW 2005 Cortical inhibitory neurons and schizophrenia. Nat Rev Neurosci 6:312–324

Lipska BK, Khaing ZZ, Weickert CS, Weinberger DR 2001 BDNF mRNA expression in rat hippocampus and prefrontal cortex: effects of neonatal ventral hippocampal damage and antipsychotic drugs. Eur J Neurosci 14:135–144

Liu QR, Walther D, Drgon T et al 2005 Human brain derived neurotrophic factor (BDNF) genes, splicing patterns, and assessments of associations with substance abuse and Parkinson's Disease. Am J Med Genet B Neuropsychiatr Genet 134:93–103

Lou H, Kim SK, Zaitsev E, Snell CR, Lu B, Loh YP 2005 Sorting and activity-dependent secretion of BDNF require interaction of a specific motif with the sorting receptor carboxypeptidase e. Neuron 45:245–255

Lu B 2003 BDNF and activity-dependent synaptic modulation. Learn Mem 10:86–98

Lu B, Chow A 1999 Neurotrophins and hippocampal synaptic transmission and plasticity. J Neurosci Res 58:76–87

Lu B, Pang PT, Woo NH 2005 The yin and yang of neurotrophin action. Nat Rev Neurosci 6:603–614

Martinowich K, Hattori D, Wu H et al 2003 DNA methylation-related chromatin remodeling in activity-dependent BDNF gene regulation. Science 302:890–893

Minichiello L, Calella AM, Medina DL, Bonhoeffer T, Klein R, Korte M 2002 Mechanism of TrkB-mediated hippocampal long-term potentiation. Neuron 36:121–137

Molteni R, Lipska BK, Weinberger DR, Racagni G, Riva MA 2001 Developmental and stress-related changes of neurotrophic factor gene expression in an animal model of schizophrenia. Mol Psychiatry 6:285–292

Mowla SJ, Pareek S, Farhadi HF et al 1999 Differential sorting of nerve growth factor and brain-derived neurotrophic factor in hippocampal neurons. J Neurosci 19:2069–2080

Nykjaer A, Lee R, Teng KK et al 2004 Sortilin is essential for proNGF-induced neuronal cell death. Nature 427:843–848

Pang PT, Teng HK, Zaitsev E et al 2004 Cleavage of proBDNF by tPA/plasmin is essential for long-term hippocampal plasticity. Science 306:487–491

Patterson SL, Grover LM, Schwartzkroin PA, Bothwell M 1992 Neurotrophin expression in rat hippocampal slices: a stimulus paradigm inducing LTP in CA1 evokes increases in BDNF and NT-3 mRNAs. Neuron 9:1081–1088

Patterson SL, Abel T, Deuel TA, Martin KC, Rose JC, Kandel ER 1996 Recombinant BDNF rescues deficits in basal synaptic transmission and hippocampal LTP in BDNF knockout mice. Neuron 16:1137–1145

Patterson SL, Pittenger C, Morozov A et al 2001 Some forms of cAMP-mediated long-lasting potentiation are associated with release of BDNF and nuclear translocation of phospho-MAP kinase. Neuron 32:123–140

Pezawas L, Verchinski BA, Mattay VS et al 2004 The brain-derived neurotrophic factor Val66Met polymorphism and variation in human cortical morphology. J Neurosci 24:10099–10102

Szekeres G, Juhasz A, Rimanoczy A, Keri S, Janka Z 2003 The C270T polymorphism of the brain-derived neurotrophic factor gene is associated with schizophrenia. Schizophr Res 65:15–18

Takahashi M, Shirakawa O, Toyooka K et al 2000 Abnormal expression of brain-derived neurotrophic factor and its receptor in the corticolimbic system of schizophrenic patients. Mol Psychiatry 5:293–300

Teng HK, Teng KK, Lee R et al 2005 ProBDNF induces neuronal apoptosis via activation of a receptor complex of p75NTR and sortilin. J Neurosci 25:5455–5463

Timmusk T, Palm K, Metsis M et al 1993 Multiple promoters direct tissue-specific expression of the rat BDNF gene. Neuron 10:475–489

Toyooka K, Asama K, Watanabe Y et al 2002 Decreased levels of brain-derived neurotrophic factor in serum of chronic schizophrenic patients. Psychiatry Res 110:249–257

Tsai SJ, Hong CJ, Yu YW, Chen TJ 2004 Association study of a brain-derived neurotrophic factor (BDNF) Val66Met polymorphism and personality trait and intelligence in healthy young females. Neuropsychobiology 49:13–16

Tsankova NM, Berton O, Renthal W, Kumar A, Neve RL, Nestler EJ 2006 Sustained hippocampal chromatin regulation in a mouse model of depression and antidepressant action. Nat Neurosci 9:519–525

Weickert CS, Hyde TM, Lipska BK, Herman MM, Weinberger DR, Kleinman JE 2003 Reduced brain-derived neurotrophic factor in prefrontal cortex of patients with schizophrenia. Mol Psychiatry 8:592–610

West AE, Chen WG, Dalva MB et al 2001 Calcium regulation of neuronal gene expression. Proc Natl Acad Sci USA 98:11024–11031

Woo NH, Teng HK, Siao CJ et al 2005 Activation of p75NTR by proBDNF facilitates hippocampal long-term depression. Nat Neurosci 8:1069–1077

Yano H, Ninan I, Zhang H, Milner TA, Arancio O, Chao MV 2006 BDNF-mediated neurotransmission relies upon a myosin VI motor complex. Nat Neurosci 9:1009–1018

Zagrebelsky M, Holz A, Dechant G, Barde YA, Bonhoeffer T, Korte M 2005 The p75 neurotrophin receptor negatively modulates dendrite complexity and spine density in hippocampal neurons. J Neurosci 25:9989–9999

DISCUSSION

Barde: The bottom line of what I am going to say is bad news with regard to the release of pro-BDNF from neurons, as there are no clearly detectable levels of pro-BDNF in the adult brain. The reason why pro-neurotrophins are interesting is because a few years ago Barbara Hempstead and her colleagues showed that, quite unexpectedly, pro-neurotrophins can bind to p75 with high affinity. This is relevant because the activation of p75 usually does bad things to cells, so it does matter whether neurotrophins are secreted as proneurotrophins, as they would bind to p75, or as mature neurotrophins because then they would activate completely different pathways. In addition, all the work we keep hearing about on the Val-Met substitution is in pro-BDNF, so there is every reason to worry about whether or not pro-BDNF can be detected in the brain or not and is secreted from neurons. I'd like to briefly summarize unpublished work performed by Tomoya Matsumoto, using in part reagents previously generated by Roland Kolbeck and Johannes Klose, as well as Stefanie Rauskolb. The experiment is extremely simple: one takes a brain, does a western blot (after making sure that the antibodies recognize BDNF) and all that is seen is mature BDNF with no detectable pro-BDNF. This is based on two pieces of evidence: first, the band that we call mature BDNF is absent in the BDNF knockout; second, when we use a mouse that we generated in part for this purpose in which the BDNF gene has been replaced in a knock-in approach by a tagged version, BDNF-Myc (giving rise to a mouse that we call the Mickey Mouse!), and then use Myc antibodies we find a slight shift indicating that the tag is still there. Again, only mature BDNF is seen with no evidence for significant quantities of pro-BDNF in the normal brain. What these studies also revealed is part of the explanation for what I consider a confusion in the field: that is, in all these mice all BDNF antibodies detect a band slightly bigger than pro-BDNF, which is equally present both in the knockout BDNF animals and the Myc mouse BDNF without alterations of the size of BDNF in extracts of the latter animals. We think then that a contaminant has been mistaken for pro-BDNF. The classical view of why neurotrophins are first synthesized as proneurotrophins is because of the disulfide bridging of the neurotrophins. As many of you probably know, there are four different proteins in this family and all are first synthesized as pro-neurotrophins. This gives a 1:1 ratio with regard to the mature protein, providing an appropriate environment allowing correct disulfide bridging which is quite complex, 1–4, 2–5, 3–6 giving rise to the 'cysteine knot'. In my opinion, this is the 'raison d'être' of the pro-neurotrophins. However, this doesn't mean that cells other than neurons may not store or secrete proneurotrophin. A second reason as to why there has been so much confusion in the field is that there is very little neurotrophin to work with. It is just not easy to do protein chemistry with very little protein. Many people, including ourselves, initially transfected cells with neurotrophins cDNAs. If COS cells, 293 cells or even neurons are used, pro-BDNF pours out of these cells, presumably because these cells have a limited capacity to process pro-neurotrophin. But as I said, when we analyse normal, intact brain, we can only detect mature BDNF. Lastly, I am not questioning that proneurotrophins can come out of cells others than neurons. For example, there is good evidence that microglial cells, when activated, secrete pro-NGF. After lesion of the adult brain there is nice work showing that quite a lot of pro-NGF is present in the CSF (see for example Harrington et al 2004). This is relevant because p75 is often overexpressed after lesion. This is part of a mechanism for eliminating cells. In sum then, I think that the release of proneurotrophins is part of a pathological phenomenon that has nothing to do with the function of the normal brain. This is further supported by recent, unpublished work, again by Tomoya Matsumoto who did classical pulse-chase studies with neurotrophins and primary neuron cultures labelled with radioactive amino acids. We found that pro-BDNF is cleaved rapidly and the only thing that remains stored in neurons is mature BDNF.

Lu: To a certain extent I disagree. First, early work by Margaret Fahnestock in Canada has shown a prominent pro-BDNF band on a western blot using tissues from several human brain regions. This band is decreased in the Alzheimer's brain (Michalski & Fahnestock 2003). One may argue about how good the antibodies are and whether they detect a non-specific protein with the same size as proBDNF. Second, we have now generated a monoclonal antibody specific for pro-BDNF and performed the same western blot analysis as described by Yves Barde. We detected a prominent band with the same size as recombinant pro-BDNF in the cortex, hippocampus, cerebellum, basal forebrain, but not in striatum and spinal cord of young wild-type mice. This band is completely absent in the same brain regions of littermates of BDNF homozygous mutant (BDNF$^{-/-}$) mice (Nagappan and Lu, unpublished observation). Third, we and Barbara Hempstead and her colleagues found that pro-BDNF is quite fragile and easily cleaved by intracellular proteases when cell membranes are broken down, e.g. during the process of cell homogenization, which is a required step in western blot or pulse-chase experiments. It is therefore critical to ensure that intracellular proteases are completely inhibited by using a cocktail of freshly prepared protease inhibitors during the process of cell homogenization. Fourth, the protein extraction procedure used to prepare lysates from different brain regions could selectively enrich mature BDNF thereby altering the interpretation. Another point I want to make is regarding the BDNF antibodies. Most of the commercial antibodies are raised against domains in the mature BDNF, and therefore should recognize both pro-BDNF and mature BDNF. Some antibodies may have higher affinities to mature BDNF, and therefore give the impression that there is more mature BDNF in the cells. Finally, I am not sure whether the BDNF-Myc in the knock-in mice behaves the same way as native pro-BDNF in terms of its folding, trafficking, cellular expression and cleavage.

Which cells have it? Work by Cheryl Dreyfus showed that cultured astrocytes produce primarily pro-BDNF. Neurons can also produce and secrete pro-BDNF. In Richard Murphy's published work, when neurons are transfected with the BDNF construct there is a lot of secreted pro-BDNF. However, this could be due to overexpression. I think it is important to determine the expression and secretion of pro-BDNF in neurons from different parts of the brain, at different developmental stages, in normal, physiologically relevant conditions. I do agree with Yves that you can see a lot of pro-BDNF in pathological conditions such as stress, stroke and depression, when the system has to produce a lot of BDNF. Under these circumstances there is just not enough enzymatic activity inside the cells to process the newly synthesized pro-BDNF, and the result is a lot of pro-BDNF secretion. I also wanted to mention a specific case, LTD. In the normal situation in the adult you don't see LTD in the hippocampus, and there is very little p75 in the adult brain. There is one reproducible way of inducing LTD in the adult, which is simply to put the mouse or the rat on a small, elevated platform 1 metre above the ground for 30 min. The animal becomes scared. If we take a brain slice we can then induce LTD, which can be neutralized by blocking pro-BDNF-p75 interactions. In situations with stress or pathology, the system jacks up pro-BDNF, and under these circumstances proBDNF will be highly expressed and can work.

Chao: It is clear that p75 is not highly expressed in the adult brain except in the basal forebrain. However, this receptor is rapidly elevated after inflammation, injury or nerve damage.

Akil: What is the change in sequence of the cleavage site from pro to mature: is it Lys-Lys, Lys-Arg or Arg-Arg?

Barde: There are three basic amino acids out of four in the presumed furin-type of cleavage site.

Akil: I am an old pro-opiomelanocortin person who attempted to take the pituitary data and ATT20 and all of that, and apply it to brain. I was humbled by that task. It is regulatable, but the only time where it is really regulatable is if it is slow. In a Lys-Lys cleavage site, it is very sensitive to levels of precursor expression because it is a slow process, but in a quick cleavage it is very hard to overcome. My bias would be to think a little more about the kinetics of changes of gene expression, precursor protein and enzyme activity in the tissue. I can see it happening but I would like to understand it more mechanistically.

Tongiorgi: Yves Barde, have you looked in the peripheral nervous system to see whether your ideas about the pro-BDNF are still valid in the mouse under normal conditions?

Barde: No. I was talking about normal, uninjured neurons in the adult brain. I am open to the idea that cells that are not neurons may secrete proneurotrophins.

Tongiorgi: So even in the spinal cord you don't see pro-BDNF?

Barde: No.

Tongiorgi: Is tPA regulated in animals with depression-like symptoms?

Lu: There are reports of this.

Tongiorgi: Could this be another step in regulation that could be altered in pathology?

Lu: Yes. There was a correlation of plasmin down-regulation and Alzheimer's disease (Ledesma et al 2000).

Lee: Bruce McEwen and Steve Strickland have published studies in which they have stressed the tPA knockout mouse and found blunted anxiety responses (Pawlak et al 2003)

Tongiorgi: I have a concern about the protein levels. Results can be completely different when looking at mRNA regulation in various systems and then looking at the protein. In your knockout mouse in which exon III was deleted (the new nomenclature by Aid et al 2007 is exon 4), the protein levels seem to be normal. What I expect here, is that there could be compensatory effects so that other BDNF exons could be up-regulated. For instance, the sequences for Ca^{2+} responsive transcription factors are not only in front of exon III, but also exons IV and V (exons 4, 5 and 6, in Aid et al 2007). The idea I want to put forward is that by blocking one part of the entire regulation you may have an up-regulation of other compensatory mechanisms. My concern is whether you have checked what happens in terms of possible up and down regulation by other systems. In addition, from the studies by the group of Margaret Fahnenstock, I remember the opposite (Peng et al 2005): the pro-BDNF in the prefrontal cortex was actually down-regulated. There is probably a completely different regulation depending on the neuroanatomical location. We need to think about gene regulation not in terms of the entire brain, but rather in terms of neuronal systems and connectivity. So we need to bring the wiring of the different systems into this discussion.

Lu: I want to pick up on this issue in terms of regulation by different promoters. In fact, there is a compensatory regulation. In different brain regions we saw different promoter 3 regulation. In the cortex, the most obvious thing was that the promoter 3 knockout mice exhibit no activity-dependent expression of BDNF while the total BDNF level was exactly the same as the wild type control. In other words, perhaps promoter 3 contributes a small fraction of the total BDNF. This raises an interesting issue. Why would the brain design such a complex scheme that generates multiple RNAs coding for the same protein? An important consequence is that different exon-containing mRNAs are expressed in different types of cells, brain regions and even different subcellular compartments, such as dendrites versus cell bodies. Different transcripts are regulated by different environmental factors such as activities, hormones, epigenetic factors, etc.

Buonanno: You showed a figure in which the Trk receptors were both pre and post-synaptic, and p75 was also pre- and post-synaptic. But when you showed the model, you only showed pro-BDNF working on the post-synaptic side. Is the effect both pre- and post-synaptic, and is it possible that in different areas it is more of a presynaptic effect?

Lu: It depends on the timescale. For example, LTP is regulated by mature BDNF and TrkB at different time windows. In the initial stages BDNF facilitates synaptic vesicle docking to the presynaptic site. Shortly after this there may be a regulation of the NMDA receptor on the postsynaptic side. Then, at a slightly different timescale, in a few hours, there is what is called spine morphing, which BDNF is involved in. Over 10–24 h BDNF also regulates postsynaptic spine formation. We are only looking at one synapse here.

Buonanno: I was interested in pro-BDNF.

Lu: Electron microscopic localization showed that p75 was in both pre and post synaptic sites. In terms of effects, we saw that it was primarily on the NMDA-dependent form of LTD, and is mediated through NR2B, so it has to be postsynaptic.

Walsh: There are now pharmacological tools that can assist in deciphering the role of these protease cascades. You mentioned that the level of plasmin is low. We find this level can be increased at the level of tPA. There is a negative regulator of tPA called PAI 7. We now have nanomolar potent brain-penetrant PAI 7 inhibitors that act to increase the level of plasmin. One of these compounds is now in phase 1 clinical trials for Alzheimer's disease. It is not just pro-BDNF that is a substrate, but also amyloid Aβ. We are very interested in modulating Aβ levels. In some of the models you showed we know that our PAI 7 inhibitors have positive effects. My point is that there are now agents that can modulate the amyloid Aβ pathway and also the BDNF pathway.

Lu: We have explored this a bit, using PAI1 and exploring BDNF regulation and cleavage by tPA. In addition, there is work by Huntley and colleagues (Nagy et al 2006), which implicates the metalloprotease system and MMP9 in addition to tPA.

Spedding: There you have to be careful about the metalloproteases breaking down the extracellular matrix and changing growth factor disposition.

Hen: Do your promoter 3 knock-ins still respond to antidepressants?

Lu: We haven't done this yet, but it's on our agenda. I'd predict that they won't respond to antidepressants.

Barde: I have a short comment regarding the role of p75 and LTD. Both Martin Korte and Bai Lu and colleagues found that in the absence of p75 LTD cannot be established any more. However, regarding any role of pro-BDNF, we are sceptical. We performed experiments with the BDNF knockout and found that LTD is still present, just as in wild-type. The bottom line is that while p75 is important for LTD, at least in the hippocampus, BDNF is not.

Lu: When BDNF is knocked out, both pro- and mature BDNF are removed. We know that mature BDNF inhibits LTD while pro-BDNF facilitates it. So the result from BDNF knockout mice is hard to interpret. The right experiment is to express uncleavable pro-BDNF selectively in the hippocampus to see whether there is more LTD. Normally we don't see LTD in adult animals.

Flint: Has anyone looked to see what transcription factors are binding in different tissues? Have people done chip on chip to see whether that differentiates the expression patterns?

Lu: Not a whole screen, but the promoter 3 has been well characterized by Mike Greenberg's group. There is a CREB binding site, CBP and SRE. There are also NF-κB binding sites and multiple factors binding to this. Also, Eric Nestler's group has recently identified the binding of HDACs to this promoter (Tsankova et al 2006).

Flint: If you look in the nucleus accumbens and compare that to hippocampus, what different patterns do you see in transcription factor binding sites?

Lu: That hasn't been done yet. It's intriguing why BDNF elicits opposite effects in the hippocampus and nucleus accumbens.

References

Aid T, Kazantseva A, Piirsoo M, Palm K, Timmusk T 2007 Mouse and rat BDNF gene structure and expression revisited. J Neurosci Res 85:525–535

Harrington AW, Leiner B, Blechschmitt C 2004 Secreted proNGF is a pathophysiological death-inducing ligand after adult CNS injury. Proc Natl Acad Sci USA 101:6226–6230

Ledesma MD, Da Silva JS, Crassaerts K, Delacourte A, De Strooper B, Dotti CG 2000 Brain plasmin enhances APP alpha-cleavage and Abeta degradation and is reduced in Alzheimer's disease brains. EMBO Rep 1:530–535

Michalski B, Fahnestock M 2003 Pro-brain-derived neurotrophic factor is decreased in parietal cortex in Alzheimer's disease. Brain Res Mol Brain Res 111:148–154

Nagy V, Bozdagi O, Matynia A et al 2006 Matrix metalloproteinase-9 is required for hippocampal late-phase long-term potentiation and memory. J Neurosci 26:1923–1934

Pawlak R, Magarinos AM, Melchor J, McEwen B, Strickland S 2003 Tissue plasminogen activator in the amygdala is critical for stress-induced anxiety-like behavior. Nat Neurosci 6:168–174

Peng S, Wuu J, Mufson EJ, Fahnestock M 2005 Precursor form of brain-derived neurotrophic factor and mature brain-derived neurotrophic factor are decreased in the pre-clinical stages of Alzheimer's disease. J Neurochem 93:1412–1421

Tsankova NM, Berton O, Renthal W, Kumar A, Neve RL, Nestler EJ 2006 Sustained hippocampal chromatin regulation in a mouse model of depression and antidepressant action. Nat Neurosci 9:519–525

Functions and mechanisms of BDNF mRNA trafficking

Enrico Tongiorgi and Gabriele Baj

BRAIN Centre for Neuroscience, University of Trieste, Via Giorgieri, 10-34127 Trieste, Italy

Abstract. Long-lasting changes in the basis of memory storage require delivery of newly synthesized proteins to the affected synapses. While most of these proteins are generated in the cell body, several key molecules for plasticity can be delivered in the form of silent mRNAs at synapses in extra-somatic compartments where they are locally translated in response to specific stimuli. One such mRNA encodes brain derived neurotrophic factor (BDNF), a key molecule in neuronal development that plays a critical role in learning and memory, and which displays abnormal levels in several neuropsychiatric disorders. BDNF mRNA accumulates in distal dendrites in response to stimuli that trigger activation of NMDAR and TrkB receptors. A single BDNF protein is produced from several splice variants having different 5'UTRs. We have shown that these mRNA variants have a different subcellular localization (soma, proximal or distal dendritic compartment) and that the protein is co-localized with the transcript from which it originated. As these splice variants are also differentially expressed in response to various stimuli and antidepressants, we propose that they represent a spatial and temporal code to regulate BDNF protein expression locally.

2008 Growth factors and psychiatric disorders. Wiley, Chichester (Novartis Foundation Symposium 289) p 136–151

One of the most fascinating challenges of neuroscience is to understand the molecular processes that mediate learning and memory. Advances in this field have direct relevance to the understanding of the pathophysiology of devastating forms of cognitive impairment found in neuropsychiatric diseases and mental retardation.

Long-term memory is the result of biochemical events that convert transient activity-dependent changes in neuronal activity into long-lasting alterations in synaptic responsiveness. Several studies have provided compelling evidence that long-lasting changes in synaptic efficacy are dependent on delivery of newly synthesized proteins to the post-synaptic compartment of affected synapses (Nguyen et al 1994, Reymann & Frey 2007). This line of research has yielded unexpected insights suggesting that the step of protein synthesis that is essential for long-term memory may occur locally in dendrites instead of the soma, as generally assumed

(Steward & Schuman 2001). Indeed, local mRNA translation in dendrites was shown to be important for maintaining long-term changes in synaptic strength (Kang & Schuman 1996, Reymann & Frey 2007). In support of this view, detailed immunohistochemical analysis indicates the presence of every component of the translation machinery in dendrites, including rRNAs, translation factors, endoplasmic reticulum and Golgi apparatus (reviewed in Sutton & Schuman 2005). Moreover, the frequent location of polyribosomes at the base of dendritic spines suggests that protein synthesis might be regulated, locally, by activity at individual synapses (Steward & Levy 1982).

The recent demonstration that cognitive impairment found in patients with the Fragile X syndrome of mental retardation is caused by defects in dendritic translation has underscored the central role of this process in learning and memory (Willemsen et al 2004). Accordingly, there have been several studies aimed at determining which mRNAs can actually be transported into the dendrites and then locally translated. The data available indicate that dendrites of hippocampal neurons can contain about 150–400 different mRNAs coding for all classes of proteins that were previously know to be involved in synaptic plasticity as well as house keeping proteins (Eberwine et al 2002, Zhong et al 2006, see Table 1). As a mammalian neuron can typically express between 15 000 and 30 000 different mRNAs, it can be estimated that dendritic mRNAs may represent about 1–2% of the whole neuronal transcriptome.

Although most studies on RNA targeting in neurons concern mainly the dendritic transport, increasing evidence indicates that mRNAs are also present in the axonal compartment (Giuditta et al 1991). It seems, however, that this mechanism

TABLE 1   Categories of dendritic mRNAs

Category of mRNAs in CA1 dendrites	Percentage
Receptors, ion channels, and postsynaptic molecules	7.8%
Cytoskeleton	7.8%
Extracellular matrix, cell adhesion, and immuno-molecules	20.1%
Signal transduction and protein modification	16.9%
Translation factors and RNA-binding proteins	4.5%
Ribosomal proteins	16.2%
Peptide processing and degradation	7.8%
Protein transport, membrane trafficking, endocytosis, and exocytosis	6.5%
Molecular motor	0.6%
Growth factors	2.6%
Other	9.1%

Groups represent dendritic RNA candidates that have dendritic signal vs. cell body signal ratios equal or greater than 2 and their relative abundance in dendrites of hippocampal CA1 neurons in adult rats. Adapted from Zhong et al (2006).

is more of an exception than a rule, and that it is present only in restricted populations of mature neurons, located mostly in the peripheral nervous system. In more general terms, targeting RNAs to a given cellular compartment is a phenomenon that is widely diffused in organisms as different as plants, fungi, insects, molluscs and vertebrates, and represents a mechanism extremely well conserved during evolution to segregate the production of proteins in highly polarized cells (Kloc et al 2002). Thus, it is not surprising that mRNA transport along the microtubules, one possible modality of cellular transport in eukaryotes, is driven even in neural cells by evolutionary conserved mechanisms involving formation of 'transporting granules' (Kritchevski & Kosik 2001). These large complexes contain mRNAs, non-coding RNAs and RNA binding proteins (RBPs) most of which are conserved from *Drosophila* to human. Examples of such RNA binding factors are Staufen, Barentz, Pumilio and the protein families of the Fragile-X, hn-RNP and CPEB (Kanai et al 2004).

BDNF is a dendritically targeted mRNA

Brain-derived neurotrophic factor (BDNF) is a member of the neurotrophin family that has been implicated in multiple aspects of neuronal plasticity and recent studies suggest that its local translation in dendrites may play a key role in establishing long-lasting forms of synaptic plasticity (Pang et al 2004). In addition, through activation of its receptor, TrkB, BDNF can control activation of local protein synthesis during long-term potentiation (LTP, Bramham & Messaoudi 2005). The prominent role of BDNF in synaptic plasticity and in memory formation has suggested that any genetic or environmental influences on its activity or expression may interfere with brain function. Accordingly, reduced levels of BDNF have been found in a variety of human neuropsychiatric conditions, including Alzheimer's disease, schizophrenia and mood disorders (Chao et al 2006). A human single nucleotide polymorphism (Val66Met) that reduces BDNF secretion and localization of the protein in dendrites was found associated with reduced memory performance (Egan et al 2003) and bipolar disorder.

The first clear evidence that BDNF and TrkB mRNAs are located in dendrites was found in primary cultures of rat hippocampal neurons where, under basal conditions, these two mRNAs are localized in the initial dendritic compartment (an average of 31.5 μm from the cell soma considering all types of dendrites and within a range of 30–100 μm from the cell soma, when considering apical dendrites only). However, in response to tetanic electrical activity induced by elevated concentrations of KCl (10 or 20 mM) in the culture medium, these mRNAs extended to the distal dendrites (further than 100 μm) (Tongiorgi et al 1997). Interestingly, depolarization induced an accumulation of BDNF and TrkB mRNAs in secondary and tertiary dendritic branchings of large calibre dendrites but rarely in the very fine, distal process endings. Later, we found that the BDNF and TrkB mRNAs are localized in the dendrites of various types of neurons including hippocampal, cortical and basal forebrain neurons (Molnar et al 1998, Capsoni et al 1999) and that *in vivo* they are strongly accumulated into distal dendrites in response to visual activity (Capsoni et al 1999) or seizures (Tongiorgi et al 2004).

The first step in the cascade of events leading to this phenomenon appears to be the activation of NMDA receptors. *In vitro* and *in vivo* evidence support this idea: (1) in culture, electrical activity-dependent dendritic targeting of both BDNF and TrkB mRNA can be completely abolished by blockers of glutamate receptors (Tongiorgi et al 1997); (2) *in vivo*, the NMDA receptor antagonist (MK801) blocks seizure-induced dendritic targeting of BDNF mRNA (Tongiorgi et al 2004). Dendritic targeting of BDNF mRNA does not appear to depend upon an increase in gene transcription, because NMDA receptor agonists do not induce BDNF mRNA expression (Zafra et al 1990), and because activity-dependent BDNF and TrkB mRNA targeting *in vitro* occurs without new mRNA transcription (Tongiorgi et al 1997). Accumulation of BDNF and TrkB mRNAs in distal dendrites requires the presence of Ca^{2+} in the external culture medium and Ca^{2+} influx into the cell through glutamate receptors (NMDA-type) and voltage-gated L-type Ca^{2+} channels (Tongiorgi et al 1997, 2004, Righi et al 2000). We also found that BDNF itself contributes to the redistribution of its own mRNA into the dendrites and that it does so through activation of a TrkB-mediated PI3 kinase intracellular signalling cascade (Righi et al 2000). Exogenous application of BDNF induced a targeting of BDNF or TrkB mRNAs to a distance which was about half of that observed in KCl-stimulated neurons, suggesting activation of only one component of the targeting mechanism.

A brief depolarization by KCl was able to increase the endogenous protein levels of both BDNF and TrkB in distal dendrites. Since this increase occurred within 10 minutes, up to distances greater than $100\,\mu m$ from the cell soma and BDNF protein trafficking is $0.1\,\mu m/s$ (equivalent to $6\,\mu m/min$) it is unlikely that the protein level increase was due to transport of BDNF or TrkB from the cell soma. In addition, protein up-regulation occurred even under conditions in which microtubule-mediated transport was disrupted by application of nocodazole. Thus, this study strongly suggested that BDNF and TrkB mRNAs localized to the distal dendrites can to be locally translated into protein (Tongiorgi et al 1997).

This first study however, did not address the important question of whether the mRNA for BDNF is present in distal dendrites constitutively. Through high resolution *in situ* hybridization on rat brain sections at the electron microscopy level, BDNF mRNA was also found to be localized in apical dendrites of CA1 neurons of untreated animals, at distances greater than $70\,\mu m$ from the soma (Tongiorgi et al 2004). Most interestingly, in the dendritic compartment it was associated with polyribosomes (Tongiorgi et al 2004), suggesting active translation. TrkB mRNA was also found localized in the proximal somato-dendritic compartment of unstimulated hippocampal neurons *in vitro* (Tongiorgi et al 1997), and of basal forebrain neurons *in vivo* in untreated animals, while the mRNAs for the other neurotrophin receptors TrkA, TrkC and p75 were restricted to the cell soma (Tongiorgi et al 2000). In agreement with these findings, BDNF and TrkB mRNAs have been amplified from dendritic mRNA prepared from synapto-neurosomes (Eberwine at al 2002). It is therefore conceivable that, in dendrites, the local availability of BDNF and TrkB is controlled through regulation of both dendritic targeting and local translation of their mRNAs. Evidence that this might be the case has come from our recent studies on epileptogenesis and visual cortex.

Epileptogenic stimuli trigger accumulation of dendritic BDNF mRNA

Epileptogenic limbic seizures cause a dramatic accumulation of BDNF and TrkB mRNAs in the dendrites (Simonato et al 2002, Tongiorgi et al 2004). BDNF mRNA dramatically accumulates in the distal dendrites of all principal hippocampal neurons after pilocarpine administration in the rat, with a peak at 3 h after onset of status epilepticus. Accumulation of BDNF mRNA was also observed in two other models of temporal lobe epilepsy (kainate and kindling) and occurred during epileptogenesis (i.e. after pilocarpine- and kainate-induced status epilepticus, or after the initial seizures induced by kindling stimulation), but not after epileptic seizures in chronic animals. This suggests that the phenomenon is associated with the development, and not with the maintenance, of epilepsy. Non-epileptogenic stimuli, i.e. stimuli that are not followed by spontaneous seizures or by a decreased seizure threshold, such as single maximal electroshock seizures or continuous perforant path stimulation for 2 hours, did not induce accumulation of BDNF mRNA into the dendritic compartment (Tongiorgi et al 2004). The latter type of stimulus is known to induce a robust LTP at synapses between the entorhynal cortex (perforant path axons) and the apical dendrites of dentate gyrus granules cells. The lack of accumulation of BDNF mRNA in dendrites at 2 hours following this type of hippocampal LTP induction does not exclude the possibility that enhanced mRNA trafficking might occur later, e.g. during the consolidation phase or in response to other types of LTP-induction protocols. On the other hand, accumulation of BDNF mRNA in dendrites might not represent one event that occurs during LTP induction, which is different from another dendritic mRNA, encoding Arc, which is both targeted and translated in dendrites within the first hour following the same protocol for LTP-induction (Steward et al 1998).

Several features of the pilocarpine seizure-induced accumulation of BDNF mRNA in the dendrites have been identified (Tongiorgi et al 2004). First, epileptogenic seizures cause BDNF mRNA to localize selectively at particular sets of synapses. For example, after pilocarpine-induced seizures, BDNF mRNA localizes in CA3 stratum lucidum that corresponds to the terminal fields of the mossy fibres (originating from the granule cells) or in the inner third of the dentate gyrus molecular layer that contains all terminations of the associational-commissural projection system originating from neurons in the hilus of the dentate gyrus. These neurons are highly activated during the seizures and, therefore, the selective targeting of BDNF mRNA to the sites of their terminations coincides with the set of synapses that are most active. Second, dendritic accumulation of BDNF mRNA appears to be co-ordinately regulated with TrkB mRNA in both the expression pattern and the dendritic localization (Simonato et al 2002). Third, BDNF protein is preferentially localized in cell bodies and axons under basal conditions (Conner et al 1997), but it accumulates in dendrites after pilocarpine-induced seizures, with a distribution and a time-course that match those of its mRNA (Tongiorgi et al 2004).

Visual experience induces BDNF mRNA targeting in the visual cortex

By analogy with the hippocampus, in the visual cortex BDNF mRNA is expressed in the soma of pyramidal cells as well as in their dendrites (Capsoni et al 1999). This is particularly visible in layer V neurons of adult rats, while during an early stage of postnatal development BDNF mRNA is localized in a few cell perykaria but not in dendrites (Pattabiraman et al 2005). Thus, not only the cellular expression throughout cortical layers but also the subcellular localization of BDNF mRNA is modified during postnatal development.

Visual experience regulates the sub-cellular distribution of BDNF mRNA. Accordingly, BDNF mRNA targeting in pyramidal cell dendrites is abolished by dark rearing but resumes after 2 h of exposure to normal light (Capsoni et al 1999). Similarly, in rat primary cortical cultures, decrease of neuronal activity, as obtained by tetrodotoxin (TTX), induces a restriction of BDNF mRNA to cell bodies, whereas an increase of neuronal activity after treatment with KCl augments dendritic targeting of BDNF mRNA (Pattabiraman et al 2005).

BDNF mRNA splice variants

All genes encoding neurotrophins have basically a similar structure, but among these the genomic structure of the BDNF gene is unusually complex. The complete structural organization of mouse, rat and human BDNF gene has been characterized in detail only recently (Liu et al 2005, Aid et al 2007). This gene contains multiple promoters that drive the expression of transcripts bearing different non-coding exons spliced upstream of a common 3' exon that encompasses the entire encoding sequence (Fig. 1). In particular, the BDNF gene encodes eight two-part transcripts that have been termed BDNF1, 2A, 2B, 2C, 3, 4, 5 and 6A (Fig. 2).

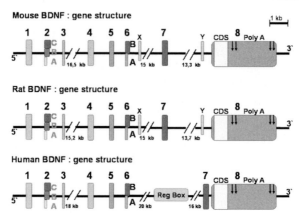

FIG. 1. BDNF gene structures for rodents and human as reported from NCBI in April 2007.
X and Y are two possible exons recently updated by Aid et al (2007). The box in the human
BDNF gene seems to be the site of an antisense gene called BDNFOS that is a candidate regulator RNA for human BDNF translation. Interestingly, this is the only part of the gene not
present in rodent genes.

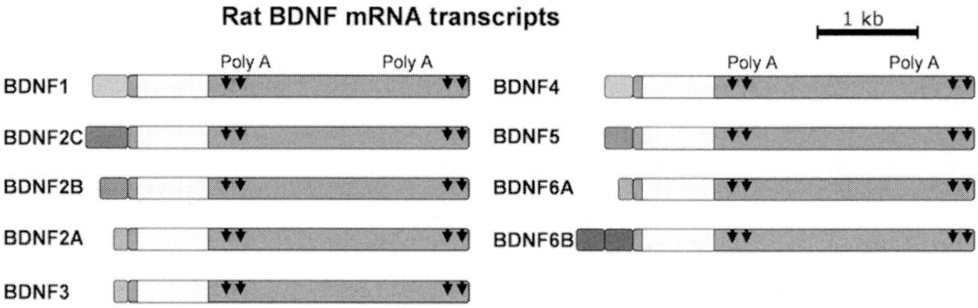

FIG. 2. Rat BDNF splicing variant transcripts expressed in brain as reported by Liu et al
(2006).

For each, the exon that encodes a different 5′-untranslated region begins transcripts that are spliced to a major peptide-encoding exon 8. In addition, a three-
part transcript, BDNF6B, is the result of splicing events that incorporate exons
6B, 7 and 8. Each BDNF exon is flanked by consensus splice acceptor (AG) and
donor (GT) sites. The most abundant splice variants in rodents corresponding to
the variants 1, 2, 4 and 5 were previously known (Aid et al 2007; variants I, II, III
and IV, respectively) and characterized in different organs. However, it must be
emphasized that the function of the different BDNF transcripts remains
obscure.

All BDNF transcripts initiated from different BDNF exons are anticipated (Liu
et al 2005) to produce four different proBDNF precursor products (proBDNF1–4;

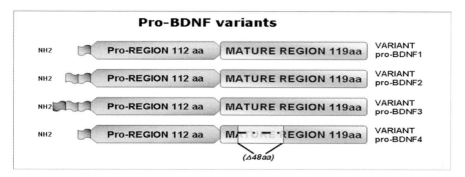

FIG. 3.   BDNF pre-pro-protein variants encoded by the human BDNF gene. The different protein variants differ only in the length of the signalling peptide (flags at *N*-terminus). The presence of a variant (pro-BDNF4) with a 48aa deletion in the mature region of the protein as suggested by Liu et al (2006) has not been confirmed *in vivo*.

Fig. 3) with molecular weights 28–32 kDa, which in turn produce a 14 kDa mature BDNF protein through proteolytic cleavage (Mowla et al 2001). ProBDNF2 encoded by BDNF1 and proBDNF3 encoded by BDNF6B contain 8 and 15 additional N-terminal amino acids, respectively, in comparison with proBDNF1. ProBDNF4 differs from the other isoforms in that it presents a deletion of 48 amino acids inside the mature region (Liu et al 2005).

Remarkably, different isoforms of BDNF are expressed in different subcellular compartments: exon 5 (IV, old nomenclature)-containing mRNAs have been detected both in the soma and dendrites while exon 4 (III) expression is restricted to the cell body (Pattabiraman et al 2005). Dark rearing *in vivo* (Capsoni et al 1999) and blockade of spiking activity *in vivo* and *in vitro* prevents translocation of BDNF mRNAs to the dendrites, specifically of those encoded by exon 5 (IV) (Pattabiraman et al 2005), resulting in their accumulation in the soma. Among the different BDNF transcripts we studied the localization of the most expressed in hippocampus by cloning the rat BDNF coding sequence (rCDS), in frame with the green fluorescent protein (GFP) reporter gene, alone or preceded by one of four rat BDNF 5'UTR (exon1, exon2C, exon3 and exon4). Results suggest that mRNA and protein are precisely co-localized (see Fig. 4)

Function of the differential localization of BDNF splice variants: a novel paradigm

One attractive hypothesis is that the different BDNF mRNA isoforms may contribute to the local expression of BDNF in different cellular compartments at different times during postnatal life and in response to different stimuli. Activity-dependent transcription, distinct turnover properties or translational

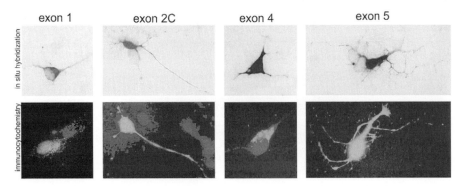

FIG. 4.   mRNA and protein co-localization in hippocampal neurons. Hippocampal neurons were transfected with different BDNF–GFP chimeras encoding for the most expressed BDNF mRNA transcripts (BDNF 1, 2C, 4, 5) under physiological condition in the hippocampus. The mRNAs of the splice variants were localized through *in situ* experiments using a riboprobe against the region encoding GFP. Furthermore, the localization of the chimeric BDNF–GFP protein was detected through specific immunocytochemistry using a primary antibody against GFP and a fluoresceinated secondary antibody.

competence of the different BDNF isoforms may account for differences in the availability of BDNF at specific subcellular districts. More specifically, exon 4 (III, old nomenclature) transcripts, being present only in the soma, could be involved in maturation of interneurons through a trans-synaptic route: indeed, a subset of cortical inhibitory neurons, the basket parvalbuminergic cells, as well as in the dentate gyrus of the hippocampus, make synapses almost exclusively with the soma of the pyramidal neurons and express TrkB (reviewed in Tongiorgi et al 2006). On the other hand, there are other neurons, mainly excitatory, which form synapses with dendrites, and whose synaptic maturation might be regulated by local release of BDNF produced by translation of exon 5 (IV)-containing mRNAs targeted to dendrites. Importantly, dendritic release of BDNF acting on a local scale has been reported to affect nearby dendrites of recipient cells (Horch & Katz 2002).

   Thus, targeting of BDNF mRNA to different districts of cortical and hippocampal neurons may be necessary for local release of BDNF in order to confer spatial and temporal specificity to the process of synaptic strengthening/depression.

Outcome for neuropsychiatric disorders

According to this novel paradigm it is of great interest to reconsider the effects of pharmacological treatments on BDNF gene expression (Castren 2004). Many recent studies have shown that different BDNF mRNA splice variants are

TABLE 2   Summary of exon-specific effects of antidepressant in chronic treatments

	BDNF mRNA transcripts in hippocampus after chronic treatment			
	ex1	ex2	ex4	ex5
ECS	▲ + 75%	=	▲ + 10%	▼ −20%
Fluoextine	▲ + 60%	=	▲ + 30%	=
Desipramine	▲ + 20%	=	▲ + 70%	▼ −20%
Tranylcypromine	▲ + 50%	=	=	▼ −20%

ECS, electro convulsive seizure; Fluoxetine, selective serotonin reuptake inhibitor; Desipramine, nore-pinephrine selective reuptake inhibitor; Tranylcypromine, non-hydrazine reversible monoamine oxidase inhibitor. The expression of different BDNF exon-specific transcripts was quantified trough real time PCR experiments and shows a differential regulation of BDNF gene.

modulated by antidepressants differently and in a region-specific manner (Dias et al 2003), suggesting that diverse antidepressants have directed actions on specific BDNF exon promoters. These results clearly suggest that diverse classical antidepressant treatments (Fluoxetine, Desipramine, Tranylcypromine) and atypical treatments (electro convulsive seizure) produce long-lasting specific changes in BDNF transcripts expression in brain areas related to mood regulation (Table 2). On this basis we propose that the different BDNF mRNA transcripts may follow or represent a spatial and temporal code for BDNF protein expression both in the developing brain and during mature life.

Acknowledgements

This work has been supported by the Italian Ministry of University and Research (PRIN 2005) and Telethon grant E0954 to E.T.

References

Aid T, Kazantseva A, Piirsoo M, Palm K, Timmusk T 2007 Mouse and rat BDNF gene structure and expression revisited. J Neurosci Res 15:525–535

Bramham CR, Messaoudi E 2005 BDNF function in adult synaptic plasticity: the synaptic consolidation hypothesis. Prog Neurobiol 76:99–125

Capsoni S, Tongiorgi E, Cattaneo A, Domenici L 1999 Differential regulation of brain-derived neurotrophic factor mRNA cellular expression in the adult rat visual cortex. Neuroscience 93:1033–1040

Castren E 2004 Neurotrophic effects of antidepressant drugs. Curr Opin Pharmacol 4:58–64

Chao MV, Rajagopal R, Lee FS 2006 Neurotrophin signalling in health and disease. Clin Sci (Lond) 110:167–173

Conner JM, Lauterborn JC, Yan Q, Gall CM, Varon S 1997 Distribution of brain-derived neurotrophic factor (BDNF) protein and mRNA in the normal adult rat CNS: evidence for anterograde axonal transport. J Neurosci 17:2295–2310

Dias BG, Banerjee SB, Duman RS, Vaidya VA 2003 Differential regulation of brain derived neurotrophic factor transcripts by antidepressant treatments in the adult rat brain. Neuropharmacology 45:553–563

Eberwine J, Belt B, Kacharmina JE, Miyashiro K 2002 Analysis of subcellularly localized mRNAs using in situ hybridization, mRNA amplification, and expression profiling. Neurochem Res 27:1065–1077

Egan MF, Kojima M, Callicott JH et al 2003 The BDNF Val66Met polymorphism affects activity-dependent secretion of BDNF and human memory and hippocampal function. Cell 112:257–269

Giuditta A, Menichini E, Perrone Capano C et al 1991 Active polysomes in the axoplasm of the squid giant axon. J Neurosci Res 28:18–28

Horch HW, Katz LC 2002 BDNF release from single cells elicits local dendritic growth in nearby neurons. Nat Neurosci 5:1177–1184

Kanai Y, Dohmae N, Hirokawa N 2004 Kinesin transports RNA: isolation and characterization of an RNA-transporting granule. Neuron 43:513–525

Kang H, Schuman EM 1996 A requirement for local protein synthesis in neurotrophin-induced hippocampal synaptic plasticity. Science 6:1402–1406

Kloc M, Zearfoss NR, Etkin LD 2002 Mechanisms of subcellular mRNA localization. Cell 108:533–544

Krichevsky AM, Kosik KS 2001 Neuronal RNA granules: a link between RNA localization and stimulation-dependent translation. Neuron 32:683–696

Liu QR, Walther D, Drgon T et al 2005 Human brain derived neurotrophic factor (BDNF) genes, splicing patterns, and assessments of associations with substance abuse and Parkinson's Disease. Am J Med Genet B Neuropsychiatr Genet 134:93–103

Liu QR, Lu L, Zhu XG, Gong JP, Shaham Y, Uhl GR 2006 Rodent BDNF genes, novel promoters, novel splice varicants, and regulation by cocaine. Brain Res 1067:1–12

Molnar M, Tongiorgi E, Avignone E et al 1998 The effects of anti-nerve growth factor monoclonal antibodies on developing basal forebrain neurons are transient and reversible. Eur J Neurosci 10:3127–3140

Mowla SJ, Farhadi HF, Pareek S et al 2001 Biosynthesis and post-translational processing of the precursor to brain derived neurotrophic factor. J Biol Chem 276:12660–12666

Nguyen PV, Abel T, Kandel ER 1994 Requirement of a critical period of transcription for induction of a late phase of LTP. Science 265:1104–1107

Pang PT, Teng HK, Zaitsev E et al 2004 Cleavage of proBDNF by tPA/plasmin is essential for long-term hippocampal plasticity. Science 15:487–491

Pattabiraman PP, Tropea D, Chiaruttini C, Tongiorgi E, Cattaneo A, Domenici L 2005 Neuronal activity regulates the developmental expression and subcellular localization of cortical BDNF mRNA isoforms in vivo. Mol Cell Neurosci 28:556–570

Reymann KG, Frey JU 2007 The late maintenance of hippocampal LTP: requirements, phases, 'synaptic tagging', 'late-associativity' and implications. Neuropharmacology 52:24–40

Righi M, Tongiorgi E, Cattaneo A 2000 Brain-derived neurotrophic factor (BDNF) induces dendritic targeting of BDNF and tyrosine kinase B mRNAs in hippocampal neurons through a phosphatidylinositol-3 kinase-dependent pathway. J Neurosci 1:3165–3174

Simonato M, Bregola G, Armellin M et al 2002 Dendritic targeting of mRNAs for plasticity genes in experimental models of temporal lobe epilepsy. Epilepsia 43:153–158

Steward O, Levy WB 1982 Preferential localization of polyribosomes under the base of dendritic spines in granule cells of the dentate gyrus. J Neurosci 2:284–291

Steward O, Schuman EM 2001 Protein synthesis at synaptic sites on dendrites. Annu Rev Neurosci 24:299–325

Steward O, Wallace CS, Lyford GL, Worley PF 1998 Synaptic activation causes the mRNA for the IEG Arc to localize selectively near activated postsynaptic sites on dendrites. Neuron 21:741–751

Sutton MA, Schuman EM 2005 Local translational control in dendrites and its role in long-term synaptic plasticity. J Neurobiol 64:116–131
Tongiorgi E, Righi M, Cattaneo A 1997 Activity-dependent dendritic targeting of BDNF and TrkB mRNAs in hippocampal neuorons. J Neurosci 17:9492–9505
Tongiorgi E, Armellin M, Cattaneo A 2000 Differential somato-dendritic localization of TrkA, TrkB, TrkC and p75 mRNAs in vivo. Neuroreport 28:3265–3268
Tongiorgi E, Armellin M, Giulianini PG et al 2004 BDNF mRNA and protein are targeted to discrete dendritic laminae by events that trigger epileptogenesis. J Neurosci 30:6842–6852
Tongiorgi E, Domenici L, Simonato M 2006 What is the biological significance of BDNF mRNA targeting in the dendrites? Clues from epilepsy and cortical development. Mol Neurobiol 33:17–32
Willemsen R, Oostra BA, Bassell GJ, Dictenberg J 2004 The fragile X syndrome: from molecular genetics to neurobiology. Ment Retard Dev Disabil Res Rev 10:60–67
Zafra F, Hengerer B, Leibrock J, Thoenen H, Lindholm D 1990 Activity dependent regulation of BDNF and NGF mRNAs in the rat hippocampus is mediated by non-NMDA glutamate receptors. EMBO J 9:3545–3550
Zhong J, Zhang T, Bloch LM 2006 Dendritic mRNAs encode diversified functionalities in hippocampal pyramidal neurons. BMC Neurosci 7:7

DISCUSSION

Chao: The analysis of BDNF mRNA you presented is quite extensive. Is there any common theme or thread in terms of mechanism with other RNAs that are locally translated?

Tongiorgi: In terms of trafficking of the mRNA, there are some RNA-binding proteins that function as a general binder. Staufen is one of these; it is present in all RNA transporting granules and therefore is likely to mediate trafficking of any dendritic mRNA. This would be a target if you wanted to modulate the entire pool of dendritic proteins. Most likely, the composition of the granules might change according to specific pools. One of the hypotheses that I put forward is that each granule represents a small programme, because it includes a series of mRNAs to make each synapse bigger or depressed. The other side of the story is the protein translation. Clive Bramham in Norway (Soulé et al 2006) has demonstrated that BDNF is a key molecule in activating local protein synthesis. Also, the studies in fragile X suggest that other signalling pathways are involved, such as the metabotropic glutamate receptor. But the regulatory mechanisms of protein translation appear to be more simple. Perhaps the endpoint is that trafficking is more specific for a specific mRNA, and translation is more generalized.

Lee: We think that there is another trafficking protein called sortilin (Chen et al 2005). It is possible to have both of these defects in the same neuron: an mRNA defect and a sorting into the regulating pathway, such that there's a defect at the Golgi and a defect at the mRNA level in the dendrites. It will be a lot of work to figure out under what conditions each one is predominant. It is early days.

Tongiorgi: I'm pretty sure that the two mechanisms should coexist. I don't think this tiny change in trafficking can completely support the deficits in memory.

Akil: This whole area of synthesis in the dendrites has been new to me over the last couple of years. I am confused about the meaning of it. If I understand correctly, NMDA blockade increases spine protein synthesis. Is that correct?

Tongiorgi: Well, not really. Activation of NMDA receptor activates local translation of CaMKII-α through a mechanism dependent on Aurora-kinase/CPEB activation and polyadenylation (Wu et al 1998, Wells et al 2001). On the other hand, if you give convulsant agents to rats and then block the NMDA receptor by administering MK801, a general blocker of NMDA receptors, you don't see targeting of BDNF mRNA. This means that activation of the NMDA receptor is important for stimulating mechanisms of increased transport. Transport of RNA transporting granules can be induced by activation of the NMDA receptor, activation of the TrkB receptor through BDNF, and activation of TrkC receptor through NT3. NGF has no effect, at least in the hippocampus.

Buonnano: The new story is that spontaneous release of glutamate, which elicits mini excitatory postsynaptic currents, keeps the translation at bay. Then when you have a stimulus, you translate proteins at dendrites. Spontaneous activity is suppressing, in a continuous fashion, the local translation.

Tongiorgi: Along these lines, Erin Schuman is proposing that there is a bunch of different neurotransmitters, including dopamine and acetylcholine, which are able to stimulate local protein synthesis (Sutton & Schumann 2005). You may think of this in terms of coincidence of stimuli. This can also be translated into behavioural coincidence of cues. Thinking in terms of neuroanatomy, there may be an intrinsic hippocampal glutamatergic fibre and then an extra-hippocampal stimulus from other regions that form synapses on the same hippocampal neuron. Their coincident or sequential activation induces formation of specific signals that activate local translation of dendritic mRNAs. It is important to have this neuroanatomical correlation.

Lu: I am going to play devil's advocate. Let's say that activity drives mRNA to go further distal. The simplistic idea would be that whatever synapse is closer to the cell body will get more BDNF when BDNF mRNAs are produced in the cell nucleus. The reality in synaptic modulation is that sometimes the more distal synapses get potentiated. If BDNF regulates synaptic potentiation, then your model would not work. Whatever synapse is closest to the cell body will get more BDNF, so the proximal synapses will always get more BDNF than the distal ones.

Tongiorgi: That's a nice question that allows me to introduce another variable. In brain there isn't simply spatial and neuroanatomical distribution, there is also time. In LTP there are different timings. The first event that occurs is a rapid release of vesicles. Then there is local activation of synaptic machinery in terms of protein modification of kinases. Then, within the first two to four hours there is no new mRNA synthesis. The only thing that is needed is a local translation of proteins, or translation of proteins from other parts of the cell. The trafficking of the mRNA comes only 6 h after the favourable stimulus. It is also important to consider time in terms of age of the animals. Most of the studies that have been done on the role of BDNF in LTP were in juvenile animals, not the adult. It is important to compare studies in which people have looked at LTP in adult animals. There is plenty of room to have a second wave of mRNA trafficking later on, during a consolidation phase. The two things are not in conflict.

Lu: Conceptually, it is difficult to think how a synapse more distal to the cell body might be potentiated while the proximal one is not, if BDNF mRNAs all come from the cell body in an activity-dependent manner.

Tongiorgi: The mRNA for BDNF is there: we have shown it through *in situ* hybridizations at the electron microscopy level in our paper published in 2004 (Tongiorgi et al 2004). However, at the early stage of LTP induction, you simply need to have the proteins present. You need first of all secretion, which occurs immediately. Then within the first half an hour you need to have a round of protein synthesis. This can occur in dendrites. Then later on during consolidation signals travel to the nucleus and activate mRNA transcription. It is like synapses are calling the nucleus, saying something happened here and we need more RNA.

Lu: I have a bigger conceptual problem, which has to do with the new concept postulated by Mike Ehlers on Golgi outposts (Horton et al 2005). I can understand local translation for cytosolic proteins, because it does not require Golgi and vesicles. But for BDNF, what is needed is not only mRNA and ribosomes being present. The protein synthesized in the ER will need to be processed in Golgi before it is packed in the vesicle and released. According to Mike Ehlers there are very few Golgi outposts in neurons. One neuron has only one or two Golgi outposts in the branch point of a major dendrite. If this is the case, all the BDNF proteins synthesized locally in the dendrites will have to come back down to the Golgi outposts for processing and making vesicles, and then go back to dendrites again.

Tongiorgi: I agree with you. We and others have found that the mRNA is not located everywhere, but rather in hotspots. I also showed in our paper published in 1997 (Tongiorgi et al 1997) that if we block protein transport with nocodazole, we also see local hotspots of protein increase. These correspond to dendritic branching and varicosities. This is not in contrast with Mike Ehlers work (Horton et al 2005). It is not necessary for BDNF and other dendritic proteins to be synthesized in close proximity to one specific synapse (although this might happen). They might also be synthesized at Golgi guideposts and then delivered to neighbouring synapses through a short-range protein transport. So, 'private' protein synthesis for single synapses and 'shared' synthesis for multiple synapses may well coexist. We don't have to think in terms of black and white: nature is made up of a continuous series of greys.

Lu: If you think local translation of BDNF contributes to a synapse-specific regulation, there is a problem here.

Tongiorgi: Tobias Bonhoeffer has shown that synapses that are co-regulated in a BDNF-dependent manner are spanning a stretch of dendrites that is between 50 and 80 μm (Engert & Bonhoeffer 1997). This means that a group of synapses are regulated together. This makes sense: in the brain coincidence is needed for a signal that matters.

Chao: Is this an example of synaptic tagging, or does this reflect a different event?

Tongiorgi: Synaptic tagging may also be part of the story, for instance by anchoring translation factors or mRNA to a stimulated synapse. However, synaptic tagging might not involve a single synapse but a group.

Lu: In the field of synaptic plasticity and memory, the concept of synaptic specificity is very important. Although there is local diffusion, if you potentiate all the synapses you cannot form memory.

Tongiorgi: There are only specific places in which a cell can make proteins. Some of the proteins might be synthesized at synapses, but most of the proteins are not so specific. There is a larger distribution. You may have RNAs that are at synapses, but in my opinion only large synapses, not all of them. Additionally, you may have protein synthesis at Golgi outposts, which would imply that proteins need to be transported until their final destination at specific (tagged) synapses. If I produce BDNF in one site I can influence a series of synapses in this area.

Lee: Mike Ehlers' paper (Horton & Ehlers 2003) didn't have electron microscopy studies that looked for real Golgi-like structures.

Lu: There is more general work now showing that there is only one Golgi outpost. If this is correct and there is only one Golgi in one of the dendrites, whatever BDNF is produced locally in a dendrite has to come back down and get processed, and then move back to the dendrite to modulate the synapse.

Kahn: How solid is the evidence that there is only one Golgi guidepost?

Lu: Quite solid. This is why the idea is provocative.

Tongiorgi: The answer may be simpler. There is no evidence that mRNAs can go to the very distal part of the dendrites. They stop at a certain point. Our mRNA, even if it is overexpressed, doesn't get over 75% of the entire length.

Lu: This means that trafficking of mRNA is less important in terms of contributing to local translation, if it stays closer to the cell body.

Tongiorgi: Sometimes 5% or 10% in nature could be a huge difference, so I don't say what is more important or what is less—just what we found.

Buonnano: You are strongly proposing this because of the synaptic tagging issue, I would imagine. But the point is that synaptic tagging really remains a hypothesis.

There is evidence from electrophysiology that indicates that there is a memory left. This is done with two-pathway stimulation, which doesn't have single synapse resolution.

Lu: No. Local protein synthesis in the dendrites means you don't need a synaptic tag, which is used to catch proteins synthesized in the cell body, to achieve synapse (or dendritic branch) specificity. Local protein synthesis and synaptic tagging are two independent ideas to explain how late-phase LTP can be synapse-specific.

Chao: We need more cell biological studies to resolve this question.

References

Chen ZY, Ieraci A, Teng H et al 2005 Sortilin controls intracellular sorting of brain-derived neurotrophic factor to the regulated secretory pathway. J Neurosci 25:6156–6166

Engert F, Bonhoeffer T 1997 Synapse specificity of long-term potentiation breaks down at short distances. Nature 388:279–284 (erratum: 1997 Nature 388:698)

Horton AC, Ehlers MD 2003 Dual modes of endoplasmic reticulum-to-Golgi transport in dendrites revealed by live-cell imaging. J Neurosci 23:6188–6199

Horton AC, Racz B, Monson EE, Lin AL, Weinberg RJ, Ehlers MD 2005 Polarized secretory trafficking directs cargo for asymmetric dendrite growth and morphogenesis. Neuron 48:757–771

Soulé J, Messaoudi E, Bramham CR 2006 Brain-derived neurotrophic factor and control of synaptic consolidation in the adult brain. Biochem Soc Trans 34:600–604

Sutton MA, Schuman EM 2005 Local translational control in dendrites and its role in long-term synaptic plasticity. J Neurobiol 64:116–131

Tongiorgi E, Righi M, Cattaneo A 1997 Activity-dependent dendritic targeting of BDNF and TrkB mRNAs in hippocampal neurons. J Neurosci 17:9492–9505

Tongiorgi E, Armellin M Giulianini PG et al 2004 Brain-derived neurotrophic factor mRNA and protein are targeted to discrete dendritic laminas by events that trigger epileptogenesis. J Neurosci 24:6842–6852

Wells DG, Dong X, Quinlan EM et al 2001 A role for the cytoplasmic polyadenylation element in NMDA receptor-regulated mRNA translation in neurons. J Neurosci 21:9541–9548

Wu GY, Wells D, Tay J et al 1998 CPEB-mediated cytoplasmic polyadenylation and the regulation of experience-dependent translation of alpha-CAMKII mRNA at synapses. Neuron 21:1129–1139

Hippocampal neurogenesis and depression

Amar Sahay and René Hen

Departments of Neuroscience and Psychiatry, Columbia University, New York, NY 10032, USA

Abstract. Various chronic antidepressant treatments increase adult hippocampal neurogenesis, but the functional importance of this phenomenon remains unclear. Using radiological and genetic methods, we show that disrupting neurogenesis blocks behavioural responses to antidepressants. X-irradiation of a restricted region of mouse brain containing the hippocampus prevented the neurogenic and behavioural effects of two classes of antidepressants. Similarly, a genetic strategy that ablates adult progenitor cells resulted in a lack of effect of antidepressants. In addition, we have identified a form of long-term potentiation in the dentate gyrus that is dependent on the presence of young neurons and which is stimulated by antidepressants. These findings suggest that the behavioural effects of chronic antidepressants require hippocampal neurogenesis and are mediated by an increased synaptic plasticity in the dentate gyrus.

2008 Growth factors and psychiatric disorders. Wiley, Chichester (Novartis Foundation Symposium 289) p 152–164

Adult hippocampal neurogenesis is a robust phenomenon that is capable of conferring previously unrecognized forms of plasticity to the dentate gyrus. The progression from neural stem cell to mature dentate granule neuron can be divided into discrete stages, each of which is defined by distinct physiological and mor-phological properties (Esposito et al 2005, Song et al 2005) and influenced by a plethora of factors including growth factors, neurotrophins and chemokines (Lledo et al 2006). These factors act in concert with network activity to regulate the balance between proliferation, differentiation and survival of neural stem cells *in vivo*. It is through this general mechanism that levels of adult hippocampal neurogenesis change in response to aversive and enriching experiences, such as stress and learning, respectively, and the physiological state of the organism. Recent studies relying on experimental approaches that ablate adult hippocampal neurogenesis in rodents have shed some light on the contribution of neurogenesis to emotional reactivity and learning.

Experimental approaches to probe the role of adult hippocampal neurogenesis in behaviour

Preclinical studies have proven tremendously informative in bridging the 'causality gap' between adult hippocampus neurogenesis and behaviour. To date, three different loss-of-function approaches have been used to ablate adult hippocampal neurogenesis. These approaches rely on either a pharmacological intervention (MAM), X-ray and gamma-ray irradiation, or a pharmaco-genetic approach (GFAP-TK, Nestin-TK) to target the dividing stem cells in the subgranular zone. Briefly, MAM (methylazoxymethanol acetate) is a methylating agent that blocks neurogenesis by interfering with cell division (Shors et al 2001). While some studies have succeeded in using MAM effectively, the interpretation of the findings is encumbered by the deleterious side-effects associated with MAM. A second method used to abolish adult hippocampal neurogenesis is by focal application of ionizing radiation to the animal's head or only at a narrow region that includes the hippocampus, as done in our laboratory (Santarelli et al 2003, Wojtowicz 2006). Exposure to low-dose irradiation is sufficient to arrest neurogenesis completely and irreversibly.

Electrophysiological recordings reveal that mature neurons within the hippocampal formation (Snyder et al 2001, Santarelli et al 2003, Saxe et al 2006) are unaffected by the procedure. Furthermore, many hippocampus-dependent behaviours are unchanged by irradiation, indicating a relatively high degree of specificity of the focal X-ray irradiation protocol (Saxe et al 2006). One limitation inherent to this method is the increased inflammatory response elicited by irradiation, which, although transient, may have long lasting effects on the stem cell niche (Monje et al 2003). Finally, a third and alternative method for arresting neurogenesis is a transgenic mouse model in which the herpes-simplex virus thymidine kinase (HSV-TK) is expressed under the control of the GFAP promoter (Garcia et al 2004). GFAP is expressed in neural stem cells located in the SGZ and SVZ (Doetsch et al 1999, Seri et al 2001, Filippov et al 2003). The presence of HSV-TK in dividing cells confers sensitivity to the cytotoxic effects of the antiviral drug ganciclovir. Recently, a Nestin-TK mouse line has also been developed, which allows for ablation of nestin-positive non-quiescent stem cells using ganciclovir (Parent et al 2006). The TK system does not completely abolish neurogenesis as quiescent stem cells are unaffected. None of the above described approaches spare gliogenesis in the adult SGZ. Despite limitations inherent to the irradiation and TK-dependent systems, considerable advances have been made using these strategies to understand the role of neurogenesis in behaviour. It remains essential, however, to replicate findings using more specific approaches. To this end, experiments are underway in our laboratory using inducible genetic systems in combination with the Doublecortin promoter to selectively manipulate adult neurogenesis without affecting glial cell production (Sahay & Hen, unpublished data).

Assessing the role of baseline neurogenesis in emotional reactivity and learning

Using X-ray irradiation and GFAP-TK, our laboratory has investigated the contribution of baseline-adult hippocampal neurogenesis to a number of different behavioural paradigms that measure emotional reactivity and hippocampal-dependent learning. To date, there is no evidence implicating adult hippocampal neurogenesis in the pathogenesis of anxiety or depression-like behaviour. Ablation of hippocampal neurogenesis does not impact anxiety-related behaviour as assessed in conflict based tests such as the open field, light-dark choice test, and elevated plus-maze (Saxe et al 2006). Hippocampal irradiation also fails to affect behaviour in two other anxiety tests that are also used to screen for antidepressants (ADs), the novelty suppressed feeding and novelty induced hypophagia (Santarelli et al 2003, Meshi et al 2006, unpublished data). Finally, blocking neurogenesis does not affect behaviour in the forced swim test and the chronic unpredictable stress paradigm, two tests used to assess antidepressant-like behaviour (Santarelli et al 2003 and unpublished data). Taken together, these studies indicate that abolishing hippocampal neurogenesis *in adult wild-type* animals does not result in altered anxiety or depression-like behaviour.

Studies of hippocampal dependent learning, in contrast to emotional reactivity, have revealed specific requirements for adult generated dentate granule cells. Reducing or blocking SGZ neurogenesis in rats or mice has been reported to cause impairments in a hippocampus-dependent form of classical conditioning (trace conditioning; Shors et al 2001, 2002), long-term spatial memory (Snyder et al 2005), working memory (Winocur et al 2006) and contextual fear conditioning (Saxe et al 2006, Winocur et al 2006). Recently, there has also been one report of improved performance in a specific working memory paradigm after neurogenesis ablation (Saxe et al 2007). While there are some inconsistencies in these findings, which may reflect differential behavioural requirements for adult hippocampal neurogenesis in mice and rats or variations germane to methodology, it is clear that neurogenesis contributes to adult dentate gyrus function in a behaviorally relevant way. Perhaps the most significant of these observations is the requirement of neurogenesis for contextual fear conditioning, which has been demonstrated in both rats and mice, using three different methods for arresting neurogenesis (Saxe et al 2006, Winocur et al 2006). Studies from our laboratory using both focally X-ray irradiated mice and the GFAP-TK system, have shown that blocking neurogenesis prior to training reduces the amount of contextual fear expressed when rodents are re-exposed to the training context (Saxe et al 2006). Importantly, blocking neurogenesis does not impair fear conditioning to a discrete tone stimulus, indicating that shock sensitivity and motor control of the fear response are not impaired. The impairment of contextual fear conditioning may thus reflect a requirement of neurogenesis for the encoding of novel contexts, consistent with the well-recognized role of the dentate gyrus in pattern separation.

In contrast, hippocampal neurogenesis does not appear to be required for other hippocampal dependent behaviours such as spatial learning, assessed in both the Morris Water Maze and the Y-Maze (Shors et al 2001, Saxe et al 2006, Winocur et al 2006).

Investigations in our laboratory into a role for adult generated dentate granule cells in hippocampal dependent working memory tasks has revealed, unexpectedly, an enhancement in working memory in both X-ray irradiated and GFAP-TK mice (Saxe et al 2007). Mice lacking hippocampal neurogenesis performed better than controls in a delayed non-matching-to-place task on a radial eight-arm maze, but only when the inter trial interval exceeded 15 seconds (consistent with when the hippocampus becomes engaged in working memory tests) and when there was interference from earlier trials. Thus, it appears that with sufficient memory loading and presentation of repetitive information, neurogenesis may handicap the ability of the dentate gyrus to ignore conflicting information from previous trials. Whether this is true for all working memory paradigms is not clear. For example, a recent study using a non-spatial working memory task showed that whole-brain irradiated rats perform worse as a function of delay (Winocur et al 2006).

Much work is still required to understand how and under what conditions neurogenesis is required for specific kinds of learning. Studies are underway to assess the differential contribution of adult generated neurons in different stages of learning such as acquisition, consolidation and retrieval. Finally, it is conceivable that young neurons have different functions depending on their state of maturation. Intriguingly, one report using rats has even suggested a functional role for 10 day old neurons in learning (Shors et al 2001). We predict that the novel genetic approaches mentioned earlier will provide the flexibility and specificity needed to test these hypotheses and help resolve existing inconsistencies.

Behavioural effects associated with increased neurogenesis

It is widely recognized that all major classes of antidepressants (ADs) have a delayed onset of therapeutic efficacy (often several weeks). One form of structural plasticity within the hippocampus that is consistent with this long delay is the birth and subsequent integration of newly generated neurons in the adult dentate gyrus (Esposito et al 2005, Overstreet-Wadiche & Westbrook 2006). Moreover, almost all ADs known to date including serotonin and noradrenaline selective reuptake inhibitors (SSRIs and SNRIs), tricyclics, monoamine oxidase inhibitors, phosphodiesterase inhibitors and electroconvulsive shock therapy increase neurogenesis (Madsen et al 2000, Malberg et al 2000, Manev et al 2001, Nakagawa et al 2002). Therefore, the idea that ADs may work through enhancing neurogenesis has received abundant attention and recent preclinical studies have tested this hypothesis (Santarelli et al 2003, Jiang et al 2005, Meltzer et al 2006). Our laboratory first demonstrated that neurogenesis is required for the effects of both imipramine, a classic tricyclic AD, and fluoxetine (SSRI) in two mouse behavioural screens for AD activity, the novelty-suppressed feeding (NSF) test and a chronic stress procedure (Santarelli et al 2003). Importantly, this study has since been replicated in our laboratory using the GFAP-TK mice (unpublished results). More recently, and in a series of experiments conducted by another laboratory, the synthetic cannabinoid HU210 was shown to have AD-like behavioural effects in the NSF paradigm, which, interestingly, was lost following X-ray irradiation (Jiang et al 2005). In addition, a recent preliminary report (Meltzer et al 2006) showed that irradiation blocks the behavioural effects of fluoxetine in the forced swim test. Thus, a neurogenic dependence for the behavioural effects of ADs has been revealed for three different drugs in three different AD screens and using two different ways to ablate neurogenesis. Together, these studies identify a previously unrecognized role for neurogenesis in the adult hippocampus in mediating the behavioural effects of SSRIs.

The work described above suggests that enhancing neurogenesis confers AD-like behavioural responses in several tests of chronic AD action. Given the pleiotropic effects of ADs and the limitations inherent in the AD screens (Nestler et al 2002, Duman & Monteggia 2006, Warner-Schmidt & Duman 2006), it is likely that some clinically important features of these treatments are neurogenesis-independent. Three studies from our laboratory confirm this notion and suggest that the net effects of increasing neurogenesis on behaviour are likely to be influenced by factors such as levels of network activity and the genetic make-up of the organism (Scharfman & Hen 2007). One study examined the effects of fluoxetine on behaviour and DG neurogenesis in the Balb/C mouse strain, a strain that exhibits high anxiety in behavioural tests (Holick et al 2007). In this strain, chronic fluoxetine treatment reduced anxiety-like and depressive-like behaviour in the novelty-induced hypophagia and forced-swim paradigms but failed to increase neurogenesis. Not surprisingly, these behavioural effects were unaffected by hippocampal irradiation. Thus, in Balb/C mice the behavioural effects of fluoxetine are mediated through a neurogenesis-independent mechanism. A second study has found that environmental enrichment and exercise, which are known to increase neurogenesis, improved learning and had anxiolytic-like effects independent of neurogenesis (Meshi et al 2006). Finally, a third study showed that the anxiolytic and antidepressant-like effects of a novel melanin-concentrating receptor hormone receptor antagonist were also independent of it's neurogenic effects (David et al 2007). These studies indicate that AD-like effects can be achieved through at least two different pathways, one that is neurogenesis-dependent and one that is neurogenesis-independent. Moreover, they illustrate that the requirement for neurogenesis to mediate the behavioural effects of ADs is revealed only in certain biological contexts and not others. An outstanding and unanswered question in this regard is whether increasing neurogenesis is *sufficient* to confer the behavioral effects of ADs. Addressing the sufficiency hypothesis is central to our endeavour to understand the contribution of increasing neurogenesis to different behaviours and assessment of its potential as a target for novel non-monoamine based therapeutics.

Neurogenesis-dependent and -independent mechanisms of AD action

Considerable efforts have been directed at dissecting the molecular mediators of the neurogenic effects of ADs with an emphasis on the serotonin and neurotrophin systems. The serotonin system is comprised of 15 different 5HT receptors that are expressed in a variety of cell types, making it possible that SSRIs act both directly and indirectly, through regulation of network properties, on neurogenesis. A recent study has shed some light on this subject, showing that only a specific proliferative cell type, the transiently amplifying neural progenitor (ANP) (Filippov et al 2003, Tozuka et al 2005, Encinas et al 2006) directly responds to fluoxetine. Moreover, this study confirmed that once exposure to fluoxetine ends, the rate of progenitor cell division is restored to baseline and that the increase in ANPs translates into a net increase in the number of new neurons. Thus, it appears that expansion of the neural progenitor pool may underlie the AD-induced neurogenic response. The identity of 5HT receptors required for the expansion of ANPs is unknown. Signalling through multiple post-synaptic 5HT receptors can impact adult hippocampal neurogenesis (Radley & Jacobs 2002, Santarelli et al 2003, Banasr et al 2004). Indirect evidence for the 5HT1A receptors as mediators of the neurogenic effects of ADs comes from a study done in our laboratory that showed a failure of 5HT1A knockout mice to respond to the neurogenic and behavioural effects of ADs (Santarelli et al 2003). Whether this lack of response to ADs reflects an acute requirement for 5HT1A is not known. Characterization of 5HT receptor expression in the subgranular zone (SGZ) and within mature cell types of the hippocampal formation is underway in our laboratory. These studies combined with cell type restricted manipulation of specific 5HT receptors will help identify mechanisms recruited by SSRIs for their neurogenic and behavioural effects.

A number of studies have shown that AD treatments, both pharmacological and non-pharmacological, increase neurotrophin levels within the hippocampal formation. Gene expression profiling in the rat has shown that chronic electro-convulsive therapy (ECT) and AD drug treatments upregulate expression of the mRNAs for brain-derived neurotrophic factor (BDNF), TrkB and vascular-endothelial growth factor (VEGF) in the hippocampus (Nibuya et al 1995, Newton et al 2003). Functional antagonism of VEGF and BDNF signalling has revealed that these pathways are necessary for mediating the neurogenic effects of ADs (Sairanen et al 2005, Warner-Schmidt & Duman 2006). While BDNF and VEGF signalling may both be important for the neurogenic effects of ADs, they are likely to act at different stages in the maturation cascade. For example, BDNF, unlike VEGF, is thought to primarily increase survival of immature neurons and not proliferation of neural progenitors (Sairanen et al 2005). As with the 5HT system, much work is still needed to define precisely how these two neurotrophic factors are recruited *in vivo* by ADs. Given the large repertoire of biological functions subserved by neurotrophins and growth factors, it is very likely that the enhance-ment in growth factor signalling following AD treatment results in changes in levels of neurogenesis, structural and electrophysiological properties of synapses and even alterations in the vasculature. The use of cell type specific conditional knockouts will help define the contribution of the neurogenic and non-neurogenic effects of VEGF and BDNF to the AD-mediated behavioural response.

The complex pathophysiology of depression underscores the possibility that new AD treatments may rely on modulation of neural circuits within different brain regions such as the HPA axis, prefrontal cortex, nucleus accumbens and the hippo-campus. The prominent role of the HPA axis in depression has fuelled considerable investigation into strategies that dampen increased HPA reactivity. These efforts have resulted in the identification of CRF and vasopressin system antagonists with antidepressant potential (Berton & Nestler 2006). Other examples of novel candi-date antidepressant drugs include melatonin receptor agonists (agomelatine), CB1 and galanin receptor ligands (Berton & Nestler 2006). Future studies will reveal how disparate brain regions impacted by these different signalling systems relate to the behavioural responses associated with successful AD treatments.

References

Banasr M, Hery M, Printemps R, Daszuta A 2004 Serotonin-induced increases in adult cell proliferation and neurogenesis are mediated through different and common 5-HT receptor subtypes in the dentate gyrus and the subventricular zone. Neuropsychopharmacology 29:450–460

Berton O, Nestler EJ 2006 New approaches to antidepressant drug discovery: beyond mono-amines. Nat Rev Neurosci 7:137–151

David DJ, Klemenhagen KC, Holick KA et al 2007 Efficacy of the MCHR1 antagonist N-[3-(1-{[4-(3,4-difluorophenoxy)phenyl]methyl} (4-piperidyl))-4-methylphenyl]-2-methylpropanamide (SNAP 94847) in mouse models of anxiety and depression following acute and chronic administration is independent of hippocampal neurogenesis. J Pharmacol Exp Ther 321:237–248

Doetsch F, Caille I, Lim DA, Garcia-Verdugo JM, Alvarez-Buylla A 1999 Subventricular zone astrocytes are neural stem cells in the adult mammalian brain. Cell 97:703–716

Duman RS, Monteggia LM 2006 A neurotrophic model for stress-related mood disorders. Biol Psychiatry 59:1116–1127

Encinas JM, Vaahtokari A, Enikolopov G 2006 Fluoxetine targets early progenitor cells in the adult brain. Proc Natl Acad Sci USA 103:8233–8238

Esposito MS, Piatti VC, Laplagne DA et al 2005 Neuronal differentiation in the adult hippocampus recapitulates embryonic development. J Neurosci 25:10074–10086

Filippov V, Kronenberg G, Pivneva T et al 2003 Subpopulation of nestin-expressing progenitor cells in the adult murine hippocampus shows electrophysiological and morphological characteristics of astrocytes. Mol Cell Neurosci 23:373–382

Garcia AD, Doan NB, Imura T, Bush TG, Sofroniew MV 2004 GFAP-expressing progenitors are the principal source of constitutive neurogenesis in adult mouse forebrain. Nat Neurosci 7:1233–1241

Holick KA, Lee DC, Hen R, Dulawa SC 2007 Behavioral effects of chronic fluoxetine in BALB/cJ mice do not require adult hippocampal neurogenesis or the serotonin 1A receptor. Neuropsychopharmacology in press

Jiang W, Zhang Y, Xiao L et al 2005 Cannabinoids promote embryonic and adult hippocampus neurogenesis and produce anxiolytic- and antidepressant-like effects. J Clin Invest 115:3104–3116

Lledo PM, Alonso M, Grubb MS 2006 Adult neurogenesis and functional plasticity in neuronal circuits. Nat Rev Neurosci 7:179–193

Madsen TM, Treschow A, Bengzon J et al 2000 Increased neurogenesis in a model of electroconvulsive therapy. Biol Psychiatry 47:1043–1049

Malberg JE, Eisch AJ, Nestler EJ, Duman RS 2000 Chronic antidepressant treatment increases neurogenesis in adult rat hippocampus. J Neurosci 20:9104–9110

Manev H, Uz T, Smalheiser NR, Manev R 2001 Antidepressants alter cell proliferation in the adult brain in vivo and in neural cultures in vitro. Eur J Pharmacol 411:67–70

Meltzer LA, Roy M, Parente V, Deisseroth K 2006 Hippocampal neurogenesis is required for lasting antidepressant effects of fluoxetine. Abstr Soc Neurosci

Meshi D, Drew MR, Saxe M et al 2006 Hippocampal neurogenesis is not required for behavioral effects of environmental enrichment. Nat Neurosci 9:729–731

Monje ML, Toda H, Palmer TD 2003 Inflammatory blockade restores adult hippocampal neurogenesis. Science 302:1760–1765

Nakagawa S, Kim JE, Lee R et al 2002 Regulation of neurogenesis in adult mouse hippocampus by cAMP and the cAMP response element-binding protein. J Neurosci 22:3673–3682

Nestler EJ, Barrot M, DiLeone RJ, Eisch AJ, Gold SJ, Monteggia LM 2002 Neurobiology of depression. Neuron 34:13–25

Newton SS, Collier EF, Hunsberger J et al 2003 Gene profile of electroconvulsive seizures: induction of neurotrophic and angiogenic factors. J Neurosci 23:10841–10851

Nibuya M, Morinobu S, Duman RS 1995 Regulation of BDNF and TrkB mRNA in rat brain by chronic electroconvulsive seizure and antidepressant drug treatments. J Neurosci 15:7539–7547

Overstreet-Wadiche LS, Westbrook GL 2006 Functional maturation of adult-generated granule cells. Hippocampus 16:208–215

Parent J, Lichtenwalner RJ, Velander AJ, Fuller CL, Burant CF 2006 Conditional suicide gene ablation of neural progenitors in the adult mouse forebrain subventricular zone. Abstr Soc Neurosci

Radley JJ, Jacobs BL 2002 5-HT1A receptor antagonist administration decreases cell proliferation in the dentate gyrus. Brain Res 955:264–267

Sairanen M, Lucas G, Ernfors P, Castren M, Castren E 2005 Brain-derived neurotrophic factor and antidepressant drugs have different but coordinated effects on neuronal turnover, proliferation, and survival in the adult dentate gyrus. J Neurosci 25:1089–1094

Santarelli L, Saxe M, Gross C et al 2003 Requirement of hippocampal neurogenesis for the behavioral effects of antidepressants. Science 301:805–809

Saxe MD, Battaglia F, Wang JW et al 2006 Ablation of hippocampal neurogenesis impairs contextual fear conditioning and synaptic plasticity in the dentate gyrus. Proc Natl Acad Sci USA 103:17501–17506

Saxe MD, Malleret G, Vronskaya S et al 2007 Paradoxical influence of hippocampal neurogenesis on working memory. Proc Natl Acad Sci USA 104:4642–4646

Scharfman HE, Hen R 2007 Neuroscience. Is more neurogenesis always better? Science 315:336–338

Seri B, Garcia-Verdugo JM, McEwen BS, Alvarez-Buylla A 2001 Astrocytes give rise to new neurons in the adult mammalian hippocampus. J Neurosci 21:7153–7160

Shors TJ, Townsend DA, Zhao M, Kozorovitskiy Y, Gould E 2002 Neurogenesis may relate to some but not all types of hippocampal-dependent learning. Hippocampus 12:578–584

Shors TJ, Miesegaes G, Beylin A, Zhao M, Rydel T, Gould E 2001 Neurogenesis in the adult is involved in the formation of trace memories. Nature 410:372–376

Snyder JS, Kee N, Wojtowicz JM 2001 Effects of adult neurogenesis on synaptic plasticity in the rat dentate gyrus. J Neurophysiol 85:2423–2431

Snyder JS, Hong NS, McDonald RJ, Wojtowicz JM 2005 A role for adult neurogenesis in spatial long-term memory. Neuroscience 130:843–852

Song H, Kempermann G, Overstreet Wadiche L, Zhao C, Schinder AF, Bischofberger J 2005 New neurons in the adult mammalian brain: synaptogenesis and functional integration. J Neurosci 25:10366–10368

Tozuka Y, Fukuda S, Namba T, Seki T, Hisatsune T 2005 GABAergic excitation promotes neuronal differentiation in adult hippocampal progenitor cells. Neuron 47:803–815

Warner-Schmidt JL, Duman RS 2006 Hippocampal neurogenesis: opposing effects of stress and antidepressant treatment. Hippocampus 16:239–249

Winocur G, Wojtowicz JM, Sekeres M, Snyder JS, Wang S 2006 Inhibition of neurogenesis interferes with hippocampus-dependent memory function. Hippocampus 16:296–304

Wojtowicz JM 2006 Irradiation as an experimental tool in studies of adult neurogenesis. Hippocampus 16:261–266

DISCUSSION

Javitt: One treatment that you didn't mention is ketamine challenge. Can you say something about this?

Hen: Whether it is the ketamine story, the ECT story or the deep-brain stimulation study, all these lead to acute effects where the patients feel something within minutes to an hour. With such a time frame we are not talking about neurogenesis. We are probably dealing with neurogenesis-independent mechanisms. Whether ketamine can have fast non-neurogenesis-dependent effects and then more sustained neurogenesis-dependent effects is unclear. It is a possibility because it does stimulate neurogenesis. The same applies to ECT, where there are rapid effects and more sustained ones. No one has yet done the definitive experiment to see whether the behavioural effects of ECT can be blocked by irradiation.

Talmage: Is the increase in neurogenesis protective? If long-term pharmacological interventions are done before you put them through their anxiety/depression behavioural tasks, does it lessen the impact?

Hen: No. This is interesting. We thought that in the chronic and unpredictable stress paradigm we would get more of a deterioration in animals that don't have neurogenesis. This is one of the paradoxes we are dealing with. In all these conditions, radiation or transgenic ablation doesn't change the behaviour in any anxiety or stress response test. Neurogenesis ablation doesn't make them more vulnerable to stress. This suggests a two-hit effect of antidepressants. It doesn't just stimulate neurogenesis: it recruits the young neurons and does something else; so if you just get rid of neurogenesis you don't see anything. In the anxiety-related tests getting rid of neurogenesis produces no effect.

Talmage: If you start with a higher level of neurogenesis, does this make a difference?

Hen: If we start with a higher level, for example after exposure to an enriched environment, you see a little effect in the anxiety test, but this isn't blocked by irradiation.

Talmage: Is there a dorsoventral gradient in neurogenesis that might explain why some behaviours are dorsal dependent?

Hen: In our hands things like antidepressants and enriched environments stimulate neurogenesis both dorsally and ventrally. A few papers coming from a Danish group (Jayatissa et al 2006) show that chronic stress decreases neurogenesis more in the ventral part than the dorsal. If we start looking at the serotonin receptors, their pattern of expression goes in a gradient. 5HT1A, one of the targets of fluoxetine has an interesting pattern: it is in dorsal CA1 but not ventral CA1, and ventral dentate but not dorsal dentate.

Castrén: My niece had a recurrent leukaemia. She had bone marrow transplantation which was preceded by a really harsh treatment, with the idea that at the level of the bone marrow you ablate every stem cell. I don't know what the impact is of this kind of treatment on hippocampal neurogenesis. There might be reduced neurogenesis. If people who have experienced this get depressed, are they less likely to be helped by antidepressants?

Hen: The idea is an interesting one. There is some literature on the effects of local radiotherapy in the brain. After radiotherapy there is a profound cognitive impairment, to the extent that it is no longer given to adolescents or children. The problem with these studies is that there is not just a lack of neurogenesis in post-mortem brains, but also a lot of inflammation which will have long lasting effects. In mice, we use the minimum dose that kills the neurons without inducing too much inflammation.

Akil: One issue in the dendritic arborization work, and which might apply to neurogenesis, is that there is a kind of pool or store of flexibility that is available, and once this is spent it can't be spent again. My colleague Terry Robinson has shown (Kolb et al 2003) that if animals are exposed to cocaine this can enhance dendritic arborization. It looks as if you are doing something good for the animal, like an antidepressant. But afterwards they stop profiting from an enriched environment. If you now expose them to an enriched environment you have abrogated their ability to profit from a positive experience. Have you thought about these sequential models? Is there a capital that you spend with neurogenesis?

Hen: If we do chronic treatment with antidepressants over a much longer period, for the first couple of months there is an increase in neurogenesis. Then homeostasis kicks in, in a way that we don't understand, and neurogenesis goes down to a baseline level. If the treatment is then stopped and you re-treat later you can still get an increase because of the homeostatic decrease. The same thing occurs with ageing. There is a massive decrease in neurogenesis, but you can still stimulate it with an enriched environment. It looks like the system rapidly reaches homeostasis, which keeps it available for further stimulation. The paradigms that are more dramatic, for example those that involve seizure induction, result in all sorts of abnormal connections being established in the hippocampus. It is not clear whether these can be reversed.

Akil: Have you looked at the morphology of the remaining hippocampus in terms of dendritic volume, suprapyramidal/infrapyramidal laminae and so on?

Hen: Yes, and after antidepressant treatment we don't see any difference, nor do we see any after irradiation. The volume of the hippocampus doesn't change after irradiation even a year later. Our idea is that homeostasis takes place between death and birth of neurons. If the birth of young neurons is reduced, then this will also reduce cell death in other layers. We haven't proven this.

Akil: To me, it seems that one of the things you are differentiating is classical conditioning to context and instrumental learning: one is affected and the other isn't. This is another dimension to consider.

Hen: We are trying to find out from a psychological perspective what our results mean. So far, one of the ideas is the one you have proposed. Another would be that it is only when you have very brief exposure, which is what is happening in fear-conditioning paradigms, that you need these young neurons as a novelty detection system. This would fit with ideas that the dentate gyrus serves as a pattern separation device. In the Morris water maze where there is repeated training and plenty of time to learn it doesn't make a difference. Emotional memories are a good example: it is a flashback to a fast acquisition time in a salient, loaded context. This could be where the role of the young neurons is most prominent.

Raff: If one looks at post-mortem brains of humans (with glioblastomas, for example) who had their heads irradiated years before, so that the reactive inflammation is gone, does one see that cell proliferation in the hippocampus is still absent?

Hen: There are just a few papers that look at neurogenesis in old people (Reif et al 2006). In old people there are very low levels anyway, so it would be hard to see whether there's a lower level in people who had received irradiation. In younger people we can detect neurogenesis with markers such as Ki67. If we have the postmortem tissue in sufficient quality this can be measured. There is one paper that reports no change after antidepressants (Reif et al 2006) using some of these markers. The promise now is that there are a few imaging studies that may address this better (Pereira et al 2007).

Brandon: There are different pharmacological mechanisms that increase neuro-genesis. Are there any sort of quantitative or qualitative differences with these different mechanisms?

Hen: Some of these compounds act on proliferation and differentiation, others act on just one of these processes. We lack knowledge of which is more effective in terms of antidepressant effects.

Brandon: I know that Rolipram (standard PDE4 inhibitor) isn't the most specific of PDE4 inhibitors, but there are data out there that show antidepressants increase PDE4 expression. Have you any thoughts on this, in particular as PDE4 inhibitors have been suggested to be antidepressant? Is regional specificity and differential expression of PDE4 important?

Hen: There is the whole cAMP pathway that gets activated by antidepressants. cAMP levels rise, phosphorylated CREB rises, and many of the targets of phos-phorylated CREB also rise. I would say that in this case the increase in PDE4 is just to establish homeostasis in the system. There are also a few genetic studies looking at specific PDE4 knockouts, and their response to antidepressants (Zhang et al 2002).

Castrén: I was interested in the enriched environment followed by irradiation experiment. Are you sure that the enriched environment didn't protect from the X-rays, or did not allow the cells to recover?

Hen: The way this was done was by irradiating the mice, then enriching them, and then testing them. There was no effect on proliferation. Were there other effects that we didn't measure in the hippocampus? That's a possibility.

References

Jayatissa MN, Bisgaard C, Tingstrom A, Papp M, Wiborg O 2006 Hippocampal cytogenesis correlates to escitalopram-mediated recovery in a chronic mild stress rat model of depression. Neuropsychopharmacology 31:2395–2404
Kolb B, Gorny G, Li Y, Samaha AN, Robinson TE 2003 Amphetamine or cocaine limits the ability of later experience to promote structural plasticity in the neocortex and nucleus accumbens. Proc Natl Acad Sci USA 100:10523–10528

Pereira AC, Huddleston DE, Brickman AM et al 2007 An in vivo correlate of exercise-induced
    neurogenesis in the adult dentate gyrus. Proc Natl Acad Sci USA 104:5638–5643
Reif A, Fritzen S, Finger M et al 2006 Neural stem cell proliferation is decreased in schizo-
    phrenia, but not in depression. Mol Psychiatry 11:514–522
Zhang HT, Huang Y, Jin SL et al 2002 Antidepressant-like profile and reduced sensitivity to
    rolipram in mice deficient in the PDE4D phosphodiesterase enzyme. Neuropsychopharma-
    cology 27:587–595

Neuregulins and neuronal plasticity: possible relevance in schizophrenia

Andrés Buonanno, Oh-Bin Kwon, Leqin Yan, Carmen Gonzalez, Marines Longart, Dax Hoffman* and Detlef Vullhorst

*Section on Molecular Neurobiology, and *Molecular Neurophysiology and Biophysics Unit, National Institute of Child Health and Human Development, NIH, 9000 Rockville Pike, Bethesda, MD 20892, USA*

Abstract. Polymorphisms in the Neuregulin 1 (NRG1) and ErbB4 receptor genes have been associated with schizophrenia in numerous cohort and family studies, and bio-chemical measurements from postmortem prefrontal cortex homogenates suggest that NRG/ErbB signalling is altered in schizophrenia. Moreover, recent work from our group, and from others, indicates that NRG/ErbB signalling has a role in regulating glutamatergic transmission—an intriguing finding given that glutamatergic hypofunction has been proposed to be involved in the pathogenesis underlying schizophrenia. Here we will provide a brief background of the complexity of the NRG/ErbB signalling system. We will then focus on how NRG1 reverses (depotentiates) long-term potentiation (LTP) at hippocampal Schaeffer collateral–CA1 glutamatergic synapses in the adult brain. Specifically, we found that NRG1 depotentiates LTP in an activity- and time-dependent manner. A role of endogenous NRG for regulating plasticity at hippocampal synapses is supported by experiments demonstrating that ErbB receptor antagonists completely block LTP depotentiation by brief theta-pulse stimuli, a subthreshold stimulus paradigm that reverses LTP in live animals. Preliminary results indicate that NRG1-mediated LTP depotentiation is NMDA receptor independent, and manifests as an internalization of GluR1-containing AMPA receptors. The importance of the NRG/ErbB signalling pathway in regulating homeostasis at glutamatergic synapses, and its possible implications for schizophrenia, will be discussed.

2008 Growth factors and psychiatric disorders. Wiley, Chichester (Novartis Foundation Symposium 289) p 165–179

In the nervous system, the neuregulin (NRG)/ErbB signalling network is best known for its important role in developmental processes that rely on proper communication between neurons and glial cells, such as migration of neuronal progenitors along radial or Bergmann glia, or myelination of peripheral nerves by Schwann cells, and possibly of CNS axons by oligodendrocytes (Lemke 2001, Nave & Salzer 2006). However, ErbB receptors and their ligands continue to be expressed at high levels in the adult brain, suggesting that they have additional functions in the developed nervous system. In fact, a rapidly accumulating body of evidence indicates that this pathway is involved in the regulation of synaptic plasticity at central glutamatergic synapses. The purpose of this paper is to present an overview of recent studies by us and other laboratories that were instrumental in the development of this exciting field, and to discuss scenarios that could relate the genetic linkage of NRGs and ErbB4 to schizophrenia and neuropathological changes implicated in the disease process.

The neuregulin-ErbB signalling pathway

Neuregulin diversity—different genes and RNA processing

NRGs are a group of growth and differentiation factors characterized by a conserved epidermal growth factor (EGF)-like domain of ~55 amino acids featuring three sets of conserved disulfide bonded-cysteines and a pair of anti-parallel β-sheets. The EGF-like motif is both necessary and sufficient to elicit autophosphorylation of their cognate ErbB2–4 receptors that mediate many of NRG's biological effects. NRGs are transcribed from four genes that generate a large repertoire of mRNAs by differential promoter usage and splicing. Due to space limitations, we will focus our discussion on NRG1.

The human *NRG1* locus on chromosome 8q21–23, which is structurally similar in rodents, extends over 1.5 Mb. As shown in Fig. 1A, the gene is believed to be comprised of 25 exons (Falls 2003, Steinthorsdottir et al 2004). Alternative promoter usage gives rise to type I (ARIA, NDF, heregulin), type II (GGF) and type III (SMDF/CRD) transcripts. In addition, differential splicing of exons encoding the immunoglobulin-like, EGF-like (α and β) and spacer domains, as well as exons encoding distinct cytoplasmic domains, give rise to a plethora of transcripts—at least 15 bona fide NRG1 polyadenylated mRNAs have been reported (Fig. 1B). Steinthorsdottir et al (2004) recently identified six new NRG1 exons by 5′-RACE and RT-PCR, that appear to give rise to three novel types of NRG1 (IV–VI) (Fig. 1C). Transcripts originating from the proposed type IV promoter encode a novel 13 amino acid N-terminus. Recently, a polymorphism mapping close to the type IV exon E187 has been the centre of great attention for its genetic association with schizophrenia and reduced cognitive function (see below).

Postnatal expression, processing and subcellular distribution of neuregulin 1

After birth, the overall levels of NRG1 transcripts are highest during early development and decrease with age. They are found in most cholinergic nuclei, including septal neurons that project to the hippocampus (Corfas et al 1995). In addition,

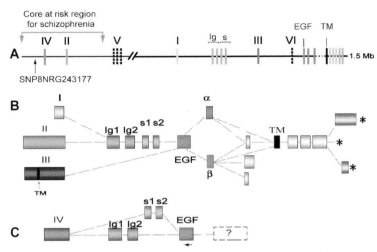

FIG. 1. *NRG1* gene structure and splice variants. (A) Exon-intron structure of the human *NRG1* gene locus. The locations of the core at-risk region for schizophrenia and SNP8NRG-243177 are indicated. (B) Schematic view of splicing events underlying NRG1 isoform diversity (adapted from Falls 2003). (C) Partial exon structure of NRG1 type IV transcripts.

NRG1 mRNAs are expressed, albeit at considerably lower levels, by all hippocampal principal cells with the exception of CA1 pyramidal neurons (Corfas et al 1995, Law et al 2004). Pro-NRG1 has been shown to be anterogradely transported down axons (Fischbach & Rosen 1997). Processing of NRG1 pro-forms by matrix metalloproteinases generates soluble (type I and II) or membrane-bound (type III) forms. Studies in cerebellar granule cell cultures and on the neuromuscular junction indicate that soluble NRG1 can be released from presynaptic nerve terminals in response to activity (Fischbach & Rosen 1997, Fernandez et al 2000, Ozaki et al 2004).

The ErbB signalling pathway

Neuregulins signal via ErbB2–4 transmembrane tyrosine kinases related to the EGF receptor (ErbB1) (Gassmann & Lemke 1997). ErbB receptors are expressed throughout the adult rodent (Gerecke et al 2001, Fox & Kornblum 2005) and primate brain (Bernstein et al 2006, Thompson et al 2007), but each protein has a distinct distribution in neurons and glia. In the forebrain, ErbB2 is expressed in most cells, ErbB3 is found predominantly in glia and subpopulations of neurons, and ErbB4 is restricted to neurons and oligodendrocytes. ErbB4 mRNA and protein levels are highest in GABAergic subtypes (Lai & Lemke 1991, Huang et al 2000, Gerecke et al 2001, Ghashghaei et al 2006, Longart et al 2007).

NRGs bind preferentially to ErbB3 and ErbB4, which then form homo- or heterodimers by recruiting either ErbB1 or ErbB2 as co-receptors to initiate signalling. Downstream signalling cascades activated by ErbB receptor stimulation are diverse and depend on the specific configuration of the ligand-activated receptor complex and recruited adapter proteins (Citri & Yarden 2006). They include MAP kinases (Erk1/2, Jun-terminal kinase, P38), PI3 kinase / protein kinase B, phospholipase C/PKC, and members of the *Src* family of non-receptor tyrosine kinases. It is noteworthy that all of these signalling pathways have also been implicated in the regulation of synaptic plasticity.

The postsynaptic density (PSD), an electron-dense area right underneath the postsynaptic membrane, is an important structural element of glutamatergic synapses and serves as a scaffold to organize the intricate meshwork of receptors, ion channels and signalling proteins. A variety of PDZ domain-containing proteins are enriched at the PSD, in particular those that belong to the family of membrane-associated guanylate kinases (MAGUKs) such as PSD95, SAP102 and PSD93 (Kim & Sheng 2004). They interact with proteins whose carboxyl terminal sequence ends in S/T-X-V, most prominently the 2A and 2B subunits of the NMDA receptor. ErbB4 interacts with PSD95 and other MAGUKs via its C-terminal T-V-V sequence (Garcia et al 2000, Huang et al 2000). The targeting of ErbB4 to glutamatergic synapses immediately suggested that NRG/ErbB signalling could be involved in the acute regulation of glutamatergic transmission.

NRG–ErbB signalling in synaptic plasticity

Synaptic plasticity is the use-dependent modulation of synaptic strength and as such is believed to represent a substrate for cognitive processes such as learning and memory. The hippocampal Schaeffer collateral-to-CA1 (SC-CA1) glutamatergic synapse is one of the most widely used models to study plasticity mechanisms at the electrophysiological and molecular levels. At this synapse, AMPA and NMDA subtype glutamate receptors are functionally linked to mediate synaptic plasticity. Long-lasting changes in synaptic strength are induced by NMDA receptors and expressed as changes in the amount and channel properties of postsynaptic AMPA receptors. Long-term potentiation (LTP) and long-term depression (LTD), opposing mechanisms suggested to bidirectionally maintain glutamatergic synapses within a dynamic range, can be elicited by distinct stimulation protocols, and both require calcium influx through NMDA receptors (Malenka & Bear 2004). LTP depotentiation is another mechanism that regulates synaptic homeostasis. It can be triggered by sub-threshold theta-pulse stimuli (TPS) and has been successfully used in hippocampal slices and in freely moving rats to reverse LTP during a 'labile' period of <30 minutes (Staubli & Chun 1996, Staubli & Scafidi 1999). Depotentiation may therefore serve to counterbalance increases in synaptic strength to keep synaptic responses within a physiological range. Because of its time dependence, it may also serve as an early filter for erasure of LTP before consolidation.

Because of its physical association with the PSD of hippocampal glutamatergic synapses (see above), we and others postulated that ErbB4 receptors may acutely alter postsynaptic signalling events that control the efficacy of synaptic transmission. In fact, Huang et al showed that continuous perfusion of hippocampal slices with a NRG peptide that encompasses the EGF-like domain blocks the induction and/or expression of LTP by theta-burst stimulation ('TBS', 5 brief high-frequency trains) (Huang 2000). However, the mechanism by which NRG-1 exerted this effect remained unclear—in particular, whether it blocked the induction or expression of LTP.

Neuregulin 1 depotentiates LTP at SC-CA1 glutamatergic synapses

To address this question, we began by perfusing hippocampal slices with 0.1 nM NRG1 peptide after LTP induction by TBS. Typically, this protocol elicits stable LTP that lasts for at least 1 h. However, LTP was rapidly reversed upon the onset of NRG1 treatment, effectively returning synaptic strength back to pre-LTP baseline levels (Kwon et al 2005) (Fig. 2). Importantly, NRG1 did not affect baseline transmission in unpotentiated slices, nor did it depotentiate LTP below baseline levels. Pretreatment of slices with the specific ErbB receptor inhibitor PD158780 prior to NRG1 addition blocked NRG1-mediated LTP depotentation, thus demonstrating that this effect was mediated via the stimulation of ErbB receptors. Moreover, application of the ErbB receptor antagonist to slices 20 minutes after TBS caused a small but significant increase in LTP, suggesting that endogenous NRG signalling regulates the strength of potentiated synapses.

As discussed earlier, LTP can also be reversed by TPS, a very brief and weak stimulation paradigm (5 Hz for 1 min) that has no short- or long-term effects on basal synaptic transmission. To test if TPS-dependent depotentiation requires ErbB receptor activation, presumably by endogenous ligands, we used the 'two-pathway' stimulation configuration. This method allows the monitoring of LTP at different dendrites stimulated by distinct afferent pathways (S1 and S2) projecting to the same neurons. As shown in Fig. 3A, when slices were perfused with PD158780 immediately after induction of LTP in the first pathway (S1), the TPS were not effective at depotentiating LTP. While the amplitude of fEPSPs were reduced transiently after TPS, these effects were not sustained and LTP increased to approximately 175% of baseline by 10 min after LTP induction. The levels of LTP in S1 were indistinguishable from those in the second independent pathway (S2). These results strongly suggested that both activity- and NRG-1-induced depotentiation in the hippocampus require signalling through ErbB receptors.

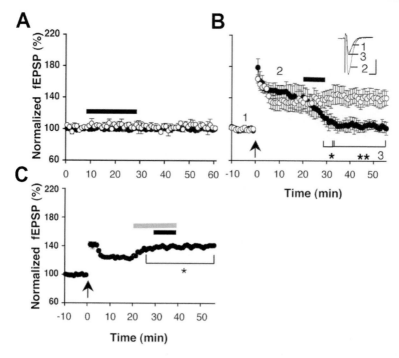

FIG. 2. NRG1 depotentiates LTP at SC-CA1 synapses. Black bars indicate time of NRG1 treatment. (A) Basal synaptic transmission is not modified by 0.1 (black circles) or 1.0 nM (open circles) NRG1 peptide. (B) Effects of 0.1 nM NRG1 (black circles) or vehicle (open circles) on LTP analysed 20 min following TBS (arrow). Values are normalized to mean fEPSP slopes recorded 10 min prior to TBS ($N = 10$). (C) 10 μM PD158780 (grey bar) blocks LTP depotentiation by NRG1 and augments its expression. From Kwon et al (2005), copyright 2005 by the Society for Neuroscience.

Another hallmark of TPS-induced LTP depotentiation is its time-dependence. The capacity of TPS to reverse LTP diminishes when delivered at increasing times after LTP induction. Consistent with the notion that TPS- and NRG1-dependent depotentiation share common features, and perhaps pathways, we found that NRG1 effectively depotentiated LTP when delivered up to 30 minutes after LTP induction, but that it was ineffective when applied 50 minutes post-induction (Fig. 3B). These results are consistent with the idea that NRG1 targets selective AMPAR subtypes (see below), and is ineffective to reverse the process once consolidated.

Molecular pathways that underlie NRG1-dependent depotentiation

To begin delineating the molecular mechanisms by which NRG1 regulates LTP, we determined the contributions of NMDA and AMPA receptors to the reversal of LTP by measuring normalized evoked postsynaptic receptor currents at

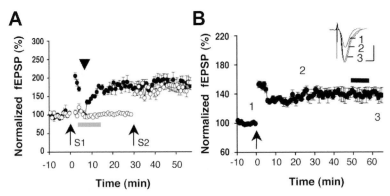

FIG. 3. NRG1-mediated LTP reversal shares similarities with activity-dependent depotentiation. (A) TPS-induced depotentiation (arrowhead) was tested in a two-pathway stimulation
protocol. The effects of TPS on TBS-induced LTP (arrows) are blocked by ErbB receptor
inhibition with PD158780 (grey bar) in pathway S1, while pathway S2 is unaffected. (B) NRG1
reverses LTP in a time-dependent manner. Slices were perfused with NRG1 peptide 50 min
after LTP stabilization. Insets are as in Fig. 2. From Kwon et al (2005), copyright 2005 by the
Society for Neuroscience.

different times before and after LTP induction, and after depotentiation. In agreement with the idea that depotentiation represents a reversal of LTP, we found
that AMPA receptor currents, selectively enhanced after the induction of LTP,
were down-regulated during NRG1 application, while NMDA receptor currents
remained unchanged throughout the experiment (Fig. 4A). Regulated trafficking
in and out of the postsynapse is believed to be a major mechanism by which AMPA
receptors affect synaptic strength. We therefore investigated at the cellular level
whether AMPA receptor trafficking is regulated by NRG1/ErbB signalling. We
transfected cultured hippocampal neurons with GluR1 fused at its extracellular
N-terminal domain to a pH-sensitive variant of GFP (pHluorin, or superecliptic
[se]GFP). While fluorescence of this variant is normal when exposed to the neutral
pH of the extracellular space or tissue culture medium, it is diminished by more
than 90% in acidic endosomal vesicles, thereby allowing for the selective visualization of surface receptors on dendrites.

We recorded GFP fluorescence in transfected live cells after the induction of
LTP by a chemical protocol. Two minutes after the onset of NRG1 perfusion,
surface seGFP-GluR1 fluorescence decreased to ~50% of baseline levels, while
untreated cells or cells pre-incubated with PD158780 exhibited stable fluorescence
throughout the duration of the experiment (Fig. 4B, C). These results were confirmed by immunofluorescence of surface expression of native GluR1 and NMDA
R1 receptors. Based on these findings, we concluded that NRG1/ErbB mediates
LTP reversal by a mechanism that selectively impinges on AMPA, but not on
NMDA receptors, and that manifests as the removal of GluR1-containing AMPA

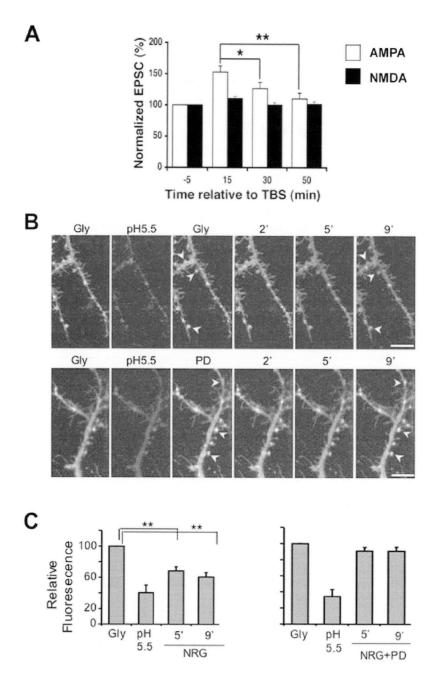

FIG. 4. NRG1 acts on AMPA receptors to reverse LTP. (A) AMPA receptor excitatory post-synaptic currents (EPSC) are selectively reduced after NRG1 stimulation in potentiated hippocampal slices. (B) Supercleiptic GFP-GluR1 surface fluorescence in cultured hippocampal neurons subjected to chemical LTP. Micrographs in the upper panel show a dendritic process undergoing seGFP-GluR1 internalization following NRG1 treatment whereas pre-incubation with PD158780 blocks receptor endocytosis (lower panel). Data from several experiments are summarized in (C). From Kwon et al (2005), copyright 2005 by the Society for Neuroscience.

receptors from the synapse. In this regard it is interesting to note recent evidence indicating that GluR2-lacking, calcium-permeable AMPA receptors are transiently inserted at hippocampal SC-CA1 synapses immediately after LTP induction, and are later replaced by GluR2-containing receptors (Plant et al 2006). It is tempting to speculate that depotentiation may specifically act on this transient, presumably GluR1-homomeric population of synaptic AMPA receptors. Given that the highest ErbB4 expression in the CNS is observed in GABAergic interneurons (see above), the observed effects of NRG1 on LTP reversal in pyramidal CA1 neurons could involve signals from local inhibitory interneurons.

It should be emphasized that while the effects of NRG1/ErbB signalling on hippocampal synaptic plasticity are clearly different from LTD (Huang et al 2000, Kwon et al 2005), it has been reported that NRG1 treatment of cultured prefrontal cortical neurons reduces baseline synaptic transmission via a process that involves the removal of NMDA receptors from the synapse (Gu et al 2005). Whether these differences are due to the different experimental strategies employed, or whether they reflect distinct downstream effects of NRG1/ ErbB signalling on synaptic plasticity in different brain areas, needs further investigation.

NRG1/ErbB4 and schizophrenia

The glutamate hypofunction hypothesis in schizophrenia

Two neurotransmitter systems, dopaminergic and glutamatergic, have classically been implicated in schizophrenia. The glutamate hypofunction hypothesis of schizophrenia originated from the observation that NMDA receptor antagonists, such as phencyclidine (PCP), MK-801 and ketamine, elicit cognitive deficits in healthy individuals that are similar to the positive (i.e. hallucinations) and negative (i.e. social withdrawal) symptoms observed in persons diagnosed with schizophrenia (see Coyle 2006). In addition, non-competitive NMDA receptor antagonists exacerbate positive symptoms in persons with schizophrenia. Because of these findings, rodent models for schizophrenia were based on these NMDA receptor antagonists. Interestingly, NMDA receptor NR1 subunit hypomorphic mice, expressing only 5% of normal levels of NR1 (Mohn et al 1999), and NR2A null mice (Miyamoto et al 2001) manifest a series of behaviours that are shared by rodents that have been administered PCP or ketamine. These include hyperactivity, stereotypic behaviours and memory impairment. Although these pharmacological and genetic findings primarily implicate NMDA receptors, it is important to note that, because of the intimate functional interactions between NMDA and AMPA receptors (see above), perturbations in both receptor systems are likely to contribute to glutamate hypofunction.

While glutamatergic hypofunction and schizophrenia share many properties, there is as yet no demonstration of a direct genetic link between glutamate receptor genes and schizophrenia. However, genes encoding for proteins involved in the regulation of glutamatergic transmission could have important implications for the pathophysiology underlying schizophrenia.

Behavioural abnormalities in NRG and ErbB hypomorphs: links to neurological disease

Direct correlates of synaptic plasticity and behaviour have been established in numerous mouse models (Tonegawa 1995). Interestingly, heterozygous NRG1 and ErbB4 mutant mice exhibit behavioural abnormalities in numerous tasks that may result from hyperactivity and abnormalities in sensory gating, behavioural phenotypes shared with the NMDAR NR1 hypomorphic mice mentioned earlier. Consistent with this observation, NRG1 heterozygotes express lower levels of NMDA receptors (Stefansson et al 2002, Hall et al 2006). Treatment of NMDA receptor NR1 hypomorphs, as well as NRG1 and ErbB4 heterozygotes, with the antipsychotic drug clozapine used to treat schizophrenia, partially restores their normal behaviour (Stefansson et al 2002). Importantly, ErbB2 and ErbB3 heterozygous mice do not exhibit behavioural abnormalities (Gerlai et al 2000), indicating a selective role for NRG1 and ErbB4 signalling in the regulation of glutamatergic function. These results are particularly interesting given the genetic association of *NRG1* and *ErbB4* with schizophrenia (see below).

Possible implications of the NRG/ErbB signalling pathway in schizophrenia

Stefansson and colleagues identified a haplotype for NRG1 that increases the risk of schizophrenia (Stefansson et al 2002), and this initial finding was later replicated in many other population and family studies (see Owen et al 2005, Harrison & Law 2006). Linkage analyses and meta-analyses also implicate ErbB4 (Nicodemus et al 2006, Silberberg et al 2006) in schizophrenia. NRG1 type I mRNA levels are elevated in postmortem prefrontal cortex and hippocampus of persons with schizophrenia (Hashimoto et al 2004); however, no interaction between the at-risk haplotype and the elevated NRG1 mRNA levels was found in these initial studies. Therefore, it is currently not clear if the reported changes in NRG1 mRNA levels result from compensatory mechanisms.

More recently, Weinberger and colleagues reported elevated mRNA levels of NRG1 type IV in schizophrenia patients and healthy controls homozygous for SNP8NRG243177 (C/T), which is part of the at-risk haplotype (see Fig. 1A) and maps near the first exon (E187) of NRG1 type IV (Law et al 2006). Importantly, SNP8NRG243177 is associated with the development of psychotic symptoms, impaired frontal and temporal lobe activation and deficits in cognitive function in a group of young people at high risk of developing schizophrenia (Hall et al 2006).

Functional evidence for an involvement of NRG1/ErbB4 signalling in schizophrenia comes from a recent study in which a decrease in the association of ErbB4 with PSD-95 was measured in prefrontal cortex lysates from postmortem brains of persons with schizophrenia as compared to controls (Hahn et al 2006). Interestingly, this change was accompanied by a decrease in NR2A tyrosine phosphorylation in response to NRG1 stimulation, suggesting that this NMDA receptor subunit may be a downstream target of ErbB4.

Summary

The NRG1/ErbB signalling network has emerged as a potentially important regulator of plasticity of glutamatergic synapses in the adult brain. The ability to reverse recent LTP at hippocampal SC-CA1 synapses suggests that this pathway could serve as an early point of control to limit the extent to which synapses become stably potentiated, and may thereby contribute to synaptic homeostasis. As perturbation of glutamatergic function is increasingly recognized as an important factor in the pathophysiology underlying schizophrenia, it is highly encouraging to see that the genetic evidence implicating NRG1 in schizophrenia is backed by a plausible biological rationale for a role of the NRG1/ErbB signalling pathway in the regulation of glutamatergic transmission. Further progress in understanding this complex system will without doubt result from the convergence of basic neuroscience and molecular psychiatry approaches.

Acknowledgements

This research was supported by the intramural research programme of the NIH, NICHD.

References

Bernstein HG, Lendeckel U, Bertram I et al 2006 Localization of neuregulin-1alpha (heregulin-alpha) and one of its receptors, ErbB-4 tyrosine kinase, in developing and adult human brain. Brain Res Bull 69:546–559
Citri A, Yarden Y 2006 EGF-ErbB signalling: towards the systems level. Nat Rev Mol Cell Biol 7:505–516
Corfas G, Rosen KM, Aratake H, Krauss R, Fischbach GD 1995 Differential expression of ARIA isoforms in the rat brain. Neuron 14:103–115
Coyle JT 2006 Glutamate and schizophrenia: beyond the dopamine hypothesis. Cell Mol Neurobiol 26:363–382
Falls DL 2003 Neuregulins: functions, forms, and signaling strategies. Exp Cell Res 284:14–30
Fernandez PA, Tang DG, Cheng L, Prochiantz A, Mudge AW, Raff MC 2000 Evidence that axon-derived neuregulin promotes oligodendrocyte survival in the developing rat optic nerve. Neuron 28:81–90

Fischbach GD, Rosen KM 1997 ARIA: a neuromuscular junction neuregulin. Annu Rev Neurosci 20:429–458

Fox IJ, Kornblum HI 2005 Developmental profile of ErbB receptors in murine central nervous system: implications for functional interactions. J Neurosci Res 79:584–597

Garcia RA, Vasudevan K Buonanno A 2000 The neuregulin receptor ErbB-4 interacts with PDZ-containing proteins at neuronal synapses. Proc Natl Acad Sci USA 97:3596–3601

Gassmann M, Lemke G 1997 Neuregulins and neuregulin receptors in neural development. Curr Opin Neurobiol 7:87–92

Gerecke KM, Wyss JM, Karavanova I, Buonanno A, Carroll SL 2001 ErbB transmembrane tyrosine kinase receptors are differentially expressed throughout the adult rat central nervous system. J Comp Neurol 433:86–100

Gerlai R, Pisacane P, Erickson S 2000 Heregulin, but not ErbB2 or ErbB3, heterozygous mutant mice exhibit hyperactivity in multiple behavioral tasks. Behav Brain Res 109: 219–227

Ghashghaei HT, Weber J, Pevney L et al 2006 The role of neuregulin–ErbB4 interactions on the proliferation and organization of cells in the subventricular zone. Proc Natl Acad Sci USA 103:1930–1935

Gu Z, Jiang Q, Fu AK, Ip NY, Yan Z 2005 Regulation of NMDA receptors by neuregulin signaling in prefrontal cortex. J Neurosci 25:4974–4984

Hahn CG, Wang HY, Cho DS et al 2006 Altered neuregulin 1-ErbB4 signaling contributes to NMDA receptor hypofunction in schizophrenia. Nat Med 12:824–828

Hall J, Whalley HC, Job DE et al 2006. A neuregulin 1 variant associated with abnormal cortical function and psychotic symptoms. Nat Neurosci 9:1477–1478

Harrison PJ, Law AJ 2006 Neuregulin 1 and schizophrenia: genetics, gene expression, and neurobiology. Biol Psychiatry 60:132–140

Hashimoto R, Straub RE, Weickert CS, Hyde TM, Kleinman JE, Weinberger DR 2004 Expression analysis of neuregulin-1 in the dorsolateral prefrontal cortex in schizophrenia. Mol Psychiatry 9:299–307

Huang YZ, Won S, Ali DW et al 2000 Regulation of neuregulin signaling by PSD-95 interacting with ErbB4 at CNS synapses. Neuron 26:443–455

Kim E, Sheng M 2004 PDZ domain proteins of synapses. Nat Rev Neurosci 5:771–781

Kwon OB, Longart M, Vullhorst D, Hoffman DA, Buonanno A 2005 Neuregulin-1 reverses long-term potentiation at CA1 hippocampal synapses. J Neurosci 25:9378–9383

Lai C, Lemke G 1991 An extended family of protein-tyrosine kinase genes differentially expressed in the vertebrate nervous system. Neuron 6:691–704

Law AJ, Lipska BK, Weickert CS et al 2006 Neuregulin 1 transcripts are differentially expressed in schizophrenia and regulated by 5′ SNPs associated with the disease. Proc Natl Acad Sci USA 103:6747–6752

Law AJ, Shannon Weickert C, Hyde TM, Kleinman JE, Harrison PJ 2004 Neuregulin-1 (NRG-1) mRNA and protein in the adult human brain. Neuroscience 127:125–136

Lemke G 2001 Glial control of neuronal development. Annu Rev Neurosci 24:87–105

Longart M, Chatani-Hinze M, Gonzalez CM et al 2007 Regulation of ErbB-4 endocytosis by neuregulin in GABAergic hippocampal interneurons. Brain Res Bull 73:210–219

Malenka RC, Bear MF 2004 LTP and LTD: an embarrassment of riches. Neuron 44:5–21

Miyamoto Y, Yamada K Noda Y, Mori H, Mishina M, Nabeshima T 2001 Hyperfunction of dopaminergic and serotonergic neuronal systems in mice lacking the NMDA receptor epsilon1 subunit. J Neurosci 21:750–757

Mohn AR, Gainetdinov RR, Caron MG, Koller BH 1999 Mice with reduced NMDA receptor expression display behaviors related to schizophrenia. Cell 98:427–436

Nave KA, Salzer JL 2006 Axonal regulation of myelination by neuregulin 1. Curr Opin Neurobiol 16:492–500

Nicodemus KK, Luna A, Vakkalanka R et al 2006 Further evidence for association between ErbB4 and schizophrenia and influence on cognitive intermediate phenotypes in healthy controls. Mol Psychiatry 11:1062–1065

Owen MJ, Craddock N, O'Donovan MC 2005 Schizophrenia: genes at last? Trends Genet 21:518–525

Ozaki M, Itoh K, Miyakawa Y, Kishida H, Hashikawa T 2004 Protein processing and releases of neuregulin-1 are regulated in an activity-dependent manner. J Neurochem 91:176–188

Plant K, Pelkey KA, Bortolotto ZA et al 2006 Transient incorporation of native GluR2-lacking AMPA receptors during hippocampal long-term potentiation. Nat Neurosci 9:602–604

Silberberg G, Darvasi A, Pinkas-Kramarski R, Navon R 2006 The involvement of ErbB4 with schizophrenia: association and expression studies. Am J Med Genet B Neuropsychiatr Genet 141:142–148

Staubli U, Chun D 1996 Factors regulating the reversibility of long-term potentiation. J Neurosci 16:853–860

Staubli U, Scafidi J 1999 Time-dependent reversal of long-term potentiation in area CA1 of the freely moving rat induced by theta pulse stimulation. J Neurosci 19:8712–8719

Stefansson H, Sigurdsson E, Steinthorsdottir V et al 2002 Neuregulin 1 and susceptibility to schizophrenia. Am J Hum Genet 71: 877–892

Steinthorsdottir V, Stefansson H, Ghosh S et al 2004 Multiple novel transcription initiation sites for NRG-1. Gene 342:97–105

Thompson M, Lauderdale S, Webster MJ et al 2007 Widespread expression of ErbB2, ErbB3 and ErbB4 in non-human primate brain. Brain Res 1139:95–109

Tonegawa S 1995 Mammalian learning and memory studied by gene targeting. Ann N Y Acad Sci 758:213–217

DISCUSSION

Chao: I have a question about the receptors. Can you rule out the involvement of other ErbB receptor members in electrophysiological studies?

Buonanno: So far we haven't been able to. All we can say is that ErbB4 is necessary for this effect but we can't say it is sufficient.

Chao: The ErbB receptors are known to heterodimerize and to homodimerize.

Buonanno: Yes. There are four ErbB receptors, 1–4. Neuregulin binds specifically to ErbB3 and ErbB4. There is a large emphasis in the literature that ErbB3s are only glial. I disagree. Although glial cells predominantly express ErbB3, there is a transient expression of ErbB4 on oligodendrocytes, and we have also found that there are certain neuronal populations that also express ErbB3. In particular, the one that may be of interest is the thalamus. There also is lots of expression of NR2C subunit at the thalamus.

Lu: I have a physiology question. My understanding is that ErbB4 is expressed primarily in GABA neurons. What you are seeing here is neuregulin modulation of synapses in excitatory neurons, so it may be an indirect effect. Second, you showed that the TPS (theta pulse stimuli) effect can be blocked in neuregulin knockout mice or by receptor antagonists. A critical experiment would be to show that TPS could induce the secretion or activation of neuregulin.

Buonanno: To address the first one, ErbB4 is at its highest levels in inhibitory neurons. We have found a disconnect for ErbB2 and ErbB4 with regard to mRNA and protein. We all agree that ErbB4 is highest in inhibitory neurons and my position is that I don't yet know whether the levels that we can detect with certain antibodies in CA1 neurons, which are much lower, are relevant here. In a section we can see it in CA1 and not in the dentate neurons. We also see a small signal with P33-labelled cRNA probes when we do *in situ* hybridization. However, this does not eliminate the idea that this could be an indirect effect.

Lu: An experiment to directly test this would be to do LTP using the whole-cell approach where you could inject inhibitor directly into the cells. If this could block your neuregulin effect then this would be a demonstration of a direct effect of neuregulin on excitatory neurons.

Buonanno: This is a difficult experiment but we are trying to do it. We tried GABA receptor inhibitors and found that the neuregulin effect is not blocked by GABAA or GABAC inhibitors.

Lu: Can you see the TPS-induced secretion of neuregulin?

Buonanno: It would be great to know that. The groups who have shown release of neuregulin due to activity have been working in synaptosomes and granule cells. This is difficult to measure because the factors are at low levels. Most of these neuregulins bind to heparins or proteoglycans, or are membrane-associated. These aren't factors that will be easily released as soluble, free proteins. To measure release of neuregulin is extremely difficult. I don't know of any antibodies that would permit this experiment, but we are developing new ones.

Flint: I have problems with this electrophysiology. It gets more complicated each time I hear about it. Now, apparently, LTD doesn't exist.

Buonanno: Low-frequency long stimulus LTD has not been shown in slices from adult animals. Spike timing-dependent LTD might occur in adult animals.

Flint: So it is even more complicated. I have a real problem relating any of the phenomena to what happens in the animals. Is TPS an artefact of the way electrodes have been stuck in?

Buonanno: No. TPS-dependent depotentiation has been shown by Ursula Staubli and Joey Scafidi to reverse LTP *in vivo* (Staubli & Scafidi 1999).

Flint: In every case this is induced. You are sticking some stuff into the animal.

Buonanno: You have the electrodes that are sitting there, but you do controls to make sure this isn't having an effect.

Flint: So this is not like LTD, which is an induced phenomenon.

Buonanno: This is what I am saying. In one case you expose the animal to a novel environment where you record, and watch LTP in the animal.

Flint: But the experiments you showed were not like this.

Buonanno: No, mine were in acute slices.

Flint: You have an observational phenomenon: you see some EPSP thing go up and down. Putting it in a slice and giving some electricity results in the same thing. How do we know that the two phenomena have any relationship?

Lu: This is using electrophysiological methods to see something happening that is essentially correlative. The experiment to do here would be to let the animals learn something and remember it. In the middle of this you give TPS and induce depotentiation, and see if you can prevent learning or memory.

Buonanno: This is what we want to do. We need perspective, here, though: neuregulins are about 10 years behind neurotrophins. This is just the start.

Javitt: So are you saying that the LTP is not neuregulin-dependent, but the depotentiation is.

Buonanno: Yes.

Javitt: So if we want to take this into patients, the most straightforward prediction would be that if we had them learn new information, this should be relatively intact. But we then give neuregulin, what effect does it have? It seems there are things that NMDA does that don't involve neuregulin. It should be possible to look at these to distinguish a primary neuregulin effect from an NMDA effect.

Talmage: It might be regional. There are data from prefrontal cortex showing that neuregulin application suppresses NMDA-mediated transmission (Gu et al 2005). In this context, aspects of learning that are prefrontal cortex dependent would be affected more than those that are hippocampal.

Javitt: This leads to my next comment. There are parts of the brain outside the hippocampus and prefrontal cortex that are worth looking at.

Buonanno: Yes, it will be important to look at different synapses to see whether the mechanisms differ. Which way do we go? If neuregulin functions this way *in vivo* are the patients in the situation where their synapses are saturated, or is it that the threshold is too high?

References

Gu Z, Jiang Q, Fu AKY, Ip NY, Yan Z 2005 Regulation of NMDA receptors by neuregulin signaling in prefrontal cortex. J Neurosci 25:4974–84
Stäubli U, Scafidi J 1999 Time-dependent reversal of long-term potentiation in area CA1 of the freely moving rat induced by theta pulse stimulation. J Neurosci 19:8712–871

Impact of genetic variant BDNF (Val66Met) on brain structure and function

Zhe-Yu Chen*, Kevin Bath*, Bruce McEwen†, Barbara Hempstead‡ and Francis Lee*§[1]

*Department of Psychiatry, Weill Medical College of Cornell University, New York, NY 10021, †Laboratory of Neuroendocrinology, The Rockefeller University, New York, NY 10021, ‡Division of Hematology, Department of Medicine and §Department of Pharmacology, Weill Medical College of Cornell University, New York, NY 10021, USA

Abstract. A common single-nucleotide polymorphism in the human brain-derived neurotrophic factor (BDNF) gene, a methionine (Met) substitution for valine (Val) at codon 66 (Val66Met), is associated with alterations in brain anatomy and memory, but its relevance to clinical disorders is unclear. We generated a variant BDNF mouse (BDNF$^{Met/Met}$) that reproduces the phenotypic hallmarks in humans with the variant allele. Variant BDNF$_{Met}$ was expressed in brain at normal levels, but its secretion from neurons was defective. In this context, the BDNF$^{Met/Met}$ mouse represents a unique model that directly links altered activity-dependent release of BDNF to a defined set of *in vivo* consequences. Our subsequent analyses of these mice elucidated a phenotype that had not been established in human carriers: increased anxiety. When placed in conflict settings, BDNF$^{Met/Met}$ mice display increased anxiety-related behaviours that were not normalized by the antidepressant, fluoxetine. A genetic variant BDNF may thus play a key role in genetic predispositions to anxiety and depressive disorders.

2008 Growth factors and psychiatric disorders. Wiley, Chichester (Novartis Foundation Symposium 289) p 180–192

Brain-derived neurotrophic factor (BDNF), a molecule known to regulate neuronal survival and plasticity, is widely expressed in the developing and adult mammalian brain (Huang & Reichardt 2001, Chao 2003). In addition to regulating neuronal survival and differentiation, BDNF participates in activity-dependent plasticity processes such as long-term potentiation, learning and memory (Lu 2003a). Recently, a common single nucleotide polymorphism (SNP) in the BDNF

---

[1] This paper was presented at the symposium by Francis Lee, to whom correspondence should be addressed.

gene leading to a valine to methionine substitution at position 66 in the prodo-main (Val66Met) has been identified and shown to influence human hippocampal volume and memory (Egan et al 2003). This BDNF SNP only exists in human and is found to be also associated with altered susceptibility to a variety of neu-ropsychiatric disorders (Momose et al 2002, Neves-Pereira et al 2002, Sklar et al 2002, Ventriglia et al 2002, Sen et al 2003). This polymorphism in the BDNF gene represents an important initial example of a role for neurotrophins in behav-ioural processes in humans. This review will focus on the behavioural conse-quences of this variant form of BDNF in humans, and compare and contrast these findings with those in a newly generated mouse model containing this variant BDNF SNP.

Molecular mechanism underlying variant $BDNF_{Met}$

The actions of BDNF are dictated by two classes of cell surface receptors, the TrkB receptor tyrosine kinase and the p75 neurotrophin receptor ($p75^{NTR}$), a member of the tumour necrosis factor (TNF) receptor superfamily (Chao 2003). BDNF binding to TrkB receptor produces neurotrophic responses through rapid activation of the PI3 kinase, Ras/MAPK and PLCγ pathways, thus influencing transcriptional events that have multiple effects on cell cycle, neurite outgrowth and synaptic plasticity (Qui & Green 1991, Traverse et al 1992, Cowley et al 1994, Mazzucchelli et al 2002, Rosenblum et al 2002, Chao et al 2006). Signal transduc-tion through p75 independently gives rise to increase in JNK (c-Jun N-terminal kinase) and NF-κB (nuclear factor κB), thus triggering apoptosis (Roux & Barker 2002). Consistent with the critical role of BDNF in synaptic plasticity, BDNF is synthesized and released in an activity-dependent manner (Lu 2003b). In the mam-malian brain, BDNF is synthesized as a precursor called proBDNF, which is pro-teolytically cleaved to generate mature BDNF. ProBDNF may preferentially bind $p75^{NTR}$, whereas mature BDNF preferentially binds TrkB receptor (Lee et al 2001, Teng et al 2005).

The molecular mechanisms underlying altered $BDNF_{Met}$ function have begun to be studied primarily in *in vitro* cell culture systems. The Met substitution in the prodomain was shown in neurosecretory cells and primary cultured neurons to lead to three trafficking defects: (1) decreased variant BDNF distribution into neuronal dendrites; (2) decreased variant BDNF targeting to secretory granules; and (3) subsequent impairment in regulated secretion (Egan et al 2003, Chen et al 2004, 2005). In addition, when expressed together in the same cell, $BDNF_{Met}$ alters the trafficking of wild-type BDNF ($BDNF_{Val}$) through the formation of heterodimers that are less efficiently sorted into the regulated secretory pathway (Chen et al 2004). These initial findings are consistent with previous studies indicating that the prodomain of neurotrophins plays an important role in regulating their intracellular trafficking to secretory pathways (Suter et al 1991). Together, these *in vitro* studies with BDNF$_{Met}$ point to the presence of a specific trafficking signal in the BDNF prodomain region encompassing the Met substitution that is required for efficient BDNF sorting.

Recently, a trafficking protein, sortilin, was shown to be necessary for the efficient sorting of BDNF to the regulated secretory pathway. Sortilin interacts specifically with BDNF in a region encompassing the Met substitution (Chen et al 2005). Replacement of Met at this position led to decreased interaction of BDNF with this trafficking protein and suggests that decreased protein–protein interaction between BDNF and the trafficking machinery is one plausible molecular model for the secretion defect observed with the variant BDNF. This variant BDNF provides an example of how appropriate trafficking of BDNF may have a significant impact on the physiological responses to neurotrophins.

However, fundamental questions remain as to how these *in vitro* effects relate to the *in vivo* consequences of this SNP in humans. The main caveat to these *in vitro* overexpression studies has been that overexpression of neurotrophins has itself led to altered trafficking fates in cultured neurons (Farhadi et al 2000). As the majority of BDNF is released from the regulated secretory pathway in neurons, impaired regulated secretion of BDNF$_{Met}$ represents a significant decrease in available BDNF.

It also remains possible that there are additional defects in BDNF$_{Met}$ processing that may contribute to the observed deficits, although *in vitro* studies in neurons suggest no defect in BDNF$_{Met}$ processing (Egan et al 2003, Chen et al 2004). It has been reported that tissue plasminogen activator, by activating the extracellular protease plasmin, converts proBDNF to the mature BDNF, and that such conversion is critical for late-phase long-term potentiation in the mouse hippocampus (Pang et al 2004). Given that proBDNF preferentially activates p75^{NTR} over TrkB receptor, it is likely that proteolytic conversion of proBDNF may be implicated in BDNF functioning.

Variant BDNF$_{Met}$ and behavioural impairments

Until recently, no genetic associations had been identified linking neurotrophin genes to human cognitive functioning. Given BDNF's established role in mediating processes related to learning and memory (Korte et al 1995, Patterson et al 1996, Desai et al 1999), this increased susceptibility to cognitive impairment suggests that the variation in BDNF may play a role in the development of neuropsychiatric disorders as well as affecting nervous system function.

However, in any study attempting to associate a gene with pathology or behavioural variation, it is often unclear how the change in genotype results in the phenotypic change. This is especially difficult when attempting to link a change in genotype with a discrete change in cognitive functioning. It is possible that the identified genetic variant has a direct effect on cognition, but it is also plausible that the genetic variation mediates an effect through some other downstream functional change, or through the regulation of some other gene. These caveats must be kept in mind during this discussion. In addition, the majority of studies that have been conducted to date have either excluded subjects not of European descent, or have removed other ethnic groups prior to data analysis.

One of the most reliable effects observed in carriers of the Met allele (Val/Met) is a difference in hippocampal morphology. In studies of brain morphometry using structural magnetic resonance imaging (MRI) scans, Val/Met individuals have repeatedly been shown to have a smaller hippocampal volume relative to controls who are homozygous for the Val allele (Val/Val) (Pezawas et al 2004, Szeszko et al 2005, Bueller et al 2006, Frodl et al 2007). This difference may be related to the role that BDNF and its receptors play in the development as well as continued plasticity of the brain (Huang & Reichardt 2001, Lu et al 2005). Despite a wealth of information on individuals heterozygous for the Met polymorphism, little information exists for individuals who are homozygous for the Met allele (Met/Met) as this genotype is rare in the general population, comprising only 4% of people in Caucasian populations (Shimizu et al 2004, Gratacos et al 2007). In addition to effects on the hippocampus, studies have also shown decreased volume in the dorsolateral prefrontal cortex, an area associated with planning and higher order cognitive functioning, as well subcortical regions such as the caudate nucleus in carriers of the Met allele (Pezawas et al 2004). Recently it was found that Met allele carriers have smaller temporal and occipital lobar grey matter volumes (Ho et al 2006).

One of the common behavioural phenotypes associated with the variant $BDNF_{Met}$ is impairment of higher cognitive abilities. Individuals with the Val/Met genotype have been shown to perform more poorly than control subjects (Val/Val) on memory tasks that rely heavily on the hippocampus (Egan et al 2003, Hariri et al 2003). On the basis of batteries of neuropsychological tests, carriers of the Met allele (Val/Met and Met/Met) were shown to perform worse on tasks that involved recalling places and events, but did not differ from Val/Val individuals on tasks that have been classically shown to be less hippocampal-dependent, such as word learning and planning tasks (Egan et al 2003, Hariri et al 2003). The pattern of brain activation in Val/Met individuals also significantly differed from that of Val/Val subjects during tasks that rely on the hippocampus. Using functional MRI (fMRI), Hariri et al (2003) showed that during a place recognition task, a task that has been shown to result in strong hippocampal activation (Gabrieli et al 1998, Schacter et al 1999, Schacter & Wagner 1999), individuals with the Val/Met genotype had significantly lower levels of activation compared to Val/Val individuals during both the encoding and retrieval portions of the task. In a similar functional imaging study, Egan et al (2003) employed a task that required individuals to remember a set of stimuli and recall the stimulus that had been presented two stimuli prior to the current stimulus (N-back task), a paradigm that typically results in suppression of the hippocampus. They found that individuals with the Met/Met genotype did not show the same level of hippocampal suppression as subjects with the Val/Val or Val/Met genotypes. These findings taken together suggest that carriers of the Met allele have a selective impairment in hippocampal-dependent memory.

Anxiety is a common symptom among most psychiatric disorders. Several recent studies have looked at the relationship between $BDNF_{Met}$ and trait anxiety. The results have been conflicting, with the Val allele associated with vulnerability in one study and the Met allele designated as the 'risk' allele in another study (Sen et al 2003, Jiang et al 2005, Lang et al 2005). Inconsistency across genetic studies may be attributable to sampling and measurement issues, genetic heterogeneity due to differential sampling of populations or low frequency of homozygous Met carriers, which may lessen the effect size of any particular association. It may also relate to a failure to take into account relevant gene-by-gene and gene-by-environment interactions. A recent investigation found an association between incident stroke and depression, with the strongest association for Met/Met genotype participants (Kim et al 2007). This study provides evidence for a gene–environment interaction with respect to the impact of stroke on depression. Another study revealed a significant three-way interaction between the BDNF genotype, 5-HTTLPR, and maltreatment history in predicting depression (Kaufman et al 2006). Children with the $BDNF_{Met}$ allele and two short alleles of 5-HTTLPR had the highest depression scores, but the vulnerability associated with these two genotypes was only evident in the maltreated children.

Variant $BDNF_{Met}$ knock-in mouse

Recently, a variant BDNF mouse ($BDNF^{Met/Met}$) was generated that reproduces the phenotypic hallmarks in humans with this BDNF SNP (Chen et al 2006). The expression of $BDNF_{Met}$ is regulated by endogenous BDNF promoters in the $BDNF_{Met}$ knock-in mouse, which fully mimic the human $BDNF_{Met}$ polymorphism. The $BDNF_{Met}$ knock-in mouse has allowed for assessment of the *in vivo* consequences of $BDNF_{Met}$ not only for biochemical but also anatomical and behavioural measures.

Initial secretion studies were performed on neurons obtained from the $BDNF_{Met}$ mice, and BDNF in the resultant media was measured by enzyme-linked immunosorbent assay (ELISA). There was a significant decrease in activity-dependent secretion of endogenous BDNF from $BDNF^{Met/Met}$ mice (~30% decrease). As the majority of BDNF is released from the regulated secretory pathway in neurons, impaired regulated secretion from BDNF$^{Met/Met}$ neurons represents a significant decrease in available BDNF.

Subsequent anatomical analyses showed that there was a significant decrease in hippocampal volume in both BDNF$^{+/Met}$ and BDNF$^{Met/Met}$ mice. Furthermore, Golgi staining was used to visualize individual dentate gyrus neurons of the hippocampus. At 8 weeks of age, there was no difference in the cell soma area among BDNF$_{Met}$ mice and their littermate controls, but a decrease in dendritic arbour complexity in BDNF$_{Met}$ mice. Behavioural studies determined that there was a specific impairment in hippocampal contextual fear conditioning in both BDNF$^{+/Met}$ and BDNF$^{Met/Met}$ mice, whereas there was no difference in cue-dependent fear conditioning. BDNF$_{Met}$ mice thus appear to replicate the two hallmark alterations in hippocampal anatomy and hippocampal-dependent learning as human carriers of the BDNF$_{Met}$ allele. These results suggest that BDNF$_{Met}$ mice are a valid animal model for the human variant BDNF SNP.

Subsequent analyses of these mice elucidated a phenotype that had not been established in human carriers: increased anxiety. When placed in conflict settings, BDNF$^{Met/Met}$ mice display increased anxiety-related behaviours in three separate tests and thus provide a genetic link between BDNF and anxiety. Human genetic association studies have been inconclusive as to the contribution of this SNP to increased anxiety (Gratacos et al 2007). Two main differences in the mouse study design probably contributed to discerning this anxiety-related phenotype. First, mice were subjected to conflict tests to elicit the increased anxiety-related behaviour, whereas human studies relied on questionnaires. Second, the anxiety-related phenotype was only present in mice homozygous for the Met allele, which suggested that association studies that focused primarily on humans heterozygous for the Met allele may not detect an association.

The form of anxiety elicited in these BDNF$^{Met/Met}$ mice was not responsive to a common selective serotonin reuptake inhibitor (SSRI). These results suggest that humans with this allele may not have optimal responses to this class of antidepressants. Currently, there are no reliable genetic or non-genetic biomarkers to predict who will respond to an SSRI. The transgenic BDNF$^{Met/Met}$ mouse may serve as a valuable model to identify novel pharmacological approaches to treating anxiety symptoms that underlie many neuropsychiatric disorders.

Conclusions

The human genetic variant BDNF (Val66Met) represents the first example of a neurotrophin family member that has been linked to anatomical and behavioural phenotypes in humans. However, its relevance to clinical disorders is unclear. A BDNF$_{Met}$ mouse model has been generated to test, in a more controlled and precise manner than in human studies, the contribution of this variant BDNF SNP to neuropsychiatric disease processes. In all, these findings indicate a new direction in therapeutic strategies to rescue anxiety symptoms in humans with this polymorphic allele. Drug discovery strategies to increase BDNF release from synapses or to prolong the half-life of secreted BDNF may improve therapeutic responses for humans with this common BDNF polymorphism.

References

Bueller JA, Aftab M, Sen S, Gomez-Hassan D, Burmeister M, Zubieta JK 2006 BDNF Val(66)Met allele is associated with reduced hippocampal volume in healthy subjects. Biol Psychiatry 59:812–815

Chao MV 2003 Neurotrophins and their receptors: a convergence point for many signalling pathways. Nat Rev Neurosci 4:299–309

Chao MV, Rajagopal R, Lee FS 2006 Neurotrophin signalling in health and disease. Clin Sci (Lond) 110:167–173

Chen ZY, Patel PD, Sant G et al 2004 Variant brain-derived neurotrophic factor (BDNF) (Met66) alters the intracellular trafficking and activity-dependent secretion of wild-type BDNF in neurosecretory cells and cortical neurons. J Neurosci 24:4401–4411

Chen ZY, Ieraci A, Teng H et al 2005 Sortilin controls intracellular sorting of brain-derived neurotrophic factor to the regulated secretory pathway. J Neurosci 25:6156–6166

Chen ZY, Jing D, Bath KG et al 2006 Genetic variant BDNF (Val66Met) polymorphism alters anxiety-related behavior. Science 314:140–143

Cowley S, Paterson H, Kemp P, Marshall CJ 1994 Activation of MAP kinase kinase is necessary and sufficient for PC12 differentiation and for transformation of NIH 3T3 cells. Cell 77:841–852

Desai N, Rutherford L, Turrigiano G 1999 BDNF regulates the intrinsic excitability of cortical neurons. Learn Mem 6:284–291

Egan MF, Kojima M, Callicott JH et al 2003 The BDNF Val66Met polymorphism affects activity-dependent secretion of BDNF and human memory and hippocampal function. Cell 112:257–269

Farhadi H, Mowla S, Petrecca K, Morris S, Seidah N, Murphy R 2000 Neurotrophin-3 sorts to the constitutive secretory pathway of hippocampal neurons and is diverted to the regulated secretory pathway by coexpression with brain-derived neurotrophic factor. J Neurosci 20:4059–4068

Frodl T, Schule C, Schmitt G et al 2007 Association of the brain-derived neurotrophic factor Val66Met polymorphism with reduced hippocampal volumes in major depression. Arch Gen Psychiatry 64:410–416

Gabrieli JD, Brewer JB, Poldrack RA 1998 Images of medial temporal lobe functions in human learning and memory. Neurobiol Learn Mem 70:275–283

Gratacos M, Gonzalez JR, Mercader JM, Cid RD, Urretavizcaya M, Estivill X 2007 Brain-derived neurotrophic factor Val66Met and psychiatric disorders: meta-analysis of case-control studies confirm association to substance-related disorders, eating disorders, and schizophrenia. Biol Psychiatry 61:911–922

Hariri AR, Goldberg TE, Mattay VS et al 2003 Brain-derived neurotrophic factor Val66Met polymorphism affects human memory-related hippocampal activity and predicts memory performance. J Neurosci 23:6690–6694

Ho BC, Milev P, O'Leary DS, Librant A, Andreasen NC, Wassink TH 2006 Cognitive and magnetic resonance imaging brain morphometric correlates of brain-derived neurotrophic factor Val66Met gene polymorphism in patients with schizophrenia and healthy volunteers. Arch Gen Psychiatry 63:731–740

Huang E, Reichardt L 2001 Neurotrophins: roles in neuronal development and function. Annu Rev Neurosci 24:677–736.

Jiang X, Xu K, Hoberman J et al 2005 BDNF variation and mood disorders: a novel functional promoter polymorphism and Val66Met are associated with anxiety but have opposing effects. Neuropsychopharmacology 30:1353–1361

Kaufman J, Yang BZ, Douglas-Palumberi H et al 2006 Brain-derived neurotrophic factor–5-HTTLPR gene interactions and environmental modifiers of depression in children. Biol Psychiatry 59:673–680

Kim JM, Stewart R, Kim SW et al 2007 BDNF genotype potentially modifying the association between incident stroke and depression. Neurobiol Aging. In press

Korte M, Carroll P, Wolf E, Brem G, Thoenen H, Bonhoeffer T 1995 Hippocampal long-term potentiation is impaired in mice lacking brain-derived neurotrophic factor. Proc Natl Acad Sci USA 92:8856–8860

Lang UE, Hellweg R, Kalus P et al 2005 Association of a functional BDNF polymorphism and anxiety-related personality traits. Psychopharmacology (Berl) 180:95–99

Lee R, Kermani P, Teng KK, Hempstead BL 2001 Regulation of cell survival by secreted pro-neurotrophins. Science 294:1945–1948

Lu B 2003a BDNF and activity-dependent synaptic modulation. Learn Mem 100:86–98

Lu B 2003b Pro-region of neurotrophins: role in synaptic modulation. Neuron 39:735–738

Lu B, Pang PT, Woo NH 2005 The yin and yang of neurotrophin action. Nat Rev Neurosci 6:603–614

Mazzucchelli C, Vantaggiato C, Ciamei A et al 2002 Knockout of Erk1 MAP kinase enhances synaptic plasticity in the striatum and facilitates striatal mediated learning and memory. Neuron 34:807–820

Momose Y, Murata M, Kobayashi K et al 2002 Association studies of multiple candidate genes for Parkinson's disease using single nucleotide polymorphisms. Ann Neurol 51:133–136

Neves-Pereira M, Mundo E, Muglia P, King N, Macciardi F, Kennedy J 2002 The brain-derived neurotrophic factor gene confers susceptibility to bipolar disorder: evidence from a family-based association study. Am J Hum Genet 71:651–655

Pang PT, Teng HK, Zaitsev E et al 2004 Cleavage of proBDNF by tPA/plasmin is essential for long-term hippocampal plasticity. Science 306:487–491

Patterson S, Abel T, Deuel T, Martin K, Rose J, Kandel E 1996 Recombinant BDNF rescues deficits in basal synaptic transmission and hippocampal LTP in BDNF knockout mice. Neuron 16:1137–1145

Pezawas L, Verchinski BA, Mattay VS et al 2004 The brain-derived neurotrophic factor Val66Met polymorphism and variation in human cortical morphology. J Neurosci 24:10099–10102

Qui M-S, Green SH 1991 NGF and EGF rapidly activate p21ras in PC12 cells by distinct, convergent pathways involving tyrosine phosphorylation. Neuron 7:937–946

Rosenblum K, Futter M, Voss K et al 2002 The role of extracellular regulated kinases I/II in late-phase long-term potentiation. J Neurosci 22:5432–5441

Roux PP, Barker PA 2002 Neurotrophin signaling through the p75 neurotrophin receptor. Prog Neurobiol 67:203–233

Schacter DL, Wagner AD 1999 Perspectives: neuroscience. Remembrance of things past. Science 285:1503–1504

Schacter DL, Curran T, Reiman EM, Chen K, Bandy DJ, Frost JT 1999 Medial temporal lobe activation during episodic encoding and retrieval: a PET study. Hippocampus 9:575–581

Sen S, Nesse RM, Stoltenberg SF et al 2003 A BDNF coding variant is associated with the NEO personality inventory domain neuroticism, a risk factor for depression. Neuropsychopharmacology 28:397–401

Shimizu E, Hashimoto K, Iyo M 2004 Ethnic difference of the BDNF 196G/A (Val66Met) polymorphism frequencies: the possibility to explain ethnic mental traits. Am J Med Genet B Neuropsychiatr Genet 126:122–123

Sklar P, Gabriel S, McInnis M et al 2002 Family-based association study of 76 candidate genes in bipolar disorder: BDNF is a potential risk locus. Mol Psychiatry 7:579–593

Suter U, Heymach J, Shooter E 1991 Two conserved domains in the NGF polypeptide are necessary and sufficient for the biosynthesis of correctly processed and biologically active NGF. EMBO J 10:2394–2400

Szeszko PR, Lipsky R, Mentschel C et al 2005 Brain-derived neurotrophic factor Val66Met polymorphism and volume of the hippocampal formation. Mol Psychiatry 10:631–636

Teng HK, Teng KK, Lee R et al 2005 ProBDNF induces neuronal apoptosis via activation of a receptor complex of p75NTR and sortilin. J Neurosci 25:5455–5463

Traverse S, Gomez N, Paterson H, Marshall C, Cohen P 1992 Sustained activation of the mitogen-activated (MAP) kinase cascade may be required for differentiation of PC12 cells. Biochem J 288:351–355

Ventriglia M, Bocchio Chiavetto L, Benussi L et al 2002 Association between the BDNF 196 A/G polymorphism and sporadic Alzheimer's disease. Mol Psychiatry 7:136–137

DISCUSSION

Flint: Can I clarify one thing about the Val66Met polymorphism in the pro-domain? In the mature animal we have heard that there is no pro-BDNF, and you have said that mature BDNF is only found in the adult. Does this mean that this effect has to be developmental?

Lee: No, I think this effect is potentially in the Golgi apparatus. The pro-domain is likely to be involved in proper protein folding and trafficking. The consensus is that the cutting might occur at the Golgi or within the secretory granule itself. We don't know where the cleavage event occurs. Perhaps what sortilin is doing is maintaining fidelity of folding. It might be needed for proper folding and sorting to occur, and once it is there, its job is done. If you have a decreased protein–protein interaction with the pro-domain and sortilin, the result could be the 25% loss of efficiency in the amount of protein that gets into the granule.

Flint: From your *in situ* hybridizations it looked like you were only seeing a lot of BDNF of protein in the adult.

Lu: That technique cannot distinguish between pro and mature BDNF.

Flint: There must be some relationship here.

Barde: You have 10 times more protein, but immunoassays do not distinguish between the pro or mature forms. I think its all mature BDNF anyway, but there is a 10-fold increase as predicted by the *in situ* hybridization and quantitative mRNA determination.

Lee: Presumably, you would agree that in some form pro-BDNF exists during the rapid biosynthetic phase.

Barde: Of course.

Flint: The trouble I have with this is that you are reporting anatomical changes in the hippocampus, which in my mind must be developmental at some stage. You are showing that the major expression of this gene is postnatal.

Lu: Expression of a gene does not always equate to expression of a protein.

Akil: The hippocampus keeps developing postnatally.

Lee: I think the question is about whether the expression of BDNF early on is enough to cause changes in hippocampal volume.

Malaspina: People can have decreased hippocampal volume even in their 20s. Many things can measurably reduce hippocampal volume without this being developmental.

Flint: He's dealing with a genetic effect.

Lee: We believe that the hippocampal volume difference is not because of a cell loss. It is most likely going to be the dendritic arborization effect: an increase in complexity of the dendritic arbours. This can occur at any time.

Hen: You took us on a surprising tangent. On the one hand, you tell us that these animals don't respond to fluoxetine. Obviously we want to know what is happening in the hippocampus, not in the olfactory bulb. If neurogenesis has anything to do with their lack of response to fluoxetine, we would expect that fluoxetine does not stimulate neurogenesis in these animals. Fluoxetine not only has effects on proliferation, but also on survival and differentiation. These are the effects I'd expect to be absent in your experiments.

Lee: We'll see.

Bothwell: The Met/Met BDNF primarily affects the regulated secretion, and not so much the constitutive secretion. You suggested that BDNF was coming from support cells. Are these glial cells? They might not have the secretory pathway.

Lee: It is possible. There is also controversy about whether BDNF is secreted in a regulated manner from glial cells, based on Cheryl Dreyfus' work (Jean et al 2006). We are not sure which cells are involved.

Lu: What other cells are in there?

Lee: Type B, but mainly gilal cells. Possibly also endothelial cells.

Castrén: So sortilin is also implicated in the interaction with the p75 receptor. What is the relationship between these effects? Is there any competition? Is this pure chance?

Lee: Sortilin probably has a binding module that binds multiple growth factors. It just happened that when Barbara Hempstead started studying pro-NGF, sortilin bound to it. 10% of sortilin is at the cell surface. It is probably doing two things. Very similarly to the mannose-6-phosphate receptor, it is probably doing a Golgi-sorting event. It gets to the cell surface and picks up pro-NGF or neurotensin and does something else. The only time when high p75 levels and high sortilin levels occur together is during injury, not in normal brain. In the normal brain there isn't much p75 around. Even if the sortilin went up there, it probably wouldn't see any p75.

Castrén: Is the site the same as pro-neurotensin?

Lee: This hasn't been mapped.

Akil: With FGF, there are some forms that are secreted, some that stay cytoplasmic and some that go to the nucleus. Is there a sorting difference, with less going into the secretory pathway if some goes somewhere else?

Lee: We think it is a secretory granule. We have done a co-localization with some secretory granule markers. It is not clear what compartment it goes to, and whether it goes to an additional compartment other than this granule-like compartment.

Akil: Are there allelic variants? Is it a matter of amount where a certain percentage goes to secretory granules and the rest dies?

Lu: Is there is a compensatory increase in constitutive secretion in the Met/Met animals?

Lee: This was a sort of overexpression siRNA experiment, but in the Met/Met animal we don't see a compensatory increase in constitutive secretion.

Akil: It is not decreasing either.

Lee: Exactly. What you have picked up on is that the levels of BDNF in the whole brain are identical. It has gone somewhere.

Akil: That's why I am asking: is it cytoplasmic, but not secretory? Is it going to the nucleus? Is it doing some other job?

Lee: I don't know. It is somewhere in suspended animation!

Akil: Is there a correlation between allelic variation and olfactory function in humans?

Lee: We don't know.

Lu: We should probably look at BDNF very differently from most of the growth factors, including FGF. Perhaps 10% of BDNF is like other growth factors, with constitutive secretion. The majority of BDNF (> 80%) is going through regulated secretion.

Raff: Are Met/Met humans anxious?

Lee: A good guidepost to this would be the serotonin transporter story. In order to have major depression you need two copies and a horrific childhood. It could be another gene–environment interaction. It just happened that by virtue of a uniform background and a controlled environment, we were able to tease out this phenotype.

Raff: Do we know if they are narcissistic and anxious?

Castrén: There is a study where neuroticism is actually increased. The problem there is that the alleles vary. The Val allele is a risk for bipolar disorder.

Lee: Margit Burmeister (Sen et al 2003) said that the Val allele was associated with neuroticism. Robert Lipsky's (Jiang et al 2005) group said that it was the Met allele. Another group in Germany said it was neither (Lang et al 2005).

Malaspina: I have a comment about the olfactory deficits. With bipolar disorder it is interesting that lithium improves olfactory discrimination. Using the available techniques people haven't been able to demonstrate any odour discrimination deficits in depression or anxiety. I am now doing olfactory ERPs in these groups. In schizophrenia there are different levels of severity of the deficit. Does this go against your hypothesis that anxious and depressed patients don't have measurable defects?

Lee: I don't know. This might be a very small effect size: there is always variation in the controls.

Malaspina: Controls do remarkably well on olfactory discrimination using the University of Pennsylvania test. The females in general score measurably better than males. These technologies have not been able to pick it up. There may be something that can rescue the BDNF effect in the anxiety and the depression disorders that is a second defect in schizophrenia.

Sendtner: We have done many experiments to localize BDNF within the cells that produce it. We have never found it in the nucleus, or evenly distributed in the cytoplasm: it was always in vesicle-like structures, at least in those cells that we investigated. Most cells in the CNS that express BDNF also express TrkB. Therefore there must be an intelligent sorting mechanism within the cell such that BDNF doesn't get into the same vesicles as TrkB. You did some interesting experiments with the phospho-TrkB antibody. Did you see evidence for abnormal sorting such that these two kinds of vesicles come together within cells?

Lee: We could do those experiments, but we'd have to get the neurons out of the mice. The phospho-TrkB antibody works with immunocytochemistry and with an epitope tag. Theoretically we should be able to follow both of these.

Akil: Is localization with both allelic variants?

Sendtner: Just wild-type.

Akil: My working hypothesis is that the interesting question is whether this changes with the Met allele variant.

Lee: Exactly.

Hen: There is a complicating factor: in the BDNF heterozygotes, there are profound changes in the serotonergic system. I wouldn't be surprised if you found quite a bit of change in the serotonergic system. You mentioned gene–environment interactions. I'd be very interested in seeing interactions between Val66Met polymorphisms and the serotonin transporter polymorphism.

Lu: This has been done to some degree.

Giedd: There are fMRI studies looking at COMT interactions (Harrison & Weinberger 2005) but I did not find any specifically addressing BDNF and serotonin. There is a paper looking at the interaction between serotonin transporter and BDNF and lithium response but it does not use fMRI (Rybakowski et al 2007).

Lu: Are the Met/Met animals aggressive?

Lee: We don't keep them long enough: if the mice are over 4 months old they get very aggressive. There have been studies with the heterozygote transporter knockout mouse and the heterozygote BDNF mice, and everything got worse.

Sklar: What happens if you give mature BDNF back to these mice? Since this is a constitutive knock-in one does not know specifically what is altered downstream or in development.

Lee: People have shown that serotonin 1A and 2A are altered in the heterozygote knockout mouse. We plan to do binding studies on this. We were talking to Rudy Jaenisch because he has the conditional BDNF over-expressor. This is the way to go: you could theoretically use a virus and inject for localized over-expression.

Tongiorgi: You mentioned a nice restriction in hippocampal volume which correlates well with the reduction in hippocampal volume in humans. Is there any neuroanatomical change so you can measure pruning of dendrites or myelin deficits?

Lee: We have looked at CA1, CA3 and dentate gyrus neurons, and they are statistically significantly smaller. They are smaller from P7.

References

Harrison PJ, Weinberger DR 2005 Schizophrenia genes, gene expression, and neuropathology: on the matter of their convergence. Mol Psychiatry 10:40–68; image 5

Jean YY, Lercher LD, Dreyfus CF 2006 Glutamate elicited increases in expression and release of BDNF in basal forebrain (BF) astrocytes influences the survival and function of BF cholinergic neurons. Society for Neuroscience Abstract.

Jiang X, Xu K, Hoberman J et al 2005 BDNF variation and mood disorders: a novel functional promoter polymorphism and Val66Met are associated with anxiety but have opposing effects. Neuropsychopharmacology 30:1353–1361

Lang UE, Hellweg R, Kalus P et al 2005 Association of a functional BDNF polymorphism and anxiety-related personality traits. Psychopharmacology (Berl) 180:95–99

Rybakowski JK, Suwalska A, Skibinska M et al 2007 Response to lithium prophylaxis: interaction between serotonin transporter and BDNF genes. Am J Med Genet B Neuropsychiatr Genet 144:820–823.

Sen S, Nesse R, Stoltenberg S et al 2003 A BDNF coding variant is associated with the NEO personality inventory domain neuroticism, a risk factor for depression. Neuropsychopharmacology 28:397–401

General discussion II

Chao: I wish to summarize several points from today's session. There is a pronounced developmental trajectory to many events in the CNS: prefrontal cortex development, grey matter development, the level of brain-derived neurotrophic factor (BDNF) expression and even the elaboration of long-term potentiation (LTP) and long-term depression (LTD), which appear to occur only during certain developmental time frames. This raises the interesting issue of critical periods and developmental time frames. I am curious to hear from the geneticists and clinicians about how they consider the data on developmental changes and timing. Theses changes present many problems in terms of clinical application and predictabilities.

Flint: The genetic approach is nice, because it can be done with no theory. But then you have no idea when and where the gene is acting. The problems the studies we have been hearing throw up are immense. If everyone agrees that a particular polymorphism is involved in depression or schizophrenia, sorting out where in the brain this is acting is going to be a huge problem.

Giedd: We have a lack of knowledge about the developmental course of these systems. Can this be mapped out?

Flint: To be heretical, I would argue that the genetics is a waste of time. Instead we need to give all the money to René Hen who can take the existing models of depression and find new mechanisms.

Malaspina: One of the values of these sorts of forums is that unless we can inform one another constantly about the pathways and the critical periods of the disease, then it's hard to make sense either one way or the other.

Hen: We need to distinguish the development time course from the therapeutic workings. If you want to design better drugs you need to understand how the current ones work. For this we don't need development that much. If you want to categorize disease and identify treatment-resistant schizophrenia, for example, then you need the genetics. It is probably based on the genetic subcategorizations that you will end up with type 1, 2, 3 and so on. The genetics enables us to categorize diseases better than just having depression and schizophrenia as big amorphous blobs, but in terms of devising treatments we need to understand how drugs such as Prozac work.

Spedding: Looking at the existing drugs is going backwards. We won't get new drugs this way. We already know that the existing drugs do not precisely target the pathophysiology.

Hen: That's not what I meant. When I am talking about understanding how Prozac works, the first thing you need to understand is what part of the brain it works on. Then you can think of new targets for that part of the brain. Currently we don't know what part of the brain it works on.

Owen: Jonathan Flint has a point, up to a point: depression is a good example of something that one seems to be able to model adequately in animals. Therefore invasive functional work can be done. I think it is different for schizophrenia and bipolar disorder, where we will have to rely on the genetics to get into the pathways. I am interested to hear that with BDNF the Val/Met findings have replicated so clearly. If this is true, it is exciting, but it suggests that it is a polymorphism in search of a pathological phenotype.

Sklar: It does not have to be a pathological phenotype. Amino acids are changed all over the genome for many reasons.

Owen: Given the other evidence we have heard here, it would be sensible to take a careful look at comparing people with the different genotypes from a psychopathological perspective.

Sklar: In psychiatry, theories have come and gone. They are useful therapeutically: the dopamine theory has resulted in drugs that have been successful. Similarly for serotonin and glutamate. The brain only has a certain number of systems that it uses to communicate. No matter what is the genetic cause, those systems are involved. The question is whether they are causally involved or not. I am not sure there is currently any way to answer this question other than genetics. The basic fact is that each of us walks around with roughly 10 million polymorphisms. Most of these set our systems in ways that are not understood. Almost all will not be causally related to disease. It will take a long time to sort all this out. We lack strong biological aetiological evidence for schizophrenia and bipolar disorder, and we thus lack great candidate hypotheses, so that some of these unbiased genetic approaches need to be pursued at least for a while. It may turn out to be impossible to find the genes. There is as yet no empirical evidence for this.

Akil: It is interesting to talk to people in other fields. They are often surprised that we have an embarrassment of riches: we have too much information in neuroscience. The trick is to figure out how to frame the questions in the face of a lot of potential questions and a lot of data. It is easy to think it is just genetics or the single nucleotide polymorphisms (SNPs) that have this problem. But from the basic science point of view there is a lot to work on. It is helpful to think about how to prioritize. I have a more convergent kind of view of how neuroscience needs to progress, where people with different styles of thinking and levels of discourse need to be allowed to bloom. We are just too stupid to know what the best way is. I don't think genetics has exhausted its possibilities in terms of technology and analysis. I don't think neuroscientists have figured out all the best ways to frame the question and image things. It is premature to decide if one approach is useless. We can't afford to throw away entire approaches. Given that money is tight and work is expensive, we should talk as we are doing here and agree what the most important problems are.

Buonanno: I agree, but if you press me for my choice, the problem I have is the plasticity of the brain itself and its tremendous interconnectivity. The way that we do science most of the time is that we all specialize because the systems are complicated. I would put my money on genetics: it has to continue moving forward because we need to get to those first effects and then be able to focus on those changes that either account for the deficits or are compensatory changes that result from the brain plasticity.

Growth and schizophrenia: aetiology, epidemiology and epigenetics

D. Malaspina, M. Perrin, K. R. Kleinhaus*, M. Opler and S. Harlap

Department of Psychiatry, New York University School of Medicine, New York, NY 10016, USA and
*Department of Psychiatry, Columbia University, New York, NY 10032, USA

Abstract. There is a strong genetic component for schizophrenia risk, but it is unclear how the illness is maintained in the population given the significantly reduced fertility of those with the disorder. One possibility is that new mutations occur in schizophrenia vulnerability genes. If so, then those with schizophrenia may have older fathers, since advancing paternal age is the major source of new mutations in humans. We found that paternal age at conception is a robust risk factor for schizophrenia, explaining perhaps a quarter of all cases. The predisposing genetic events appear to occur stochastically in proportion to advancing paternal age, and the possible mechanisms include *de novo* point mutations or defective epigenetic regulation of paternal genes. The risk might also be related to paternal toxic exposures, nutritional deficiencies, suboptimal DNA repair enzymes or other factors that influence the fidelity of genetic information in the constantly replicating male germ line. We propose that *de novo* genetic alterations in the paternal germline cause an independent and common variant of schizophrenia and that abnormal methylation of paternally imprinted genes could be the mechanism. These findings suggest exciting new directions for research into the aetiology of schizophrenia.

2008 Growth factors and psychiatric disorders. Wiley, Chichester (Novartis Foundation Symposium 289) p 196–207

Schizophrenia is commonly considered to result from the interplay between genetic susceptibility and environmental exposures, particularly those that occur during fetal development and in adolescence. A number of susceptibility genes have recently been identified, as detailed by other chapters in this book, but these are estimated to have only a small effect on the population-wide risk for the disease. Since most schizophrenia cases have no family history of psychosis, we examined the relationship between paternal age and the risk for schizophrenia to see if *de novo* genetic events could contribute to the incidence of schizophrenia. This strategy was chosen because paternal age is the major source of *de novo* mutations in the human population. The effect of paternal age on mutation rates is theorized to be due to the constant cell replication cycles that occur in spermatogenesis (Crow

196

1997). Following puberty, spermatogonia undergo some 23 divisions per year. At ages 20 and 40, respectively, a man's germ cell precursors will have undergone about 200 and 660 such divisions. During a man's life, the spermatogonia are vulnerable to DNA damage and mutations may accumulate in clones of spermatogonia as men age. In contrast, the numbers of such divisions in female germ cells is usually 24, all but the last occurring during fetal life.

We demonstrated a monotonic increase in the risk of schizophrenia as paternal age advanced in the rich database of the Jerusalem Perinatal Cohort (Malaspina et al 2001). Compared with the offspring of fathers aged 20–24 years, in well controlled analyses, each decade of paternal age multiplied the risk for schizophrenia by 1.4 (95% confidence interval: 1.2–1.7), so that the relative risk (RR) for offspring of fathers aged 45+ was 3.0 (1.6–5.5), with 1/46 of these offspring developing schizophrenia. There were no comparable maternal age effects. This finding has now been replicated in numerous cohorts from diverse populations (Sipos et al 2004, El-Saadi et al 2004, Zammit et al 2003, Byrne et al 2003, Dalman & Allebeck 2002, Brown et al 2002, Tsuchiya et al 2005). By and large, each study shows a tripling of the risk for schizophrenia for the offspring of the oldest group of fathers, in comparison to the risk in a reference group of younger fathers. There is also a 'dosage effect' of increasing paternal age; risk is roughly doubled for the offspring of men in their 40s and is tripled for paternal age >50 years. These studies are methodologically sound and most of them have employed prospective exposure data and validated psychiatric diagnoses. Together they demonstrate that the paternal age effect is not explained by other factors, including family history, maternal age, parental education and social ability, family social integration, social class, birth order, birth weight and birth complications. Furthermore, the paternal age effect is specific for schizophrenia, versus other adult onset psychiatric disorders. This is not the case for any other known schizophrenia risk factor, including many of the putative susceptibility genes (Craddock et al 2006).

There have been no failures to replicate the paternal age effect, nor its approximate magnitude, in any adequately powered study. The data support the hypothesis that paternal age increases schizophrenia risk through a *de novo* genetic mechanism. The remarkable uniformity of the results across different cultures lends further coherence to the conclusion that this robust relationship is likely to reflect an innate human biological phenomenon that progresses over ageing in the male germline, which is independent of regional, environmental, infectious or other routes.

Indeed, the consistency of these data is unparalleled in schizophrenia research, with the exception of the increase in risk to the relatives of schizophrenia probands (i.e. 10% for a sibling). Yet while having an affected first degree relative confers a relatively higher risk for illness than having a father >50 years (~10% versus ~2%), paternal age explains a far greater portion of the population attributable risk for schizophrenia. This is because a family history is infrequent among schizophrenia cases, whereas paternal age explained 26.6% of the schizophrenia cases in our Jerusalem cohort. If we had only considered the risk in the cases with paternal age >30 years, our risk would be equivalent to that reported by Sipos et al (2004) in the Swedish study (15.5%). When paternal ages >25 years are considered, the calculated risk is much higher. Although the increment in risk for fathers age 26 through 30 years is small (~14%), this group is very large, which accounts for the magnitude of their contribution to the overall risk. The actual percentage of cases with paternal germline-derived schizophrenia in a given population will depend on the demographics of paternal childbearing age, among other factors. With an upswing in paternal age, these cases would be expected to become more prevalent.

We used several approaches to examine the biological plausibility of paternal age as a risk factor for schizophrenia. First, we established a translational animal model using inbred mice. Previously it had been reported that the offspring of aged male rodents had less spontaneous activity and worse learning capacity than those of mature rodents, despite having no noticeable physical anomalies (Auroux 1983). Our model carefully compared behavioural performance between the progeny of 18–24 month old sires with that of four month old sires. We replicated Auroux's findings, demonstrating significantly decreased learning in an active avoidance test, less exploration in the open field, and a number of other behavioural decrements in the offspring of older sires (Bradley-Moore et al 2002).

Next, we examined if parental age was related to intelligence in healthy adolescents. We reasoned that if *de novo* genetic changes can cause schizophrenia, there might be effects of later paternal age on cognitive function, since cognitive problems are intertwined with core aspects of schizophrenia. For this study, we cross-linked data from the Jerusalem birth cohort with the neuropsychological data from the Israeli draft board (Malaspina et al 2005a). We found that maternal and paternal age had independent effects on IQ scores, each accounting for ~2% of the total variance. Older paternal age was exclusively associated with a decrement in non-verbal (performance) intelligence IQ, without effects on verbal ability, suggestive of a specific effect on cognitive processing. In controlled analyses, maternal age showed an inverted U-shaped association with both verbal and performance IQ, suggestive of a generalized effect.

Finally, we examined if paternal age was related to the risk for autism in our cohort. We found very strong effects of advancing paternal age on the risk for autism and related pervasive developmental disorders (Reichenberg et al 2006). Compared to the offspring of fathers aged 30 years or younger, the risk was tripled for offspring of fathers in their 40s and was increased fivefold when paternal age was >50 years. Together these studies provide strong and convergent support for the hypothesis that later paternal age can influence neural functioning. The translational animal model offers the opportunity to identify candidate genes and epigenetic mechanisms that may explain the association of cognitive functioning with advancing paternal age.

A persistent question is whether the association of paternal age and schizophrenia could be explained by psychiatric problems in the parents that could both hinder their childbearing and be inherited by their offspring. If this were so, then cases with affected parents would have older paternal ages. This has not been demonstrated. To the contrary, we found that paternal age was 4.7 years older for sporadic than familial cases from our research unit at New York State Psychiatric Institute (Malaspina et al 2002). In addition, epidemiological studies show that advancing paternal age is unrelated to the risk for familial schizophrenia (Byrne et al 2003, Sipos et al 2004). For example, Sipos found that each subsequent decade of paternal age increased the relative risk (RR) for sporadic schizophrenia by 1.60 (1.32 to 1.92), with no significant effect for familial cases (RR = 0.91, 0.44 to 1.89). The effect of late paternal age in sporadic cases was impressive. The offspring of the oldest fathers had a 5.85-fold risk for sporadic schizophrenia (Sipos et al 2004); relative risks over 5.0 are very likely to reflect a true causal relationship (Breslow & Day 1980).

It is possible that the genetic events that occur in the paternal germline are affecting the same genes that influence the risk in familial cases. However, there is evidence that this is not the case. First, a number of the loci linked to familial schizophrenia are also associated with bipolar disorder (Craddock et al 2006), whereas advancing paternal age is specific for schizophrenia (Malaspina et al 2001). Next, a few genetic studies that separately examined familial and sporadic cases found that the 'at risk haplotypes' linked to familial schizophrenia were unassociated with sporadic cases; including dystrobrevin-binding protein (Van Den Bogaert et al 2003) and neuregulin (Williams et al 2003). Segregating sporadic cases from the analyses actually strengthened the magnitude of the genetic association in the familial cases, consistent with aetiological heterogeneity between familial and sporadic groups.

Of note, the phenotype of cases with no family history and later paternal age is distinct from familial cases in many dimensions. For example, only sporadic cases showed a significant improvement in negative symptoms between a 'medication free' and an 'antipsychotic treatment' condition (Malaspina et al 2000), and sporadic cases have significantly more disruptions in their smooth pursuit eye movement quality than familial cases (Malaspina et al 1998). A recent study also showed differences between the groups in resting regional cerebral blood flow (rCBF) patterns, in comparison with healthy subjects. The sporadic group of cases had greater hypofrontality, with increased medial temporal lobe activity (fronto-temporal imbalance), while the familial group evidenced left lateralized tempero-parietal hypoperfusion along with widespread rCBF changes in cortico-striato-thalamo-cortical regions (Malaspina et al 2005b). Other data linking paternal age with frontal pathology in schizophrenia include a proton magnetic resonance spectroscopy study that demonstrated a significant association between prefrontal cortex neuronal integrity (NAA) and paternal age in sporadic cases only, with no significant NAA decrement in the familial schizophrenia group (Kegeles et al 2005). These findings support the hypothesis that schizophrenia subgroups may have distinct neural underpinnings and that the important changes in some sporadic (paternal germline) cases may particularly impact on prefrontal cortical functioning.

Several genetic mechanisms could explain the relationship between paternal age and the risk for schizophrenia (see Malaspina 2001). It could be due to *de novo* point mutations arising in one or several schizophrenia susceptibility loci. Trinucleotide repeat expansions could also underlie the paternal age effect. Repeat expansions have been demonstrated in several neuropsychiatric disorders, including myotonic dystrophy, fragile X syndrome, spinocerebellar ataxias and Huntington's disease. The sex of the transmitting parent is frequently a major factor influencing anticipation, with many disorders showing greater trinucleotide repeat expansion with paternal inheritance. Larger numbers of repeat expansions could be related to chance molecular events during the many cell divisions that occur during spermatogenesis.

However, later paternal age might also confer a risk for schizophrenia if it was associated with errors in the 'imprinting' patterns of paternally inherited alleles. Imprinting is a form of gene regulation in which gene expression in the offspring depends on whether the allele was inherited from the male or female parent. Imprinted genes that are only expressed if paternally inherited are reciprocally silenced at the maternal allele, and vice versa. Imprinting occurs during gametogenesis after the methylation patterns from the previous generation are 'erased' and new parent-of-origin-specific methylation patterns are established. Errors in erasure or re-establishment of these imprint patterns may lead to defective gene expression profiles in the offspring. The enzymes responsible for methylating DNA are the DNA methyltransferases (DNMTs). These enzymes methylate cytosine residues in CpG dinucleotides, usually in the promoter region of genes, typically to reduce the expression of the mRNA. The methylation may become inefficient for a variety of reasons; one possibility is reduced DNA methylation activity in spermatogenesis, since DNMT does diminish as paternal age increases (Benoit & Trasler 1994, La Salle et al 2004). Another possible mechanism would be if this declining DNMT activity was epigenetically transmitted to the offspring of older fathers. One of the most consistently identified molecular abnormalities in schizophrenia has been theorized to result from abnormal epigenetic mechanisms (Veldic et al 2004). This is the reduced GABA and reelin in prefrontal GABAergic interneurons. Later paternal age could be related to the abnormal regulation or expression of DNMT activity in specific cells.

Human imprinted genes have a critical role in the growth of the placenta, fetus and CNS, in behavioural development, and in adult body size. It is an appealing hypothesis that loss of normal imprinting of genes critical to neurodevelopment may play a role in schizophrenia. The prenatal exposures that influence schizophrenia susceptibility likely also entail epigenetic mechanisms, although whether these are at the same loci as paternal age effects is unknown. It should be stated that the evidence for 'fetal origins' schizophrenia is as strong or stronger that that for other adult onset chronic diseases liked to the fetal milieu (e.g. obesity, dyslipidaemia, hypertension and diabetes, i.e. 'metabolic syndrome' and its sequelae, myocardial infarction and stroke). These adult-onset disorders are thought to be related to disturbed nutrition or growth limiting exposures of the fetus in the Barker hypothesis (Barker 1994). It is proposed that prenatal experience, particularly 'a baby's nourishment before birth and during infancy,' is manifest by patterns of fetal and infant growth, such that the prenatal events 'programme' the development of risk factors for coronary heart disease, and for a host of other adult onset chronic diseases.

Maternal stress during fetal development is a plausible risk pathway for schizophrenia (Koenig et al 2002). Maternal cortisol in critical fetal periods can alter the programming of gene expression in the fetal HPA axis (Seckl & Meaney 2004), leading to lifelong changes in stress responsivity, which, among other effects, may sensitize midbrain dopamine neurons. Prenatal stress can also disrupt neurodevelopment, and is associated with preterm birth, reduced fetal growth and smaller neonatal head size (Dunkel-Schetter 1998, Wadhwa et al 1993). We probed the effects of severe circumscribed stress during pregnancy in our birth cohort in Israel. We demonstrated significant effects of prenatal exposure to maternal war stress on the risk for schizophrenia. Specifically, the risk was doubled for offspring in their 2nd month of fetal life in June 1967 (RR = 2.2, 1.1–4.6), especially in females (RR = 4.2, 1.7–10.7). The risk was strongest for those living closest to the border, where shelling of buildings occurred (33, 2.7–400), and those with chronic stress, such as lower social class (4.3, 1.7–10.5) and less educated mothers (3.2, 1.4–7.5). The increased risks were not explained by multiple potential confounding variables (Malaspina et al 2003). This result points to a 1st trimester vulnerability and suggests that maternal stress affects male and female fetuses differently.

Together, the epidemiological evidence showing a strong influence of paternal age and prenatal stress on the risk for schizophrenia supports a role for epigenetic factors in the risk for schizophrenia. These findings need to be confirmed in clinical populations and other translational studies. They suggest that genetic linkage alone is unlikely to resolve the genetic complexities of schizophrenia susceptibility.

Acknowledgments

Supported by grants from the National Institutes of Health: 1R01 MH059114 (DM); 2 K24 MH001699 (DM); 1R01 CA080197 (SH); 5K23MH066279–02 (CC) and from the National Alliance for Research of Schizophrenia and Depression (NARSAD) (DM, SH). The authors thank Ezra Susser and Caitlin Warinsky for their contributions to the intellectual and editorial components of this manuscript.

References

Auroux M 1983 Decrease of learning capacity in offspring with increasing paternal age in the rat. Teratology 27:141–148

Barker DJP 1994 Mothers, babies, and disease in later life. BMJ Publishing Group, London

Benoit G, Trasler JM 1994 Developmental expression of DNA methyltransferase messenger ribonucleic acid, protein, and enzyme activity in the mouse testis. Biol Reprod 50:1312–1319

Bradley-Moore M, Abner R Edwards T et al 2002 Modeling the effect of advanced paternal age on progeny behavior in mice. Dev Psychobiol 41:230

Breslow NE, Day NE 1980 The analysis of case-control data. In: Statistical methods in cancer research, Vol 1. World Health Organization, Lyon

Brown AS, Schaefer CA, Wyatt RJ et al 2002 Paternal age and risk of schizophrenia in adult offspring. Am J Psychiatry 159:1528–1533

Byrne M, Agerbo E, Ewald H, Eaton WW, Mortensen PB 2003 Parental age and risk of schizophrenia: a case-control study. Arch Gen Psychiatry 60:673–678

Crow JF 1997 The high spontaneous mutation rate: is it a health risk? Proc Natl Acad Sci USA 94:8380–8386

Craddock N, O'Donovan MC, Owen MJ 2006 Genes for schizophrenia and bipolar disorder? Implications for psychiatric nosology. Schizophr Bull J32:9–16

Dalman C, Allebeck P 2002 Paternal age and schizophrenia: further support for an association. Am J Psychiatry 159:1591–1592

Dunkel-Schetter, C 1998 Maternal stress and preterm delivery. Prenat Neonatal Med 3:39–42

El-Saadi O, Pedersen CB, McNeil TF et al 2004 Paternal and maternal age as risk factors for psychosis: findings from Denmark, Sweden and Australia. Schizophr Res 67:227–236

Kegeles LS, Shungu DC, Mao X et al 2005 Relationship of age and paternal age to neuronal functional integrity in the prefrontal cortex in schizophrenia determined by proton magnetic resonance spectroscopy. Schizophr Bull 31:443

Koenig JI, Kirkpatrick B, Lee PR 2002 Glucocorticoid hormones and early brain development in schizophrenia. Neuropsychopharmacology 27:309–318

La Salle S, Mertineit C, Taketo T, Moens PB, Bestor TH, Trasler JM 2004 Windows for sex-specific methylation marked by DNA methyltransferase expression profiles in mouse germ cells. Dev Biol 268:403–415

Malaspina D 2001 Paternal factors and schizophrenia risk: *de novo* mutations and imprinting. Schizophr Bull 3:379–393

Malaspina D, Friedman JH, Kaufmann C et al 1998 Psychobiological heterogeneity of familial and sporadic schizophrenia. Biol Psychiatry 43:489–496

Malaspina D, Goetz RR, Yale S et al 2000 Relation of familial schizophrenia to negative symptoms but not to the deficit syndrome. Am J Psychiatry 157:994–1003

Malaspina D, Harlap S, Fennig S et al 2001 Advancing paternal age and the risk of schizophrenia. Arch Gen Psychiatry 58:361–367

GROWTH AND SCHIZOPHRENIA

Malaspina D, Corcoran C, Fahim C et al 2002 Paternal age and sporadic schizophrenia: evidence for *de novo* mutations. Am J Med Genet 114:299–303

Malaspina D, Harlap S, Fennig S, Corcoran C, Susser E 2003 Maternal stress and offspring schizophrenia risk. Biol Psychiatry 53:168S

Malaspina D, Reichenberg A, Weiser M et al 2005a Paternal age and intelligence: implications for age-related genomic changes in male germ cells. Psychiatr Genet 15:117–1125

Malaspina D, Harkavy-Friedman J, Corcoran C et al 2005b Resting neural activity distinguishes subgroups of schizophrenia patients. Biol Psychiatry 56:931–937

Reichenberg A, Gross R, Weiser M et al 2006 Advancing paternal age and autism. Arch Gen Psychiatry 63:1026–1032

Seckl JR, Meaney MJ 2004 Glucocorticoid programming. Ann N Y Acad Sci 1032:63–84

Sipos A, Rasmussen F, Harrison G et al 2004 Paternal age and schizophrenia: a population based cohort study. BMJ 329:1070

Tsuchiya KJ, Takagai S, Kawai M et al 2005 Advanced paternal age associated with an elevated risk for schizophrenia in offspring in a Japanese population. Schizophr Res 76:337–342

Van Den Bogaert A, Schumacher J, Schulze TG et al 2003 The DTNBP1 (dysbindin) gene contributes to schizophrenia, depending on family history of the disease. Am J Hum Genet 73:1438–443

Veldic M, Caruncho HJ, Liu WS et al 2004 DNA-methyltransferase 1 mRNA is selectively overexpressed in telencephalic GABAergic interneurons of schizophrenia brains. Proc Natl Acad Sci USA 101:348–353

Wadhwa PD, Sandman CA, Porto M, Dunkel-Schetter C, Garite TJ 1993 The association between prenatal stress and infant birth weight and gestational age at birth: a prospective investigation. Am J Obstet Gynecol 169:858–865

Williams NM, Preece A, Spurlock G et al 2003 Support for genetic variation in neuregulin 1 and susceptibility to schizophrenia. Mol Psychiatry 8:485–487

Zammit S, Allebeck P, Dalman C et al 2003 Paternal age and risk for schizophrenia. Br J Psychiatry 183:405–408

DISCUSSION

Giedd: So young men should donate and store their sperm for later use.

Malaspina: Yes, the official title of this talk is 'Sperm bank and boxer shorts'!

Hen: I have an easier time understanding the mouse data than the human data! It seems that in the mice there is some kind of global dysfunction associated with late paternal age. It is what one would predict if there is a global epigenetic remodelling. How come the deficit is more specific in the human cohort, with for example schizophrenia but not bipolar disorder?

Malaspina: It is autism and schizophrenia, and there are many other diseases associated with late paternal age that are far more rare. Perhaps these would be more common in the animals. I would propose that the paternal methylation particularly protects social capacity, and the diseases in which it is strongly related, including schizophrenia and autism, are conditions where social capacity is very important. Paternal genes are differentially expressed in the limbic system, and maternal genes are differentially expressed in the cortex. The mother's genome plays a higher role in intelligence and male genes play more of a role in social functioning. This could be one reason.

Akil: A lot depends on what is being born at that time, and what you are modulating. Which diseases depend on which types of connectivity? I have a question: does the age of the male affect maternal behaviour in any way, and have you tried cross-fostering these babies from old fathers?

Malaspina: Not yet. I don't think so because of the robustness of the replications worldwide. Every single study shows this consistent tripling of the schizophrenia for the oldest fathers.

Akil: I mean in mice.

Malaspina: We have not examined the effect of paternal age on maternal behaviour. However, we have found methylation differences in the sperm of the older fathers.

Akil: A simple control would be to have a group of cross-fostered babies with different mothers that were impregnated with young sperm, just to get this fostering question out of the picture. Maternal behaviour is very important early on, including in epigenetic modulation. There is so much traffic back and forth between the pup and the mum at that early age.

Malaspina: Maternal behaviour might be protective, but we suspect that there are methylation differences in the sperm of groups of the older mice.

Haggarty: Is there a differential effect of molecules like valproate (Depakote) and tranylcypromine (Parnate) in these disorders? I ask specifically because there is evidence that these compounds affect histone acetylation as well as histone and DNA methylation events.

Malaspina: Valproate has been used in treating schizophrenia.

Chao: It is not clear exactly how valproate works.

Haggarty: It has been shown to do hundreds of different things ranging from Na^+ channels to various other ion channels. More recently, valproate and carbamazepine (Tegretol), two of the most widely used mood stabilizers for bipolar disorder, have been shown to directly inhibit the deacetylation of histones by HDACs, as do a number of other anticonvulsants (Eyal et al 2004, Beutler et al 2005). Tranylcypromine (Parnate), a monoamine oxidase inhibitor, was recently shown to be an inhibitor of the histone H3 demethylases LSD1 (Lee et al 2006). They are not potent molecules, but given the chronic nature of their administration there are some interesting possible new mechanisms. In the case of valproate, acute treatment is also known to cause a general hyperacetylation of histones in a variety of mammalian cell lines, including cultured neurons and neuronal cell lines, in a manner very similar to that of known inhibitors of HDACs, including trichostatin A and sodium butyrate (Phiel et al 2001, Eyal et al 2004, Beutler et al 2005, Dong et al 2005, Tremolizzo et al 2005). In addition to affecting gene expression (Chetcuti et al 2005, Bosetti et al 2005, Lamb et al 2006), valproate has also been shown to directly increase replication-independent DNA demethylation in concert with increased histone acetylation (Cervoni & Szyf 2001, Tremolizzo et al 2005). Valproate also reverses the behavioural and biochemical deficits induced in a rat epigenetic model of schizophrenia involving chronic administration of L-methionine, including up-regulating the mRNA levels of glutamate acid decarboxylase 67 (GAD67), the rate-limiting enzyme for γ-amino butyric acid (GABA) biosynthesis (Dong et al 2005, Tremolizzo et al 2005). In addition, valproate increases BDNF expression and inhibits the expression of the Polycomb group genes, including the histone H3 Lys27 HMT, EZH2 (Mai et al 2002, Okada et al 2004, Castro et al 2005). Growing evidence implicates a role for epigenetics in mood disorders (reviewed in Tsankova et al 2007).

Raff: Do epidemiological studies in non-concordant twins tell us whether *in utero* stresses could be relevant?

Malaspina: Twin pregnancies have high rates of glucocorticoids, which is why twins tend to be born somewhat earlier. Identical twins have a much higher rate of concordance than fraternal twins. I speculated in a previous discussion session that we may have overestimated the heritability for a number of diseases because we have based them on twin studies, which do not have the same environmental intrauterine environment as singletons.

Raff: Do the non-concordant twins provide a clue? Is it thought to be an *in utero* difference? Is it placental differences, for example? When are the relevant differences likely to be seen during gestation?

Malaspina: In identical non-concordant twins, Art Petronis (Petronis et al 2003) has found methylation differences. There is a strong understanding that gene methylation might be related to disease susceptibility. The timing of it is more difficult. One way we can look at the timing in gestation is finger ridges. There is a developmental sequence here, and it can help us see when an insult might have occurred.

Spedding: Another issue is the increased blood flow in CA1 in schizophrenics. This could indicate several things. There is a nice paper by Buszaki's group (Robbe et al 2006) showing that cannabinoids prevent ensemble activity in CA1. Ensemble activity can also be linked to how cells work together to produce LTP. If this is blocked, the activity is less effective as a whole in that group of cells. If the organism would want to drive on that activity, it would increase less efficient activity in CA1, giving increased blood flow. This has been shown for cannabinoids in CA1. This effect may not necessarily relate to increased efficient activity, but increased activity which isn't related to normal production of classically formed LTP, or classically formed cellular ensembles. Cannabinoids are thought by some to exacerbate schizophrenia. It is interesting, therefore, that these two things go in parallel on one of the main cognitive outputs for hippocampal function. I think it is quite an important finding.

Bothwell: It strikes me that the gene regulatory regions that molecular biologists tend to avoid, because they behave so peculiarly in transgenic mice, are exactly the kinds of genes we should be looking at.

Malaspina: Perhaps so.

Buonanno: At the risk of sounding neuregulin-centric, independent of the genetics, I think the biological effect I described yesterday fits well with this. It reduces the capacity to separate signal from noise, so you get a lower signal-to-noise ratio.

Tongiorgi: Is anything known about epigenetic effects associated with artificial fertilization in which women undergo induction of ovulation through intensive hormonal stimulation?

Malaspina: In vitro fertilization dramatically increases the risk of epigenetic conditions. I don't know about the effect on the ova.

McAllister: Are there any other physiological differences between these women, for example in placental weight and function?

Malaspina: Yes. We have just begun working with Carrie Salafia who is a placental pathologist. She has replicated the association of paternal age and cognition, but she has shown that a lot of this can be explained by placental changes. She also showed that the association between birthweight and IQ that is commonly reported is mediated by placenta as well.

McAllister: Is it mediated or is this just a correlation?

Malaspina: I can't say at the moment. But there was a paper published recently in Chinese (Dai et al 2007), which showed that paternal age also had a strong effect on IGF2 in the placenta.

McAllister: Does anyone know why there is such a high density of CRF1 receptors in the placenta?

Malaspina: One theory is that it becomes important to detect adversity or the perception of stress in the mother.

Brandon: You touched on the importance of oxytocin surges. How do you feel about using oxytocin agonists for treating psychiatric disorders?

Malaspina: I think it would be exciting in the right sub-group. Paternally expressed gene 3 (PEG3) in mouse affects particularly oxytocin receptors in the hypothalamus of daughters. The daughters that lack this gene look normal, but their pups die because of an inability to get off the placenta. If they are cross fostered by a knockout of PEG3 they will survive normally. There are complex behaviours that can be related to the paternal and maternal imprinted genes.

References

Beutler AS, Li S, Nicol R, Walsh MJ 2005 Carbamazepine is an inhibitor of histone deacetylases. Life Sci 76:3107–3115

Bosetti F, Bell JM, Manickam P 2005 Microarray analysis of rat brain gene expression after chronic administration of sodium valproate. Brain Res Bull 65:331–338

Castro LM, Gallant M, Niles LP 2005 Novel targets for valproic acid: up-regulation of melatonin receptors and neurotrophic factors in C6 glioma cells. J Neurochem 95:1227–1236

Cervoni N, Szyf M 2001 Demethylase activity is directed by histone acetylation. J Biol Chem 276:40778–40787

Chetcuti A, Adams LJ, Mitchell PB, Schofield PR 2005 Altered gene expression in mice treated with the mood stabilizer sodium valproate. Int J Neuropsychopharmacol 9:267–276

Dai Y, Wang Z, Li J et al 2007 Imprinting status of IGF2 in cord blood cells of Han Chinese newborns. Int J Mol Sci 8:273–283

Dong E, Agis-Balboa RC, Simonini MV, Grayson DR, Costa E, Guidotti A 2005 Reelin and glutamic acid decarboxylase 67 promoter remodeling in an epigenetic methionine induced mouse model of schizophrenia. Proc Natl Acad Sci USA 102:12578–12583

Eyal S, Yagen B, Sobol E, Altschuler Y, Shmuel M, Bialer M 2004 The activity of antiepileptic drugs as histone deacetylase inhibitors. Epilepsia 45:737–744

Lamb J, Crawford ED, Peck D et al 2006 The Connectivity Map: using gene expression signatures to connect small molecules, genes, and disease. Science 313:1929–1935

Lee MG, Wynder C, Schmidt DM, McCafferty DG, Shiekhattar R 2006 Histone H3 lysine 4 demethylation is a target of nonselective antidepressive medications. Chem Biol 13:563–567

Mai L, Jope RS, Li X 2002 BDNF-mediated signal transduction is modulated by GSK3beta and mood stabilizing agents. J Neurochem 82:75–83

Okada A, Aoki Y, Kushima K, Kurihara H, Bialer M, Fujiwara M 2004 Polycomb homologs are involved in teratogenicity of valproic acid in mice. Birth Defects Res A Clin Mol Teratol 70:870–879

Petronis A, Gottesman II, Kan P et al 2003 Monozygotic twins exhibit numerous epigenetic differences: clues to twin discordance? Schizophr Bull 29:169–178

Phiel CJ, Zhang F, Huang EY, Guenther MG, Lazar MA, Klein PS 2001 Histone deacetylase is a direct target of valproic acid, a potent anticonvulsant, mood stabilizer, and teratogen. J Biol Chem 276:36734–36741

Robbe D, Montgomery SM, Thome A, Rueda-Orozco PE, McNaughton BL, Buzsaki G 2006 Cannabinoids reveal importance of spike timing coordination in hippocampal function. Nat Neurosci 9:1526–1533

Tsankova NM, Renthal W, Kumar A, Nestler EJ 2007 Epigenetic regulation in psychiatric disorders. Nat Rev Neurosci 8:355–367

Tremolizzo L, Doueiri MS, Dong E et al 2005 Valproate corrects the schizophrenia-like epigenetic behavioral modifications induced by methionine in mice. Biol Psychiatry 57:500–509

What can we learn from the disrupted in schizophrenia 1 interactome: lessons for target identification and disease biology?

Luiz M. Camargo*, Qi Wang and Nicholas J. Brandon[1]

*Schizophrenia and Bipolar Research, Wyeth Discovery Neuroscience, CN8000, Princeton, NJ 08543 and *Merck Research Labs, Merck & Co, Boston, MA 02115, USA*

Abstract. Emerging genetic and biological data strongly supports Disrupted in Schizophrenia 1 (*DISC1*) as a schizophrenia risk gene of great significance for not only understanding the underlying causes of schizophrenia and related disorders but potentially to open up new avenues of treatment. DISC1 appeared to be a very enigmatic protein upon the initial disclosure of its protein sequence. Though it contained some well-characterized protein domains, they did not reveal anything about possible function. Recently, the identification of its binding partners has revealed an incredible diversity of potential cellular and physiological functions. In an attempt to capture this information we set out to generate a comprehensive network of protein–protein interactions (PPIs) around DISC1. This was achieved by utilizing iterative yeast-two hybrid screens, combined with detailed pathway and functional analysis. This so-called 'DISC1 interactome' contains many novel PPIs and has provided a molecular framework to explore the function of DISC1. Interrogation of the interactome has shown DISC1 to have a PPI profile consistent with that of an essential synaptic protein, which fits well with the underlying molecular pathology observed at the synaptic level and the cognitive deficits seen behaviourally in schizophrenics. Furthermore, potential novel therapeutic targets have also emerged as we have characterized in detail the interactions with the phosphodiesterase PDE4B in collaboration with the Porteous and Houslay labs, and with Ndel1-EOPA with Hayashi and colleagues. Many components of the interactome are themselves now being shown to be schizophrenia risk genes, or to interact with other risk genes, emphasising the power of protein interaction studies for revealing the underlying biology of a disease.

2008 Growth factors and psychiatric disorders. Wiley, Chichester (Novartis Foundation Symposium 289) p 208–221

[1]This paper was presented at the symposium by Nicholas Brandon, to whom correspondence should be addressed.

Schizophrenia is a severe debilitating psychiatric disorder affecting ~1% of the population worldwide that consists of three domains: positive, negative and cognitive symptoms (Tamminga & Holcomb 2005). Current therapies are effective at treating positive symptoms but treatment of the negative and cognitive domains remain unmet medical needs (Tamminga & Holcomb 2005). Amongst current theories to explain the underlying aetiology of the disease, the 'hypoglutamatergic theory' has gained much credence. An increasing amount of data from postmortem studies suggests schizophrenia is a disease of the synapse and neuronal connectivity, and in particular due to deficits in glutamate receptor containing excitatory synapses. Evidence includes pharmacological studies with N-methyl-D-aspartate receptor (NMDAR) antagonists (PCP and ketamine), which cause schizophrenic-like symptoms in normal individuals and exacerbate symptoms in patients (Stefani & Moghaddam 2005). Animal studies are also supportive with a mouse line having a reduced number of NMDA receptors showing schizophrenic-like behaviours (Mohn et al 1999). The NMDAR-containing synapse has been further implicated by the analysis of the rapidly increasing number of identified schizophrenia risk genes. In a seminal review, Weinberger and Harrison systematically reviewed the risk genes of the day and described how the functions of many of these genes converge at the site of the NMDAR (Harrison & Weinberger 2005).

We have had a long-term interest in the risk gene 'Disrupted in Schizophrenia 1' (*DISC1*). This gene was originally identified by a balanced (1;11) (q42;q14) translocation reported to co-segregate with major psychiatric illnesses in a Scottish family (Millar et al 2000). An increasing number of independent genetic studies have confirmed *DISC1* as one of the most substantiated risk factors for schizophrenia with variants of the gene linked to both psychotic and cognitive symptoms in patients (Ishizuka et al 2006, Porteous et al 2006). Until recently the biological function of DISC1 was very poorly understood. This is rapidly changing with a large number of studies linking DISC1 to cAMP signalling, axon elongation and neuronal migration. All of these breakthroughs have derived from identifying protein interaction partners of DISC1 (Ndel1, PDE4B, kinesin motor proteins) and analysing the function of the resultant complexes (Kamiya et al 2005, Millar et al 2005a, Taya et al 2007). All of these interactions, and many more besides, can be found in the DISC1 interactome which we recently published (Camargo et al 2007). The DISC1 interactome was the result of a number of years of study, starting in 2001. Upon analysis of the protein sequence of DISC1 it was clear that it contained a number of domains, which could be important for protein–protein interactions. In partnership with Hybrigenics (*www.hybrigenics.com*) we conducted a number of yeast two-hybrid (Y2H) screens with DISC1 (see Camargo et al 2007 for details on methods). These initial studies identified a large number of interactors. A number of bioinformatic and literature-driven decisions were then made to follow up a select number of these proteins with more Y2H screening and selective characterization on other biological systems as deemed appropriate. Critical to this was the assignment of a 'Predicted Biological Score' to each interaction. I encourage you to look at the full methods in the original paper for discussion of this term, but in our experience every interaction with an 'A' score in the Y2H system has been validated in a neuronal system. The result of these iterative screens is the 'DISC1 interactome', a highly connected network consisting of 127 proteins and 158 interactions (Fig. 1). A number of intriguing and potentially crucial hypotheses can be drawn from the interactome, which we will discuss further.

DISC1 is intimately linked to synapse function

Our original theory was that if DISC1 was a critical player in schizophrenia pathophysiology it had to contribute to the synaptic pathologies observed in post-mortem samples (Harrison & Weinberger 2005) and in some way to be associated with synaptic proteins at the level of protein–protein interactions. Encouragingly DISC1 translocation carriers, irrespective of clinical diagnosis, have measurable cognitive deficits, again implicating a role for DISC1 in synaptic function, plasticity and downstream behaviour (Blackwood & Muir 2004). Intriguingly, when the DISC1 interactome was interrogated in conjunction with other available protein–protein interaction datasets, many of the proteins in our network were shown to be involved in pathways critical for the formation of synapses, e.g. synaptic activity mediated by the glutamatergic AMPAR and NMDAR receptor complexes, dendritic–axonal contact, regulation of actin dynamics, cytoskeletal stability, intracellular transport, neuronal polarity and migration, dendritic growth and branching by neurotrophic factors via Trk and EGF receptors. All of these processes are critical for the development, maturation and plasticity of synapses and may also be linked to schizophrenia-related neuropathologies (Camargo et al 2007).

Since we embarked on our DISC1 interactome work the possibility that DISC1 functions as a key synaptic protein has received corroborating evidence. For example, DISC1 has been shown in a number of studies to be linked to cognitive performance, further refining the earlier finding by Blackwood and others (Burdick et al 2005, Callicott et al 2005, Cannon et al 2005). More specifically in an electron microscopic study, DISC1 has been localized at the post-synaptic density (PSD) in human brain (Kirkpatrick et al 2006). Such pieces of information are very encouraging when we review the hypotheses we generated while conducting our studies. The function of DISC1 at the PSD is not yet known but we believe that the DISC1 interactome provides an excellent starting point to explore pathways where DISC1 may impact on synaptic plasticity and function.

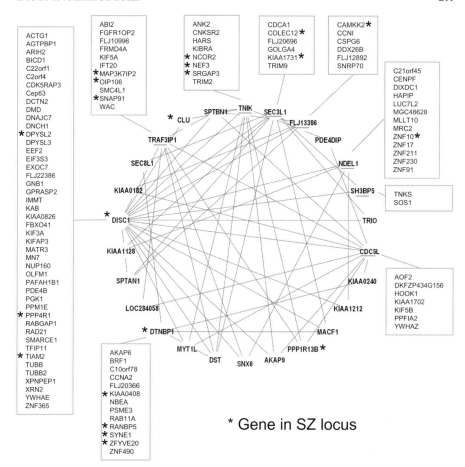

FIG. 1.   (a) The DISC1 network of protein–protein interactions (PPIs). Adapated from the original Fig. 1 in Camargo et al (2007). The shared interactions with Dysbindin (DTNBP1) have now been added. These include the shared partners SEC8L1, DST and MACF1. Underlined are proteins that interact with DISC1 and were used as baits in further yeast two-hybrid screens to derive the protein interaction network. *Indicates proteins that are located in a schizophrenia risk locus.

DISC1 is closely linked to other schizophrenia risk genes

The list of schizophrenia risk genes is expanding and though the field is being fairly rigorous in expecting replications of genetic data and relevance of biological function, the number of proteins and their diversity is still potentially overwhelming to comprehend how it fits with the disease. The protein interaction studies with DISC1 have started to suggest that perhaps things are not as complicated as they seem in that risk genes may converge functionally on the same biological process. A number of proteins in our network are in schizophrenia-associated loci, as defined by the 'Online Mendelian Inheritence in Man' database (OMIM), or are in regions of documented chromosomal aberrations linked to schizophrenia (Fig. 1) suggesting that *DISC1* and the risk genes may converge on similar biological processes. Such convergence fits very well with a recent meta-analysis of protein–protein interaction datasets. This has shown that genes in the OMIM database, associated with a certain disease, are more likely to interact with proteins associated with that same disease (Gandhi et al 2006). This suggests that protein–protein interaction studies will be a good source of potential disease candidates, though of course you will need to take other data sets and biological information into account to verify this.

The best example of this convergence to emerge directly from our studies is the interaction with the phosphodiesterase PDE4B, an enzyme which regulates levels of cAMP, and has been the subject of drug-discovery efforts for a range of other therapeutic indications (Zhang et al 2005). We identified PDE4B as a DISC1 interactor in our Y2H screens (Camargo et al 2007). In parallel Muir, Blackwood, Pickard and others had identified a schizophrenia patient with a balanced translocation in the PDE4B gene (Millar et al 2005a). These two pieces of information made it compelling to follow up the DISC1–PDE4B interaction in detail. Furthermore, pharmacological and knockout mouse data have implicated PDE4 in depression and cognition so the rationale was further strengthened. Through standard protein–protein interaction assays we were able to show that PDE4B binds to the N-terminus of DISC1 and that DISC1 binds to the conserved regulatory domain UCR2 on PDE4B (Fig. 2) (Millar et al 2005a). The UCR2 domain is important in

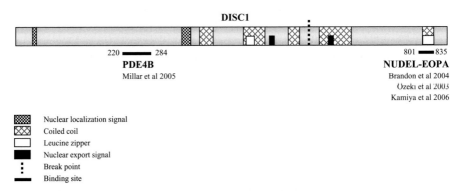

FIG. 2.   DISC1 and its key interaction domains. The annotated protein sequence of DISC1 with the binding sites identified on DISC1 for PDE4 and Ndel1 (Brandon et al 2004, Kamiya et al 2006, Millar et al 2005a, Ozeki et al 2003).

regulating enzyme activity; PKA phosphorylation of the UCR1 domain activates the enzyme through the UCR1 and UCR2 domains. In SH-SY5Y neuroblastoma cells increases in cAMP and PKA phosphorylation of UCR1 were shown to cause disassociation of the DISC1:PDE4 complex. It is clear though that there is much more to find out about this complex. In the DISC1 translocation family there is evidence of haploinsufficiancy of DISC1, which would lead to elevated PDE4 activity from the proposed models, but how does the PDE4 translocation family, with an expected decrease in activity, relate to this? There are >20 PDE4 isoforms and eleven phosphodiesterase families so the potential for compensation is great (Bender & Beavo 2006). Further studies are clearly needed to truly understand the molecular importance of the DISC1–PDE4 connection, which may help guide us in whether we need to increase or decrease cAMP levels in distinct brain regions to have therapeutically relevant effects in schizophrenia.

We also asked more directly whether DISC1 might be linked to other risk factors at the level of protein–protein interactions by running Y2H screens with other previously identified candidates including dysbindin (DTNBP1). Dysbindin has been linked to schizophrenia in a number of studies and its biology is slowly being revealed. In particular, with relevance to this discussion, it has been suggested to play a role in glutamatergic neurotransmission (Talbot et al 2004, 2006). Furthermore, Dysbindin has recently been shown to be localized at both pre- and post-synaptic sites, the latter localization suggesting it may be in close proximity to DISC1 (Talbot et al 2006). Intriguingly, like DISC1, Dysbindin interacts with microtubule cross-linking factors MACF1 and DST (BPAG1) (Fig. 1). These microtubule cross-linking factors, also known as plakins, interconnect all three cytoskeletal filament networks: actin filaments, microtubules and intermediate filaments (Jefferson et al 2004). Dysbindin also shares common interactions with other proteins in our network such as members of the exocyst complex, which play a role in trafficking of glutamate receptors to synaptic terminals, and it would be interesting to see how deficits in either DISC1 or Dysbindin affect glutamatergic transmission and receptor density. The possibility of functional convergence of schizophrenia risk genes is exciting and in many ways a potential relief as we attempt to assimilate the roles and relevance of the ever growing list of candidates.

The DISC1 and Ndel1/Nde1 partnership: the emergence of a second potential drug target

The best characterized of the DISC1 protein–protein interactions to date is that with Ndel1/Nudel/Nudel-EOPA (name utilized dependent on context and history). A number of groups identified this interaction simultaneously. This was truly an exciting time as it became evident early on that the binding domain for Ndel1 was lost in the putative truncated protein in the Scottish family (Brandon et al 2004, Ozeki et al 2003) (Fig. 2). The possibility that a molecular mechanism, underlying schizophrenia pathology was emerging was incredible. We were also able to show for the first time that DISC1 and Ndel1 interact in mouse brain and that the complex was under developmental regulation (Brandon et al 2004). The mechanism underlying this developmental control of the interaction eluded us though we had some preliminary data that phosphorylation of Ndel1 was critical (Brandon et al, unpublished). Other groups have recently focused their efforts on the characterization of the DISC1–Ndel1 complex at the centrosome, in particular by a very elegant set of experiments by Sawa and colleagues (Kamiya et al 2005). They utilized *in utero* RNAi to deplete DISC1, resulting in abnormal neuronal migration, thinning of dendritic spines, and a decreased number of dendritic arborizations (Kamiya et al 2005). These phenotypes are not dissimilar to the pathology seen in schizophrenia. Our own interests in this complex were diverted by the realization that Ndel1 was the same protein as endo-oligopeptidase A, a cysteine protease, which had been shown to degrade a wide range of important neurotransmitters *in vitro* (Hayashi et al 2005). In collaboration with Hayashi, Portera and Camargo we became interested in the possible role that DISC1 may have in regulating this enzyme. Initially we were able to show that the active site within Ndel1-EOPA was at residue cysteine 273 (C273). The relevance of this piece of data emerged as we specifically mapped the protein interaction domains of DISC1 on Ndel1. We showed that the residues leucine 266 (L266) and glutamate 267 (E267) on Ndel1 were both absolutely required for the interaction to occur. The spatial proximity of the two sites (C273 and LE266/267) suggested that the interaction may modulate enzymatic activity. Indeed, incubation *in vitro* of Ndel1/EOPA with DISC1 competitively inhibits the oligopeptidase activity (Hayashi et al 2005). The full biological relevance of this aspect of the DISC1/Ndel1 partnership is still not known. To date all the experiments have been performed *in vitro* and actual enzymatic activity in cells has not been shown. Also, for example, what role does the peptidase activity have on the better characterized role of the DISC1/Ndel1 complex in neuronal migration? If a physiological enzymatic role can be established it will be important to identify the *in vivo* substrates. The *in vitro* substrates identified to date are tantalizing in their implications for schizophrenia, with for example neurotensin suggested as an endogenous anti-psychotic. Clearly the role of the peptidase activity could also be of great importance as we look for drug-targets from within the DISC1 interactome. As an enzyme we can easily consider modulating the activity with a small molecule or potentially an antibody (as has been done *in vitro*).

Concluding remarks

The DISC1 interactome is providing a molecular framework by which the causative biological mechanisms of schizophrenia are potentially being unveiled. It has allowed critical insights into the biology of schizophrenia and provided candidate targets for drug discovery, so achieving the two key aims we set for ourselves five years ago. Now the real challenge begins as we try to translate this information into therapeutics to provide real improvements for the patient.

References

Bender AT, Beavo JA 2006 Cyclic nucleotide phosphodiesterases: molecular regulation to clinical use. Pharmacol Rev 58:488–520

Blackwood DH, Muir WJ 2004 Clinical phenotypes associated with DISC1, a candidate gene for schizophrenia. Neurotox Res 6:35–41

Brandon NJ, Handford EJ, Schurov I et al 2004 Disrupted in Schizophrenia 1 and Nudel form a neurodevelopmentally regulated protein complex: implications for schizophrenia and other major neurological disorders. Mol Cell Neurosci 25:42–55

Burdick KE, Hodgkinson CA, Szeszko PR et al 2005 DISC1 and neurocognitive function in schizophrenia. Neuroreport 16:1399–1402

Callicott JH, Straub RE, Pezawas L et al 2005 Variation in DISC1 affects hippocampal structure and function and increases risk for schizophrenia. Proc Natl Acad Sci USA 102: 8627–8632

Camargo LM, Collura V, Rain JC et al 2007 Disrupted in Schizophrenia 1 interactome: evidence for the close connectivity of risk genes and a potential synaptic basis for schizophrenia. Mol Psychiatry 12:74–86

Cannon TD, Hennah W, van Erp TG et al 2005 Association of DISC1/TRAX haplotypes with schizophrenia, reduced prefrontal gray matter, and impaired short- and long-term memory. Arch Gen Psychiatry 62:1205–1213

Gandhi TK, Zhong J, Mathivanan S et al 2006 Analysis of the human protein interactome and comparison with yeast, worm and fly interaction datasets. Nat Genet 38:285–293

Harrison PJ, Weinberger DR 2005 Schizophrenia genes, gene expression, and neuropathology: on the matter of their convergence. Mol Psychiatry 10:40–68

Hayashi MA, Portaro FC, Bastos MF et al 2005 Inhibition of NUDEL (nuclear distribution element-like)-oligopeptidase activity by disrupted-in-schizophrenia 1. Proc Natl Acad Sci USA 102:3828–3833

Ishizuka K, Paek M, Kamiya A, Sawa A 2006 A review of Disrupted-In-Schizophrenia-1 (DISC1): neurodevelopment, cognition, and mental conditions. Biol Psychiatry 59:1189–1197

Jefferson JJ, Leung CL, Liem RK 2004 Plakins: goliaths that link cell junctions and the cytoskeleton. Nat Rev Mol Cell Biol 5:542–553

Kamiya A, Kubo K, Tomoda T et al 2005 A schizophrenia-associated mutation of DISC1 perturbs cerebral cortex development. Nat Cell Biol 7:1167–1178

Kamiya A, Tomoda T, Chang J et al 2006 DISC1-NDEL1/NUDEL protein interaction, an essential component for neurite outgrowth, is modulated by genetic variations of DISC1. Hum Mol Genet 15:3313–3323

Kirkpatrick B, Xu L, Cascella N, Ozeki Y, Sawa A, Roberts RC 2006 DISC1 immunoreactivity at the light and ultrastructural level in the human neocortex. J Comp Neurol 497:436–450

Millar JK, Wilson-Annan JC, Anderson S et al 2000 Disruption of two novel genes by a trans-location co-segregating with schizophrenia. Hum Mol Genet 9:1415–1423

Millar JK, Pickard BS, Mackie S et al 2005a DISC1 and PDE4B are interacting genetic factors in schizophrenia that regulate cAMP signaling. Science 310:1187–1191

Millar JK, James R, Christie S, Porteous DJ 2005b Disrupted in schizophrenia 1 (DISC1): subcellular targeting and induction of ring mitochondria. Mol Cell Neurosci 30:477–484

Mohn AR, Gainetdinov RR, Caron MG, Koller BH 1999 Mice with reduced NMDA receptor expression display behaviors related to schizophrenia. Cell 98:427–436

Ozeki Y, Tomoda T, Kleiderlein J et al 2003 Disrupted-in-Schizophrenia-1 (DISC-1): mutant truncation prevents binding to NudE-like (NUDEL) and inhibits neurite outgrowth. Proc Natl Acad Sci USA 100:289–294

Porteous DJ, Thomson P, Brandon NJ, Millar JK 2006 The genetics and biology of DISC1—an emerging role in psychosis and cognition. Biol Psychiatry 60:123–131

Stefani MR, Moghaddam B 2005 Transient N-methyl-D-aspartate receptor blockade in early development causes lasting cognitive deficits relevant to schizophrenia. Biol Psychiatry 57:433–436

Talbot K, Eidem WL, Tinsley CL et al 2004 Dysbindin-1 is reduced in intrinsic, glutamatergic terminals of the hippocampal formation in schizophrenia. J Clin Invest 113:1353–1363

Talbot K, Cho DS, Ong WY et al 2006 Dysbindin-1 is a synaptic and microtubular protein that binds brain snapin. Hum Mol Genet 15:3041–3054

Tamminga CA, Holcomb HH 2005 Phenotype of schizophrenia: a review and formulation. Mol Psychiatry 10:27–39

Taya S, Shinoda T, Tsuboi D et al 2007 DISC1 regulates the transport of the NUDEL/LIS1/14-3-3epsilon complex through kinesin-1. J Neurosci 27:15–26

Zhang KY, Ibrahim PN, Gillette S, Bollag G 2005 Phosphodiesterase-4 as a potential drug target. Expert Opin Ther Targets 9:1283–1305

DISCUSSION

Raff: It would be very helpful to have the DISC1 sceptics tell us what they think. To some of us outside the field, the DISC1 connection in the Edinburgh family looks like a breakthrough, compared with all the other linkages, yet some geneticists seem to think DISC1 is no different from other candidates and its significance might well disappear over time. Is there something special about DISC1 in schizophrenia and depression or not?

Chao: To begin with, is your view that the normal function of DISC1 is to serve as a scaffold protein or a transport protein, or both?

Brandon: Up until January 2007 when the two new papers came out in the Journal of Neuroscience (Taya et al 2007, Shinoda et al 2007) we were saying it was a scaffold protein. In our hands at least it was binding the two enzymes I discussed in my talk (PDE4 and Ndel1-EOPA). But the new studies show binding to kinesin where it is acting as a linker molecule, taking either the Ndel1 complex or a Grb2 complex to the distal axon. I do not think we are completely convinced about what it is. With its multiple splice forms it could be a multi-functional protein doing different things in different cells and at different points in development.

Chao: Do your collaborators in Brazil know about substrates?

Brandon: In vitro they have looked at between 20 and 30 peptides. There is no consensus peptide that it cleaves. They are all unstructured small polypeptide. So far they have simply tested peptides they can get their hands on. Neurotensin and bradykinin were substrates, substance P wasn't. They showed that there was a lot of opioid processing, which they have shown it to be involved in as well. The physiological relevance is unknown.

Chao: The discovery by David Porteous of this important translocation happened a number of years ago. What has been the reaction by others? The finding has generated a great deal of interest and research.

Brandon: I have heard stories of heated exchanges about the importance and relevance of DISC1. When I first started going to psychiatric genetic meetings in 2001 it had calmed down a little but still in each lecture there were two clear opposing camps. I think it has calmed down as the biology has been worked out.

Chao: Michael, can you summarise the scepticism about DISC1?

Owen: I am a sceptic by nature, but I think this is a compelling story. Viewing it from a human geneticist's perspective, it rests very much on that single translocation family. The rest of the story is that this region of chromosome 1 is also a linkage hotspot that has been detected in a number of linkage studies. This is more supportive evidence. Then there is a whole slew of association data, which are subject to all the problems that Pamela Sklar mentioned in her paper earlier: different groups are studying different polymorphisms and there are different patterns of results, some with one diagnosis and some with another. The unanswered question is that in the translocation family, how sure are we that this is the only gene that the translocation is disrupting? People think the break point is in this gene so this must nail it to DISC1. There has to be some doubt as to that. But then you put the whole story together and it looks compelling.

Chao: How many other families have been examined at this level?

Owen: There are no other families with a translocation like that.

Brandon: People have looked. There is a Japanese study trying to identify the translocation but they couldn't find it. There is also the Johns Hopkins family with the frameshift.

Owen: Yes, there is another family with a smaller frameshift. We found exactly the same variant in a number of controls. This doesn't surprise me.

Buonanno: I like the story, but I have done Y2H and informatics before. One of the problems we find these days is that with the wealth of information out there it is easy to begin linking proteins and informatics. One of the best examples I have of this is that when we did our Y2H study we were excited and began to look at potential interacting proteins. You could build credible stories from these searches, but as the controls were performed we found that many of those proteins that made a great story turned out to be false positives.

Brandon: When we were trying to get the papers published, the final paper was pretty much *in silico*. One of the main reviewers asked us what we'd get if we did this randomly. We took a random protein set and showed specifically that our network was not random. Coupled with the methods that our collaborators and partners at Hybrigenics (see *http://www.hybrigenics.com/index.html*) use we can take out many false positives almost immediately. Hybrigenics technology classifies each Y2H interaction A–E. Every A interactor I have followed up in the lab has worked out, i.e. I have been able to show that the protein identified as binding to DISC1 in yeast also binds to DISC1 in mammalian cells or in tissue.

Buonanno: You said that you saw an overlap of immunofluorescence, but the overlap results from having expression of DISC in all types of subcellular compartments, and then the potential interacting protein is expressed in one of those compartments. What would have been your criteria to say that the overlap of immunofluorescence is not that significant?

Brandon: Now we would like to have some level of quantitation. We also did mass spectrometry approaches. I am pretty confident in the interactions I found: as confident as I can be with the technology I had at the time. There are now better ways of doing these studies.

Lu: I have one comment on this particular interactome. Years ago we joked about yeast two-hybrid: anything binds anything if you want to look for it. Physical interactions in Y2H and co-immunoprecipitation could happen when you manipulate the conditions. It depends on the affinity. The relevance to physiology is a question we need to bear in mind. Having said this, Nick Brandon has provided a conceptual framework that we can test experimentally. It points to the importance of synaptic function. In terms of protein–protein interactions *per se*, I think what Andrés is saying is that to demonstrate the interaction *in situ* at the cell level is important. Does this really happen in cells and if so in which types of cells? Is this interaction controlled by extracellular signals such as growth factors? I have another question or comment on the biological studies. In genetics you can say whether a result is replicated or not. If the results are not replicated it is bad but not fatal: it happens quite often because of environmental factors or other variables. But in cell biology, if a result cannot be replicated, it is very serious. That often means the experiments have not been done correctly or that the interpretation is wrong.

Javitt: The excitement of this field is that we never really know where the breakthroughs are coming from, and everyone is hoping that this is a breakthrough. The scepticism on the clinical side is that the diagnosis of schizophrenia is so vague, and what bothers clinicians about the pedigree is that in schizophrenia you don't see as much affective disorder and other diagnoses coming along. So when you have these pedigrees that have schizophrenia but also depression and antisocial personality, you wonder how specific it is for anything about schizophrenia and how this might just be bad brain that can express itself in different ways.

Owen: That pre-supposes that something called 'schizophrenia' exists. This is one of the most interesting things about this family: there is a range of diagnoses. There is evidence for an aetiological overlap between schizophrenia and mood disorders, which has been swept under the carpet over the years. The genetic evidence is much more supportive than has been quoted. On the molecular side, we've shown that this region of chromosome 1 is linked to schizo-affective disorders (Hamshere et al 2005). We have done linkage studies in schizophrenia and bipolar disorders, and when we take out the families who have a mixture of both from those two studies and analyse their genome, we get a very strongly significant linkage over that region. This suggests that there may be something with that region of the chromosome, be it DISC1 or another gene, that is predisposing to a form of illness that has both psychotic and affective features. We have evidence from other genes we have looked at that the phenomenological characteristics of the patients studied determine whether we see relationships with genetic findings. With G72, for example, we find evidence for association with bipolar disorder, not schizophrenia (Williams et al 2006). But, we find evidence that cases of schizophrenia who have had significant mood disorder episodes do show association. The implication of this is that the ability to 'replicate' this finding depends on the number of patients with mood disorder symptoms that have been included in the schizophrenia group. We are now going to approach this problem from the perspective of diagnostic scepticism. We'll be looking at our whole genome data from bipolar disorder *and* schizophrenia together in this way, breaking them down across the diagnostic categories.

Raff: When I ask psychiatrists about this, most tell me that they have patients who they can't tell for certain whether they are bipolar or schizophrenic.

Javitt: It is not just bipolar vs. schizo-affective vs. schizophrenia in this family. It is lots of weird stuff coming out, like alcoholism, anxiety disorders and antisocial personality, along with recurrent major depression. Very few people would argue that alcoholism is a surrogate for schizophrenia or that the diagnosis shifts between the two conditions.

Raff: Are there any individuals in this family who are classic schizophrenics or classic major depressives or classic bipolars?

Akil: I feel we are framing the question oddly. I understand the clinical constraints. If I hear about a family like this—and I am not a clinician—I would not assume it is prototypical anything. I would not expect it to be picked up in a whole genome scan. I think about it differently. I would say, this is a hotspot, and maybe we could do a better job with postmortem or in the periphery to see exactly which of the protein products are hurt. It may be a fluke of nature. At the same time, it could tell you something important about brain function. It may be that one of those changes present is the much more common problem: it may be milder, more specific, more targeted to particular cell types and so on. I wouldn't get mired into how typical or prototypical it is.

Javitt: I agree. The exciting thing is we don't know where the breakthroughs are coming from and this could lead to them. We have to be careful about the diagnosis to make sure it fits within the framework. Part of the problem is that we don't have all of the details about the features of the family, so this leads to some concern. Where this becomes diffuse is because the family is diffuse and then the pathology is diffuse. If you then go back and say now we have all these partners, let's look at the people in the family who do or don't have these features, this would be extremely interesting.

Akil: My approach would be focusing on the pathophysiology in the family to a better specificity: exactly what is messed up?

Buonanno: I like the idea, but this could just be a general malfunction of neuronal development that leads to all these issues. What is the age of onset?

Brandon: I don't know this. The investigators in Edinburgh (Douglas Blackwood, Walter Muir) indicated that they are following up the family as best they can. When we were doing the work we would have liked to get information on PD4B and Ndel1, but we were concerned about ethics. Some other groups, such as the Weinberger group (Barbara Lipska), have taken the interactome and in their patient samples they have asked whether DISC1 expression is changed. They have shown that it isn't, but when they look at their interacting partners in their schizophrenia patients, Ndel1 decreases and Fez1 decreases.

Buonanno: The picture I got from your data is that the interactions you are showing are so general, and they are affecting so many aspects of neuronal processing, that my point of view would be that it is amazing that you have normal functioning neurons. You are talking about everything from migration to elongation of neurons.

Brandon: We asked the question about whether there is a truncated protein. This is still controversial. With Y2H and bioinformatics analysis of the DISC1 interactome we see a lot of compensation in the truncation protein in terms of the *types* of proteins that are lost by the truncation (loss-of-function) but then compensated by new partners gained (gain-of-function). I don't like to talk about this too much because there is no *in vivo* evidence at the moment of the compensation. But you are right: we are not losing all the interactions in our family, but we are losing some of the critical ones, such as the attachment to the centrosome through the loss of Ndel1 binding.

Sklar: I wanted to ask a question that is the reverse of a question that I get asked all the time. I get asked, 'Is it real'? Can you summarize the evidence that DISC1 is interesting? What is consistent biochemically about DISC1? I have to make a decision about whether this is worth the significant investment in unravelling the genetics, which undoubtedly are complicated: it is a large gene, and it is complicated. What is the evidence that the truncated form is playing a biological role?

Brandon: We don't have any brain tissue, so we can't see whether the truncated form of the protein is present. David Porteous took lymphblastoid cells from the family, and showed that there seems to be only 50% of DISC1 present.

Sklar: There is some ambiguity about the antibodies in the literature?

Brandon: The antibodies are all real. As I would characterize an antibody by doing the correct controls, all of them seem to be picking up DISC1. Akira Sawa has immunoprecipitated DISC1 using his antibodies and has done mass spectrometry. DISC1 has come back. We took the Gogos antibody which showed nothing in those mice, and we saw nothing as well.

Chao: You did not mention synaptic functions in your talk. Perhaps this is a key.

Brandon: The synaptic function is amazing. In our hands, during early development DISC1 not in the synapse. But then something happens and it gets sucked into the synapse. We started to look at phosphorylation, and we have some preliminary data that it is involved.

References

Hamshere ML, Bennett P, Williams N et al 2005 Genomewide linkage scan in schizoaffective disorder: significant evidence for linkage at 1q42 close to DISC1, and suggestive evidence at 22q11 and 19p13. Arch Gen Psychiatry 62:1081–1088

Shinoda T, Taya S, Tsuboi D et al 2007 DISC1 regulates neurotrophin-induced axon elongation via interaction with Grb2. J Neurosci 27:4–14

Taya S, Shinoda T, Tsuboi D et al 2007 DISC1 regulates the transport of the NUDEL/LIS1/14-3-3epsilon complex through kinesin-1. J Neurosci 27:15–26

Williams NM, Green EK, Macgregor S et al 2006 Variation at the DAOA/G30 locus influences susceptibility to major mood episodes but not psychosis in schizophrenia and bipolar disorder. Arch Gen Psychiatry 63:366–373

Neurotrophins and cytokines in neuronal plasticity

Michael Spedding and Pierre Gressens*

Experimental Sciences, Institute of Research Servier, 11 Rue des Moulineaux, 92150 Suresnes, France and *Hôpital Robert Debré, 48 boulevard Sérurier, 75019 Paris, France

Abstract. Nerve growth factor (NGF) binds to TrkA receptors (neurotrophic) and P75^{NTR} (apoptosis or other pathways depending on the coupled adaptor proteins). Brain derived growth factor (BDNF) can bind to TrkB (neurotrophic) and P75^{NTR} receptors. BDNF is the main, activity-dependent, neurotrophin and sculpts neuronal organisation dependent on activity, thereby coupling and balancing effects on excitatory (glutamate) and inhibitory (GABA) transmission—in a synapse-specific manner. Some drugs can interact in a specific way. Positive modulators of AMPA receptors induce BDNF and favour long term potentiation (LTP) and memory processes. Some antidepressants such as tianeptine reverse stress-induced inhibition of LTP and restore neuronal plasticity in brain areas at risk. Inflammatory cytokines are produced in sickness behaviour mimicking depression. Interleukin (IL)1β can exacerbate the immediate effects of stressors, and enhance and prolong the overall effects, which may be protective in preventing overuse or by increasing conservation-withdrawal: in some synapses IL1β induces long term depression (LTD) or blocks LTP. The interactions with neurotrophins are complex and frequently reciprocal. However, NGF also contributes to inflammatory situations and mediates pain responses. This interplay is poorly understood but may be critical in cerebral palsy, neurodegenerative disorders such as amyotrophic lateral sclerosis and multiple sclerosis, and even Alzheimer's disease.

2008 Growth factors and psychiatric disorders. Wiley, Chichester (Novartis Foundation Symposium 289) p 222–237

The brain is constantly making and unmaking synapses, and many neurodegenerative diseases are disconnection disorders, as neurones need ongoing trophic input for survival. The processes of synaptogenesis and synaptic loss can be deregulated in psychiatric disorders and neurodegenerative disorders, in the new born, and in cerebral ageing, and it appears that inflammatory processes may play a role—we consider that the interplay of cytokines and neurotrophins may be critical in these disorders. Furthermore, new drug therapies may be targeted at these processes (Spedding et al 2005, Agid et al 2007).

222

Brain-derived neurotrophic factor (BDNF) is the main activity-dependent neurotrophin in the brain and also ensures scaling whereby excitatory and inhibitory transmission is balanced. BDNF binds to both TrkB (neurite extension, trophic via PI3K, MAPK, phospholipase Cγ cascades) and to P75^{NTR} which can lead to inhibition of outgrowth and in certain circumstances apoptosis. P75^{NTR} has no intrinsic activity and its signalling depends on which cytoplasmic adaptor proteins it interacts with—these are evidently cell specific.

There is a major controversy over whether proneurotrophins may yield opposite pharmacology to neurotrophins and act as molecular switches.

ProNGF and proBDNF are the predominant forms of nerve growth factor (NGF) and BDNF in the brain and may cause apoptosis via P75^{NTR}. ProNGF and proBDNF are metabolized to NGF and BDNF by metalloproteases, which may be induced and play key roles in inflammation. Furthermore, proNGF and proBDNF have opposite effects to BDNF and NGF as they have much higher selectivity for P75^{NTR} (affinity ~0.1 M) and may cause apoptosis in some systems or long term depression (LTD, particularly for proBDNF) rather than long-term potentiation (LTP). Proneurotrophins are metabolized to neurotrophins by several proteases, but particularly by tissue plasminogen (tPA) activation of plasmin (Pang et al 2004).

In this respect, Bai Lu (see Lu & Martinowich, this volume) showed that BDNF induced hippocampal late phase LTP, whereas proBDNF induced LTD. tPA was necessary for late-phase LTP expression, by BDNF formation (Pang et al 2004, Nagappan & Lu 2005). The facilitation of LTP is via TrkB/MEK-P and up-regulation of the NMDA receptor NR2B. The release of proneurotrophins is controversial but this debate (see the discussion in this volume) is critical because the balance may be changed in pathological situations. It is therefore important to resolve the debate and to model the pathophysiological situations, if we are to have drugs which can have neurotrophic effects in inflammatory situations.

Mitochondria and energy metabolism

Brain activity and energy metabolism are directly linked and BDNF is a potential candidate for this link. BDNF produced a concentration-dependent increase in the respiratory control index (RCI, a measure of the efficiency of respiratory coupling, ATP synthesis and organelle integrity) of mouse or rat brain mitochondria, co-incubated with synaptosomes containing signal transduction pathways. This effect was mediated via a MEK/MAP kinase pathway and was highly specific for oxidation of glutamate plus malate (complex I) by brain mitochondria (Markham et al 2004); oxidation by brain mitochondria of the complex II substrate succinate was unaffected by BDNF. Glial cell line-derived neurotrophic factor (GDNF) failed to modify RCI and NGF had only weak effects on RCI. BDNF, co-injected with

ibotenate, prevented the cortical and white matter lesions in a newborn mouse
model of excitotoxicity. GDNF and NGF were not neuroprotective in this
paradigm, and NGF even exacerbated lesions. This ability of BDNF to modify
brain metabolism and the efficiency of oxygen utilization is likely to be important
in relation to the development and treatment of diseases associated with the CNS.
Mitochondrial disruption, and modulation of Bcl2 may play roles in psychiatric
disorders (Einat et al 2005). Furthermore, the BDNF-mitochondria dysfunction
may be respon-sible for the metabolic disorders which are so evident in
Alzheimer's disease (Ackl et al 2005).

Therapeutic impact of neurotrophins

Neuronal plasticity models in the developing brain

The major brain lesions associated with cerebral palsy (CP) are periventricular
leukomalacia (periventricular white matter lesion) in preterm infants and cortico-
subcortical lesions in term infants. Several pre-conception, prenatal and perinatal
factors implicated in the pathophysiology of brain lesions associated with CP
include hypoxia–ischaemia and excess release of glutamate (leading to excitotoxicity), endocrine imbalances, genetic factors, growth factor deficiency, abnormal
competition for growth factors, excess free reactive oxygen species production,
maternal infection yielding excess cytokines and other pro-inflammatory agents
(Fig. 1) (Largeron et al 2001, Cai et al 2004). There is a major need for new drugs
which may help brain development under these circumstances as lasting damage
ensues, with major costs for society (Gressens & Spedding 2004).

We have developed simple high throughput *in vivo* models in newborn mice for
examining the effects of neuroplasticity in the developing brain and the interactions with cytokines and growth factors in the face of excitotoxic lesions (S-
bromowillardiine to induce lesions evoked by excess activation of AMPA or kainate
receptors; or ibotenate to induce lesions induced by NMDA and metabotropic
receptors—the agonists are injected into the white matter or cerebral cortex on
post-natal day P5 and the size of the lesions measured on P10) (Marret et al 1995,
Tahraoui et al 2001, Dommergues et al 2000, Husson et al 2005).

The interplay of cytokines and neurotrophins is complex and can have deleterious effects when compromised. For example, excessive production of inflammatory cytokines, by bacterial infection for example, causes marked extension of brain
lesions in the newborn which we have modelled (Dommergues et al 2000, Plaisant
et al 2003) (Fig 1, 2). Inflammatory cytokines markedly extend lesions of cortex
and white matter caused by ibotenate, acting on NMDA receptors. The role of
inflammatory cytokines is deleterious in extending neuronal damage, when

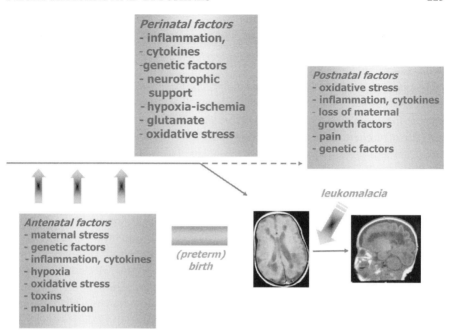

FIG. 1.   Multiple factors, including inflammatory cytokines and neurotrophic support, can modify the outcome of brain damage in the preterm infant.

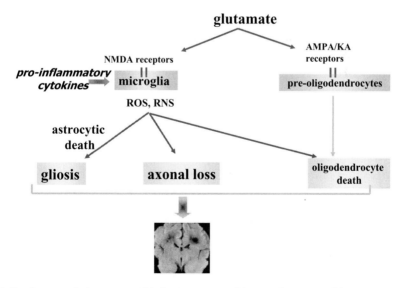

FIG. 2.   Impact of glutamate and inflammatory cytokines and neurotrophic support on the outcome of brain damage in the preterm infant.

preadministered (P0–P5) or just administered on P5. In contrast, administration of BDNF locally has neuroprotective effects against lesions induced by ibotenate, and these protective effects are mediated by MEK/MAPK pathways—whereas NGF is deleterious at P5.

Potential therapeutic agents. While NMDA receptor antagonists are acutely protective against ibotenate, the clinical use of NMDA antagonists in neonates is precluded because of a potential massive apoptotic cell death following blockade of the activity-dependent glutamatergic drive. In contrast, blockade of AMPA and kainate receptors by drugs such as Topiramate or AMPA antagonists did not produce such deleterious effects on neuronal survival, and acute neuroprotective effects were also observed (Sfaello et al 2005, Gressens et al 2005). Rather paradoxically, positive allosteric modulators of AMPA receptors (S 18986) are also neuroprotective, but this is by causing synthesis and release of neurotrophins such as BDNF (Dicou et al 2003), thus these agents may be beneficial in such circumstances.

Surprisingly, classic antidepressants (fluoxetine, venlafaxine, citalopram, imipramine) either fail to protect or are lethal when co-administered with cytokines in this model. However the antidepressant tianeptine was shown to block the deleterious effects of inflammatory cytokines on neonatal excitotoxic lesions (Plaisant et al 2003). Tianeptine is a well-tolerated antidepressant drug used in human adolescents and adults, which acts on the neuroplasticity pathways impaired by stress. Trophic factors, such as insulin-like growth factor 1 (IGF1) and BDNF, which have anti-apoptotic properties, can prevent asphyxic or excitotoxic neuronal death in animal models of perinatal damage (Gluckman et al 1998, Han & Holtzman 2000, Husson et al 2005, Bemelmans et al 2006). However, there are many difficulties involved in attempting to use drugs in neonates and children, especially where potent effects on the developing brain might be expected, and this urgently requires an open and in-depth society debate (Gressens & Spedding 2004).

Pain: nerve growth factor (NGF) is much more than neurotrophic

The interaction of neurotrophins in pain is complex. The role of NGF has expanded from a neurotrophin to being a key player in many inflammatory areas. NGF is produced in inflammatory responses and is responsible for bone pain and osteoarthritic pain, via its classic target of TrkA receptors. NGF is also responsible for shaping some of the vasculature and has marked angiogenic effects—NGF knockouts die due to misformed vasculature. However, NGF evolves from a neurotrophic role in development to a role in pain signalling from P3–P10 in the mouse (see below).

NGF yields an acute immediate allodynic effect in adult animals. Franz Hefti (Hefti et al 2006) showed a massive induction of NGF in acute injury and also in damaged joints with a unique role as an early mediator of pain. Pain (and Schwann cell gliosis) was the cause of the failure of NGF clinical trails for neurodegeneration. NGF is a pro-survival factor up to P3 in mice; but a primary mediator of pain from P9. Pain is caused by direct effects of NGF on TrkA receptors (Ugolini et al 2007), Nav1.8 sodium channels, TRPV1; on sensory nerves, secondarily on mast cells, and then causing wind up in the spinal cord. NGF is retrogradely transported to dorsal root ganglia (DRG) with TrkA receptors.

Several therapeutic approaches are being followed:

— direct NGF antagonists
— antibodies vs. NGF (Amgen phase I; Rinat RN624—phase II, Ugolini et al 2007)
— RN624—human antibodies, half-life 3 weeks.

Bone pain is very sensitive to NGF (e.g. arthritic pain in mice; cancer cells injected into bone—NGF antagonists are more potent than morphine). Antagonist peptides have been validated in humans in trials of up to 140 patients with no real side effects reported. The issue of whether NGF may be an *inflammatory* factor in Alzheimer's disease has not been explored to the author's knowledge and may well be worth investigating.

Inflammation—NGF and BDNF interplay

NGF initiates an inflammatory phenomenon via a NMDA/TrkB mechanism which can involve BDNF (Lever et al 2001). BDNF is expressed in TrkA containing neurons in dorsal root ganglia (DRG) and up-regulated in inflammatory pain, where BDNF is released and promotes glutamate release (Michael et al 1997). BDNF activates TrkB receptors, and causes pain. However, neuropathic pain is complex, apparently unresponsive to BDNF and very different from inflammatory pain (Pezet & McMahon 2006, Slack et al 2005, Zhao et al 2006).

IL1β increases BDNF secretion in pure neuronal cultures but reduces it in the presence of astrocytes (Boillee et al 2006a, b, Hauser & Oksenberg 2006); STAT3 regulates gene expression in response to neurotrophins and cytokines. Ng et al (2006) showed that NGF activated STAT3 via TrkA receptors showing interplay of signalling pathways.

The links between neurotrophins and inflammatory situations are therefore complex, but potentially of great importance. Dantzer and Kelly (2007) have reviewed their seminal contributions to the field, showing that inflammatory cytokines produced during sickness yield specific sickness behaviours which contribute to depression, and may antagonise many of the effects of neurotrophic cytokines.

Alzheimer's disease

Evidence that decreased BDNF causes Alzheimer's disease-associated cognitive decline. Margaret Fahnestock (Buttigieg et al 2007, Garzon et al 2002, Garzon & Fahnestock 2007, Peng et al 2005) has shown that BDNF mRNA and proBDNF and BDNF protein are all greatly reduced in cholinergic target tissues of Alzheimer's disease patients compared to controls. ProBDNF and BDNF levels decrease early, in the preclinical stages of Alzheimer's disease, and correlate with cognitive decline. Transgenic mice with similar decreases in BDNF levels exhibit learning and memory deficits that are rescued by BDNF administration. Three of 10 human BDNF mRNA transcripts are selectively decreased in Alzheimer's disease, indicating specific down-regulation. Transgenic mice expressing mutations in APP (and therefore with increased β-amyloid concentrations) exhibit reduced BDNF expression. This decrease correlates with cognitive deficits in both mice and men, suggesting that BDNF plays a role in synaptic loss and neuronal dysfunction underlying cognitive impairment in Alzheimer's disease. However, inflammatory cytokines can also build up in Alzheimer's disease, particularly in the perilacunar spaces in penetrating blood vessels, potentially opposing the effects of cytokines.

NGF has been used in clinical trails for Alzheimer's disease, without positive results (see below). Antonino Cattaneo has derived a transgenic mouse model (AD11 mice), based on the expression in the adult nervous system of a neutralizing recombinant anti NGF antibody (Capsoni & Cattaneo 2006, Ugolini et al 2007). AD11 mice develop a progressive neurodegenerative phenotype, that results in a severe cholinergic deficit, and in the appearance of Aβ-containing depositions and of hyperphosphorylated tau neurofibrillary tangles. AD11 mice display synaptic plasticity and behavioural deficits. The overall progressive neurodegeneration phenotype of AD11 mice is reminiscent of Alzheimer's disease. Cattaneo has proposed: the 'too little NGF, too much proNGF' hypothesis.

In middle-aged animals, LTP is impaired, partially because of excessive adenosine production, and positive allosteric modulators of AMPA receptors increase BDNF production and restore LTP (Rex et al 2005)

The neurotrophic hypotheses support the use of positive AMPA modulators which would increase the release of BDNF and have been shown to facilitate LTP and improve memory in the aged (Pawlak et al 2005). However, clinical trials in Alzheimer's disease of this class of drugs have not been reported yet.

Stress and depression

Manji et al (Manji et al 2001, Duman & Duman 2005) reviewed the data indicating that the effects of antidepressants are linked to BDNF production, particularly in the hippocampus. However the data are not clear-cut and it would be naïve to expect antidepressant therapy to be simply related to increasing the level of the main activity-dependent neurotrophin. However, whereas mild stress is trophic to almost all organisms, severe behavioural stress, associated with elevated glucocorticoid levels, blocks measures of neuronal plasticity such as LTP, in the hippocampus and the projection zones to the prefrontal cortex (Rocher et al 2004, Spedding et al 2005, Agid et al 2007). Furthermore, acute LTP changes (minutes/hours) are directly concordant with changes in dendritic arborization which change over 10 days to three weeks (Magarinos et al 1997, McEwen 2000, 2001, McEwen & Magarinos 2001, Reagan et al 2004, Vyas et al 2002, Agid et al 2007, Jay et al 2004, Spedding et al 2005). The hippocampal to prefrontal cortex pathway is the pathway where plasticity is impaired by stress and cytokines and which is the main pathway where bloodflow changes in depression—and where deep brain stimulation instantly reverses depression in treatment-resistant subjects, allowing proof of concept (Agid et al 2007, Mayberg et al 2005, Mayberg 1997). Part of the inhibition of plasticity is due to glucocorticoid release—but it is not clear to what extent this is caused by an impact on 'inflammatory' processes. In contrast, in the amygdala–orbitofrontal cortex link, increases in plasticity have been reported following stress (Vyas et al 2002). Furthermore, inflammatory cytokines can induce rage and aggressive behaviour in the periaqueductal grey (Zalcman & Siegel 2006, Bhatt & Siegel 2006). Interestingly, these plasticity changes were reversed by certain antidepressants.

AMPA, NMDA and GABA receptors may form final common pathways for the interplay of neurotrophins and cytokines as BDNF, TNFα and IL1β affect synaptic scaling but in different ways (Glazner & Mattson 2000, Leonoudakis et al 2004, Stellwagen & Malenka 2006).

Examples of ways forward for new drugs

Can drugs modulate BDNF release?

In vivo studies identified the ability of an AMPA receptor potentiator to modulate the hippocampal expression of BDNF, indicating a potential role for this type of molecule in the treatment of depression and other CNS disorders (Dicou et al 2003, Mackowiak et al 2002). *In vitro* and *in vivo* studies (Lauterborn et al 2000, 2003) have shown that different AMPA receptor potentiators can modify BDNF production in different parts of the brain indicating that regional selectivity can be achieved. As the AMPA potentiators are use-dependent then BDNF production is targeted to the appropriate brain areas. BDNF production incorporates neurotrophic (and neuroprotective) effects to the therapeutic profile of AMPA modulators (Dicou et al 2003). AMPA receptor potentiators are in development for mild cognitive impairment, and early stage Alzheimer's disease, as well as the cognitive aspects of psychiatric disorders.

Furthermore, drugs used for bipolar disorder, such as valproate and lithium, also have neurotrophic effects, mediated by GSK3 and also by the MEK/MAP kinase pathway (Hao et al 2004, Agid et al 2007, Chen & Manji 2006).

Can drugs modulate the negative effects of stress on neuronal plasticity?

Stress, and cytokines, can inhibit LTP in the hippocampus and in its projections to the ventral medial prefrontal cortex, a key cognitive pathway mediating the control of spatial and temporal context and the pathway which Mayberg has shown to be defective in depression (Agid et al 2007). The effects of stress on LTP are associated with high levels of glucocorticoid release, and are blocked by the GR antagonist, mifepristone (submitted). Tianeptine, an antidepressant, restores stress-impaired plasticity (LTP and dendritic reorganisation) (Agid et al 2007, McEwen & Olie 2005, Rocher et al 2004) and reverses the extensions of excitoxic lesions caused by cytokines (Plaisant et al 2003).

General conclusions

The neurotrophic support pathways are now mapped out and crystal structures indicate sites for mimics or antagonists with very selective interactions. Proneu-rotrophins are potentially important and may have effects which are opposite to neurotrophins—tPA and plasmin-induced metabolism of proneurotrophins put a new spin on many of the chronic neurodegenerative diseases we are interested in. The interplay of inflammation, metabolism and neurotrophic support is a key area for disease processes and the effects of drugs. It is still not worked out.

The interactions with neurotrophins are complex and frequently reciprocal. Neurotrophins also contribute to inflammatory situations. This interplay is poorly understood but may be critical in cerebral palsy, neurodegenerative disorders such as amyotrophic lateral sclerosis (ALS) (Boillee et al 2006a, b) and multiple sclerosis (Hauser & Oksenberg 2006), and even Alzheimer's disease.

References

Ackl N, Ising M, Schreiber YA, Atiya M, Sonntag A, Auer DP 2005 Hippocampal metabolic abnormalities in mild cognitive impairment and Alzheimer's disease. Neurosci Lett 384:23–28
Agid Y, Buzsaki G, Diamond DM et al 2007 How can drug discovery for psychiatric disorders be improved? Nat Rev Drug Discov 6:189–201

Bemelmans AP, Husson I, Jaquet M, Mallet J, Kosofsky BE, Gressens P 2006 Lentiviral-mediated gene transfer of brain-derived neurotrophic factor is neuroprotective in a mouse model of neonatal excitotoxic challenge. J Neurosci Res 83:50–60

Bhatt S, Siegel A 2006 Potentiating role of interleukin 2 (IL-2) receptors in the midbrain peri-aqueductal gray (PAG) upon defensive rage behavior in the cat: role of neurokinin NK(1) receptors. Behav Brain Res 167:251–260

Boillee S, Vande VC, Cleveland DW 2006a ALS: a disease of motor neurons and their non-neuronal neighbors. Neuron 52:39–59

Boillee S, Yamanaka K, Lobsiger CS et al 2006b Onset and progression in inherited ALS determined by motor neurons and microglia. Science 312:1389–1392

Buttigieg H, Kawaja MD, Fahnestock M 2007 Neurotrophic activity of proNGF in vivo. Exp Neurol 204:832–835

Cai Z, Lin S, Pang Y, Rhodes PG 2004 Brain injury induced by intracerebral injection of interleukin-1beta and tumor necrosis factor-alpha in the neonatal rat. Pediatr Res 56:377–384

Capsoni S, Cattaneo A 2006 On the molecular basis linking Nerve Growth Factor (NGF) to Alzheimer's disease. Cell Mol Neurobiol 26:619–633

Chen G, Manji HK 2006 The extracellular signal-regulated kinase pathway: an emerging promising target for mood stabilizers. Curr Opin Psychiatry 19:313–323

Dantzer R, Kelley KW 2007 Twenty years of research on cytokine-induced sickness behavior. Brain Behav Immun 21:153–60

Dicou E, Rangon CM, Guimiot F, Spedding M, Gressens P 2003 Positive allosteric modulators of AMPA receptors are neuroprotective against lesions induced by an NMDA agonist in neonatal mouse brain. Brain Res 970:221–225

Dommergues MA, Patkai J, Renauld JC, Evrard P, Gressens P 2000 Proinflammatory cytokines and interleukin-9 exacerbate excitotoxic lesions of the newborn murine neopallium. Ann Neurol 47:54–63

Duman CH, Duman RS 2005 Neurobiology and treatment of anxiety: signal transduction and neural plasticity. Handb Exp Pharmacol 305–334

Einat H, Yuan P, Manji HK 2005 Increased anxiety-like behaviors and mitochondrial dysfunction in mice with targeted mutation of the Bcl-2 gene: further support for the involvement of mitochondrial function in anxiety disorders. Behav Brain Res 165:172–180

Garzon DJ, Fahnestock M 2007 Oligomeric amyloid decreases basal levels of brain-derived neurotrophic factor (BDNF) mRNA via specific downregulation of BDNF transcripts IV and V in differentiated human neuroblastoma cells. J Neurosci 27:2628–2635

Garzon D, Yu G, Fahnestock M 2002 A new brain-derived neurotrophic factor transcript and decrease in brain-derived neurotrophic factor transcripts 1, 2 and 3 in Alzheimer's disease parietal cortex. J Neurochem 82:1058–1064

Glazner GW, Mattson MP 2000 Differential effects of BDNF, ADNF9, and TNFalpha on levels of NMDA receptor subunits, calcium homeostasis, and neuronal vulnerability to excitotoxicity. Exp Neurol 161:442–452

Gluckman PD, Guan J, Williams C et al 1998 Asphyxial brain injury–the role of the IGF system. Mol Cell Endocrinol 140:95–99

Gressens P, Spedding M 2004 Strategies for neuroprotection in the newborn. Drug Discov Today Ther Strat 1:77–82

Gressens P, Spedding M, Gigler G et al 2005 The effects of AMPA receptor antagonists in models of stroke and neurodegeneration. Eur J Pharmacol 519:58–67

Han BH, Holtzman DM 2000 BDNF protects the neonatal brain from hypoxic-ischemic injury in vivo via the ERK pathway. J Neurosci 20:5775–5781

Hao Y, Creson T, Zhang L et al 2004 Mood stabilizer valproate promotes ERK pathway-dependent cortical neuronal growth and neurogenesis. J Neurosci 24:6590–6599

Hauser SL, Oksenberg JR 2006 The neurobiology of multiple sclerosis: genes, inflammation, and neurodegeneration. Neuron 52:61–76

Hefti FF, Rosenthal A, Walicke PA et al 2006 Novel class of pain drugs based on antagonism of NGF. Trends Pharmacol Sci 27:85–91

Husson I, Rangon CM, Lelievre V et al 2005 BDNF-induced white matter neuroprotection and stage-dependent neuronal survival following a neonatal excitotoxic challenge. Cereb Cortex 15:250–261

Jay TM, Rocher C, Hotte M, Naudon L, Gurden H, Spedding M 2004 Plasticity at hippocampal to prefrontal cortex synapses is impaired by loss of dopamine and stress: importance for psychiatric diseases. Neurotox Res 6:233–244

Largeron M, Mesples B, Gressens P et al 2001 The neuroprotective activity of 8-alkylamino-1,4-benzoxazine antioxidants. Eur J Pharmacol 424:189–194

Lauterborn JC, Lynch G, Vanderklish P, Arai A, Gall CM 2000 Positive modulation of AMPA receptors increases neurotrophin expression by hippocampal and cortical neurons. J Neurosci 20:8–21

Lauterborn JC, Truong GS, Baudry M, Bi X, Lynch G, Gall CM 2003 Chronic elevation of brain-derived neurotrophic factor by ampakines. J Pharmacol Exp Ther 307:297–305

Leonoudakis D, Braithwaite SP, Beattie MS, Beattie EC 2004 TNFalpha-induced AMPA-receptor trafficking in CNS neurons; relevance to excitotoxicity? Neuron Glia Biol 1:263–273

Lever IJ, Bradbury EJ, Cunningham JR et al 2001 Brain-derived neurotrophic factor is released in the dorsal horn by distinctive patterns of afferent fiber stimulation. J Neurosci 21:4469–4477

Mackowiak M, O'Neill MJ, Hicks CA, Bleakman D, Skolnick P 2002 An AMPA receptor potentiator modulates hippocampal expression of BDNF: an in vivo study. Neuropharmacology 43:1–10

Magarinos AM, Verdugo JM, McEwen BS 1997 Chronic stress alters synaptic terminal structure in hippocampus. Proc Natl Acad Sci USA 94:14002–14008

Manji HK, Drevets WC, Charney DS 2001 The cellular neurobiology of depression. Nat Med 7:541–547

Markham A, Cameron I, Franklin P, Spedding M 2004 BDNF increases rat brain mitochondrial respiratory coupling at complex I, but not complex II. Eur J Neurosci 20:1189–1196

Marret S, Mukendi R, Gadisseux JF, Gressens P, Evrard P 1995 Effect of ibotenate on brain development: an excitotoxic mouse model of microgyria and posthypoxic-like lesions. J Neuropathol Exp Neurol 54:358–370

Mayberg HS 1997 Limbic-cortical dysregulation: a proposed model of depression. J Neuropsychiatry Clin Neurosci 9:471–481

Mayberg HS, Lozano AM, Voon V et al 2005 Deep brain stimulation for treatment-resistant depression. Neuron 45:651–660

McEwen BS 2000 Effects of adverse experiences for brain structure and function. Biol Psychiatry 48:721–731

McEwen BS 2001 Plasticity of the hippocampus: adaptation to chronic stress and allostatic load. Ann N Y Acad Sci 933:265–277

McEwen BS, Magarinos AM 2001 Stress and hippocampal plasticity: implications for the pathophysiology of affective disorders. Hum Psychopharmacol 16:S7–S19

McEwen BS, Olie JP 2005 Neurobiology of mood, anxiety, and emotions as revealed by studies of a unique antidepressant: tianeptine. Mol Psychiatry 10:525–537

Michael GJ, Averill S, Nitkunan A et al 1997 Nerve growth factor treatment increases brain-derived neurotrophic factor selectively in TrkA-expressing dorsal root ganglion cells and in their central terminations within the spinal cord. J Neurosci 17:8476–8490

Nagappan G, Lu B 2005 Activity-dependent modulation of the BDNF receptor TrkB: mechanisms and implications. Trends Neurosci 28:464–471

Ng YP, Cheung ZH, Ip NY 2006 STAT3 as a downstream mediator of Trk signaling and functions. J Biol Chem 281:15636–44

Pang PT, Teng HK, Zaitsev E et al 2004 Cleavage of proBDNF by tPA/plasmin is essential for long-term hippocampal plasticity. Science 306:487–491

Pawlak R, Rao BS, Melchor JP, Chattarji S, McEwen B, Strickland S 2005 Tissue plasminogen activator and plasminogen mediate stress-induced decline of neuronal and cognitive functions in the mouse hippocampus. Proc Natl Acad Sci USA 102:18201–18206

Peng S, Wuu J, Mufson EJ, Fahnestock M 2005 Precursor form of brain-derived neurotrophic factor and mature brain-derived neurotrophic factor are decreased in the pre-clinical stages of Alzheimer's disease. J Neurochem 93:1412–1421

Pezet S, McMahon SB 2006 Neurotrophins: mediators and modulators of pain. Annu Rev Neurosci 29:507–538

Plaisant F, Dommergues MA, Spedding M et al 2003 Neuroprotective properties of tianeptine: interactions with cytokines. Neuropharmacology 44:801–809

Reagan LP, Rosell DR, Wood GE et al 2004 Chronic restraint stress up-regulates GLT-1 mRNA and protein expression in the rat hippocampus: reversal by tianeptine. Proc Natl Acad Sci USA 101:2179–2184

Rex CS, Kramar EA, Colgin LL, Lin B, Gall CM, Lynch G 2005 Long-term potentiation is impaired in middle-aged rats: regional specificity and reversal by adenosine receptor antagonists. J Neurosci 25:5956–5966

Rocher C, Spedding M, Munoz C, Jay TM 2004 Acute stress-induced changes in hippocampal/prefrontal circuits in rats: effects of antidepressants. Cereb Cortex 14:224–229

Sfaello I, Baud O, Arzimanoglou A, Gressens P 2005 Topiramate prevents excitotoxic damage in the newborn rodent brain. Neurobiol Dis 20:837–848

Slack SE, Grist J, Mac Q, McMahon SB, Pezet S 2005 TrkB expression and phospho-ERK activation by brain-derived neurotrophic factor in rat spinothalamic tract neurons. J Comp Neurol 489:59–68

Spedding M, Jay T, Costa e Silva J, Perret L 2005 A pathophysiological paradigm for the therapy of psychiatric disease. Nat Rev Drug Discov 4:467–476

Stellwagen D, Malenka RC 2006 Synaptic scaling mediated by glial TNF-alpha. Nature 440:1054–1059

Tahraoui SL, Marret S, Bodenant C et al 2001 Central role of microglia in neonatal excitotoxic lesions of the murine periventricular white matter. Brain Pathol 11:56–71

Ugolini G, Marinelli S, Covaceuszach S, Cattaneo A, Pavone F 2007 The function neutralizing anti-TrkA antibody MNAC13 reduces inflammatory and neuropathic pain. Proc Natl Acad Sci USA 104:2985–2990

Vyas A, Mitra R, Shankaranarayana Rao BS, Chattarji S 2002 Chronic stress induces contrasting patterns of dendritic remodeling in hippocampal and amygdaloid neurons. J Neurosci 22:6810–6818

Zalcman SS, Siegel A 2006 The neurobiology of aggression and rage: role of cytokines. Brain Behav Immun 20:507–514

Zhao J, Seereeram A, Nassar MA et al 2006 Nociceptor-derived brain-derived neurotrophic factor regulates acute and inflammatory but not neuropathic pain. Mol Cell Neurosci 31:539–548

DISCUSSION

Bothwell: I am glad you talked about metabolism. It makes me wonder whether we have been missing something in the work we have been doing. You highlighted the work Moses Chao has done on transactivation, which I think will turn out to be important. We are looking at the FGF receptors which signal very much like Trk receptors. We looked at mutations of FGF receptors leading to spontaneous activation of the receptor. These are overexpression studies, but when these mutated receptors are expressed in COS or HEK293 cells, they are expressed at levels far lower than one sees in any normal cells. My student couldn't demonstrate she was expressing these receptors even though she had good antibodies, but she noticed that these cells were different and turned the medium yellow. I explained that this was the Warburg effect, which is the shutting down of mitochondrial oxidation and switching to the glycolytic pathway of oxidation. It turns out that when these spontaneously activating FGF receptors signal, they never make it to the cell surface. All their signalling comes from the biosynthetic compartment. Interestingly, when Moses transactivates receptors, much of the signalling comes from that same intracellular pathway. If FGF receptors in a non-neuronal cell line signal from this intracellular pathway, as we have with transactivation, it shuts down mitochondrial oxidation and ramps up glycolytic oxidation. The same receptors on the cell surface respond to FGF by increasing mitochondrial oxidation instead. There are opposite results with the same receptor in a different cell compartment. It's really interesting looking at some of these differing effects of transactivation versus traditional activation.

Akil: I have two comments. First, with regard to the mitochondrial story, there are glucocorticoid receptors in mitochondria. This is an interesting place for interactions. In spite of the agonal factors and pH problems, we have seen some changes in mitochondrial function which we believe survive after we clean up everything in psychiatric disorders, particularly bipolar disorder. On the basis of this we have done some preliminary work with mitochondrial altering drugs, and we see changes in emotional behaviour. I think this is an interesting direction to go in: targeting mitochondria function with drugs that specifically change mitochondrial function in classical *in vitro* assays. This could be a good target for changing affective behaviour. My second comment is about the amygdala, which we haven't talked about much in this meeting. The amygdala pops up a lot in affective disorders and in animal models of fear conditioning. Following chronic social defeats, BDNF actually goes up in the amygdala, specifically in the animals that tend to be high anxiety, and not in the others. The amygdala is at the same time a very good target for so-called 'sickness' behaviour. Interleukins and cytokines activate the amygdala and BNST (bed nucleus of the stria terminalis) in that pathway in GABA- and enkephalin-containing neurons, not CRH-containing neurons. It is an interesting interface, perhaps not part of the initial physiology, but at some point as these illnesses ramp up the combination of being activated by inflammation and turning on emotional circuitry.

Hen: I find it puzzling that you see a number of effects with tianeptine that you don't see with selective serotonin reuptake inhibitors (SSRIs), both on dendritic growth in CA3 and LTP. What is the relevance of these effects since you don't see them with more classical antidepressants?

Spedding: That's a reasonable point. We are developing two atypical anti-depressants: tianeptine and agomelatine, with Novartis. Agomelatine is a melatonin agonist that affects chronobiology. Chronobiology hasn't been mentioned in this meeting, but there are big chronobiological changes in BDNF in the hippocampus.

Hen: Are you arguing that they affect targets that are independent of the targets affected by the SSRIs?

Spedding: Yes. Neither drug blocks serotonin receptors. The problem for me is the subjectivity of the models used for depression. Forced-swim and chronic mild stress were built up on previous antidepressants, and we don't know that they are inherent to depression. You can throw away whole lines of research depending on which model you use. I wanted to go back to see which brain areas were important from imaging studies, and model these. Helen Mayberg has shown that the hippocampus and medial prefrontal cortex are critical in depression and we looked at plasticity changes in these brain areas (Mayberg et al 2005). The only impact in animal models was with stress or cytokines as an alternative approach. We need novel models, because if we go back to the old models we'll find the old drugs. New models for disease based on the pathophysiology will give us new ways forwards.

Sendtner: I'd like to come back to the effect of glucocorticoids. My question is probably for René Hen and relates to earlier experiments showing that when dexamethasone is applied to rats, there is increased apoptosis of stem cells in the dentate gyrus. These were quite significant effects. How do these effects on memory relate to the irradiation experiments? Are there similar effects or additional effects? Glucocorticoid receptors are all over the place so one could expect results in other cells and not only precursors. What is known about this?

Hen: I'd argue that the effects of stress are not limited to stem cells in the dentate gyrus. The most pronounced effect of stress is the one reported by Bruce McEwen, with reduction in the dendritic tree in CA3 and the dentate gyrus. I would not attribute the cognitive impairments seen after stress to neurogenesis. We see a bigger effect after chronic stress in terms of decreased cognitive function than what is seen when we just ablate neurogenesis.

Tongiorgi: The issue of the relationship between inflammation and brain functioning is important. There is a series of studies showing that TNF can interact with the survival mechanism. Recently, Carl Cotman has proposed that interleukin (IL)1β interferes with BDNF signalling. The idea coming out from these studies is that during ageing and in certain pathologies there is a sort of BDNF-resistant system in the brain which parallels the insulin resistance. It has been proposed that this goes through the ceramide pathway. Moses Chao has studied this pathway for many years. Is there a general consensus that there is a potentially important mechanism that can impair not only neuronal survival, but also memory? Does memory loss involve inflammation?

Spedding: I think the key ways in which neurotrophic and inflammatory aspects interact would be responsible for a variety of pathologies, such as motor neuron disease.

Chao: Enrico Tongiorgi, you referred to ceramide production after engagement of p75 receptor. This was originally proposed as a cell death mechanism. However, there has not been much work in this area over the last couple of years. It has been proposed that ceramide is a second messenger for cytokines. Since it is a lipid, it has been very difficult to study.

Tongiorgi: The end point is that no matter how much BDNF we throw at a sick brain, it won't have a positive effect on the system, because the signalling is blocked by underlying inflammatory mechanisms. Is that the general idea?

Spedding: To a certain extent, but in the main, that's too strong. It varies with the cell type and the signalling. There is good evidence indicating that the effects of neurotrophins in motor neuron disease can be modified by glial production of soluble factors.

Hen: If there is a connection between depression and inflammation, wouldn't one expect anti-inflammatory agents to have an antidepressant action?

Spedding: GSK has patented combining anti-inflammatory agents with antidepressants. I don't think it is that simple. It is not enough, because there are many factors involved. Long-term depression is associated with increase in coronary risk factors.

Malaspina: There are patients with depression who self-administer antiinflammatories and feel better with it.

Spedding: I am not saying that inflammation is the key. But there is an interesting interaction we need to sort out. It may be important for a variety of different brain disorders. There are key nodal points where inflammatory cytokines interact.

Raff: There is a problem with terminology here. The term 'inflammation', and particularly 'neuro-inflammation', is now being used to describe any condition where microglia are activated in the CNS, which includes almost all forms of neuropathology. Either one is going to need a new term for real inflammation in the CNS, where white blood cells migrate into the CNS from the blood, or one is going to have to restrict the use of the term 'neuro-inflammation' to just these conditions.

Spedding: I was referring mainly to microglial activation. It is not a full inflammation.

Castrén: Some preliminary reports showed that aspirin plus anti-depressants lead to faster onset of action. This raises another issue in this context. While I appreciate it is important to look for new drugs, it is also important to take advantage of the drugs we already have and try to optimise the use of these. I am convinced that this has not been done. The current therapy is not making the best of the treatments we have available, which could be done by combining rehabilitation with drug treatments. Perhaps there are other drugs such as aspirin that could be used in combination for a better response.

Akil: I agree the terms neuro-immunology and neuro-inflammation have taken on many meanings. I feel that interleukins and cytokines can trigger activation of certain pathways that then take on a life of their own. The inflammation need not be ongoing at that moment, but can bias circuitry. It is the circuitry that makes us feel bad when we are sick, and we can continue to turn it on and feel rotten.

Hen: What is the evidence that this persists after the inflammation subsides?

Akil: I don't know that it always does. In certain chronic repeated exposure states there is continual activation. It does need to be looked into. It may be a small part of the action, but do certain kinds of chronic illnesses or environmental exposures do this? It is part of the gene–environment formula.

Reference

Mayberg HS, Lozano AM, Voon V et al 2005 Deep brain stimulation for treatment-resistant depression. Neuron 45:651–60

Closing remarks

Moses Chao

Molecular Neurobiology Program, Skirball Institute of Biomolecular Medicine, Departments of Cell Biology, Physiology and Neuroscience, and Psychiatry, New York University School of Medicine, 540 First Avenue, New York, NY 10016, USA

At the start of this symposium, a number of key questions were posed. How strong is the link of growth factors to psychiatric disorders? What is their mechanism of action? Why do antidepressants take so long to become efficacious? Can growth factor signalling be used to design new drugs for psychiatric illnesses? Many of these questions were addressed during the meeting. A great deal of attention was paid to the genetic evidence, which indicated that psychiatric disorders are extremely complex and difficult to follow using genome-wide analysis. There was considerable molecular and cellular evidence presented that growth factors can exert an impact upon psychiatric disorders.

Since the discovery of nerve growth factor (NGF) and epidermal growth factor (EGF), there has been over 50 years of work on growth factors. Trophic factors, such as neurotrophins (NGF, brain-derived neurotrophic factor [BDNF], neurotrophin [NT]3 and NT4) and neuregulins, are potent signalling molecules which were first characterized for regulating growth and differentiation of neurons and glia during early development. These proteins are involved in many cell–cell communication events, such as myelination and the formation of synaptic structures. The absence of neurotrophins in *Caenorhabditis elegans* and *Drosophila melanogaster* indicates they have additional functions in the adult vertebrate nervous system (Chao 2000). Due to the accumulated biochemical, cell biological and genetic evidence, there are numerous insights into receptor signal transduction mechanisms. As a consequence many downstream enzymatic activities and targets have been identified. It has also become apparent that neurotrophins and neuregulins are required for synaptic transmission and neural plasticity. For example, BDNF enhances long-term potentiation (LTP) in the hippocampus. BDNF can also act as an anti-depressant. Hence, small molecular agonists that promote BDNF functions or receptor signalling may prove to be clinically relevant in the future.

There is considerable optimism that understanding the mechanism of action of growth factors will contribute greatly to the study of psychiatric illnesses, such as anxiety, depression, bipolar disorder and schizophrenia. In addition to BDNF and neuregulin, Huda Akil proposed that fibroblast growth factor (FGF) family members may be also involved. It is likely that other growth factors will be found to influence these complex disorders. An example is the association of the hepatocyte growth factor Met receptor tyrosine kinase with autism disorders (Campbell et al 2006). We need additional genetic association studies, as well as mechanistic studies to confirm these potential relationships in psychiatric disorders.

René Hen and other participants here have discussed the lengthy time course of the action of many psychotrophic drugs, asking why they take so long to become efficacious. This question addresses the core issues of the mechanism of action of growth factors, neurotransmitters, as well as the influence of neurogenesis. The actions of antidepressants in increasing levels of BDNF and the levels of key neurotransmitters such as serotonin must be interrelated and suggest that many psychiatric drugs have common actions.

Michael Spedding raised the issue of whether we may use this information to design new drugs. Psychiatry has had an advantage over other disciplines, such as neurology, in that pharmacology has provided many more effective drug treatments and drug targets. The irony is that many of these treatments were discovered by accident, and not as a consequence of hypothesis-driven studies. Though growth factor dysfunction is not directly responsible for psychiatric disorders, their diverse effects upon development of the nervous system and their activity-dependent effects upon synaptic transmission indicate that growth factors may be used as effective probes of the pathophysiology of mental illnesses.

One mechanism that was not extensively discussed is the influence of epigenetic changes. Conrad Waddington, a British scientist trained in Cambridge and a director of genetics in Edinburgh, coined the term 'epigenetics'. The definition he gave in 1942 was that epigenetics represents the 'interactions of genes with their environment that bring the phenotype into being.' The idea put forth was that genetic information alone could not explain changes in biological processes.

It has been known for decades that DNA is associated with many chromatin proteins, such as nucleosomal histones and transcription factors. Histones are modified by many enzymatic activities, including methylation, phosphorylation, acetylation and ubiquitination. These modifications have been known since the 1960s. We know there are a number of neurological syndromes that result in gene silencing by making chromatin less available for transcription. There are also many mechanisms for opening up chromatin for the transcription machinery. One question raised by a recent review issue of *Cell* devoted to epigenetics is how this information is transmitted from generation to generation (Goldberg et al 2007). Though much of the interest in epigenetic mechanisms has been in the cancer field, I propose that many of these modifications are directly relevant to psychiatric disorders. Waddington had a similar idea. He proposed that numerous cell types took on different trajectories during development, depending on epigenetic changes. Instead of individual cells, one can well imagine that the development of the brain can also probably take any number of different trajectories. This was dramatically pointed out by the studies presented by Jay Giedd. These decisions may depend on how many epigenetic modifications occur on chromatin proteins as a result of environmental changes, maternal care, injury and inflammation. Epigenetic changes are therefore highly likely to play a determining role in the progression of psychiatric disorders.

The recent identification of susceptibility genes for schizophrenia, depression and learning and memory disorders suggest that psychiatric disorders may be influenced by a discrete number of genes with multiple actions. These genes will provide clues to the biochemical mechanisms and pathways that underlie these complex disorders. There is a growing understanding of how neurotrophins and neuregulins carry out cell–cell communication in the nervous system. These mechanisms offer the opportunity to identify metabolic events that contribute to each disorder at a molecular and synaptic level.

References

Campbell DB, Sutcliffe JS, Ebert PJ et al 2006 A genetic variant that disrupts MET transcription is associated with autism. Proc Natl Acad Sci USA 103:16834–16839

Chao MV 2000 Trophic factors: an evolutionary cul-de-sac or door into higher neuronal function? J Neurosci Res 59:353–355

Goldberg AD, Allis CD, Bernstein E 2007 Epigenetics: a landscape takes shape. Cell 128:635–638

Contributor Index

Subject Index